CLINICAL TRIALS

A Practical Approach

CLINICAL TRIALS

A Practical Approach

STUART J. POCOCK

Professor of Medical Statistics and Director of Clinical Trials Research Group
London School of Hygiene and Tropical Medicine
University of London

JOHN WILEY & SONS

Chichester · New York · Brisbane · Toronto · Singapore

Library of Congress Cataloging in Publication Data:

Pocock, Stuart J.
  Clinical trials.

  Bibliography: p.
  Includes index.
  1. Medicine, Clinical—Research—Statistical methods.
2. Drugs—Testing—Statistical methods. I. Title. II. Series.
R850.A2P6 1983 615'.19'00287 83-1316
ISBN 0 471 90155 5

British Library Cataloguing in Publication Data:
  Pocock, Stuart J.
  Clinical trials: a practical approach.
  1. Medicine, Clinical—Research—Statistical
  methods 2. Drugs—Testing—Statistical methods
  I. Title
  615'.7 RS189

  ISBN 0 471 90155 5

Filmset in 'Monophoto' Times New Roman
by Eta Services (Typesetters) Ltd., Beccles, Suffolk
Printed and Bound by Bookcraft (Bath) Ltd.,
Midsomer Norton, Avon

To
Peter Armitage and Marvin Zelen
with gratitude.

Contents

Preface xi

1. **Introduction: The Rationale of Clinical Trials** 1
    1.1 Types of clinical trial. 1
    1.2 Controlled clinical trials and the scientific method 4
    1.3 An example of a clinical trial for primary breast cancer . . . 7

2. **The Historical Development of Clinical Trials** 14
    2.1 Clinical trials before 1950 14
    2.2 Clinical trials since 1950 18
    2.3 Cancer chemotherapy in the United States 21
    2.4 Treatment of acute myocardial infarction 24
    2.5 The pharmaceutical industry 26

3. **Organization and Planning** 28
    3.1 The protocol 28
    3.2 Administration, staff and finance 31
    3.3 Selection of patients 35
    3.4 Treatment schedules 38
    3.5 Evaluation of patient response 41

4. **The Justification for Randomized Controlled Trials** 50
    4.1 Problems with uncontrolled trials 51
    4.2 Problems with historical controls 54
    4.3 Problems with concurrent non-randomized controls 60
    4.4 Is randomization feasible? 63

5. **Methods of Randomization** 66
    5.1 Patient registration 66
    5.2 Preparing the randomization list 73
    5.3 Stratified randomization 80
    5.4 Unequal randomization 87

6. Blinding and Placebos 90
   6.1 The justification for double-blind trials 90
   6.2 The conduct of double-blind trials 93
   6.3 When is blinding feasible? 97

7. Ethical Issues 100
   7.1 Medical progress and individual patient care. 100
   7.2 Informed patient consent 105

8. Crossover Trials 110
   8.1 Within-patient comparisons 110
   8.2 The two-period crossover design 112
   8.3 The analysis and interpretation of crossover trials 114
   8.4 Multi-period crossover designs 119

9. The Size of a Clinical Trial 123
   9.1 Statistical methods for determining trial size 123
   9.2 The realistic assessment of trial size 130
   9.3 The inadequacy of small trials 133
   9.4 Multi-centre trials 134
   9.5 The number of treatments and factorial designs 138

10. Monitoring Trial Progress 142
   10.1 Reasons for monitoring 142
   10.2 Interim analyses 143
   10.3 Repeated significance testing: group sequential designs . . . 147
   10.4 Continuous sequential designs 155

11. Forms and Data Management 160
   11.1 Form design 160
   11.2 Data management 166
   11.3 The use of computers 168

12. Protocol Deviations 176
   12.1 Ineligible patients 176
   12.2 Non-compliance and incomplete evaluation 179
   12.3 Inclusion of withdrawals in analysis 182

13. Basic Principles of Statistical Analysis 187
   13.1 Describing the data 188
   13.2 Significance tests 197
   13.3 Estimation and confidence limits 206

14. Further Aspects of Data Analysis 211
    14.1 Prognostic factors. 211
    14.2 The analysis of survival data 221
    14.3 Multiplicity of data 228

15. Publication and Interpretation of Findings. 234
    15.1 Trial reports and their critical evaluation 234
    15.2 An excess of false-positives. 239
    15.3 Combining evidence and overall strategy 242

References   248

Index   257

Preface

There is an ever-increasing number of treatment innovations which require proper investigation to see if they are of genuine benefit to patients. The randomized controlled clinical trial has become widely regarded as the principal method for obtaining a reliable evaluation of treatment effect on patients. The purpose of this book is to explain in practical terms the basic principles of clinical trials. Particular emphasis is given to their scientific rationale, including the relevance of statistical methods, though ethical and organizational issues are also discussed in some detail.

My intention has been to present the methodology of clinical trials in a style which is comprehensible to a wide audience. I hope the book proves to be especially useful to clinicians and others who are involved in conducting trials and it would be particularly gratifying if this text encouraged more clinicians to undertake or collaborate in properly designed trials to resolve relevant therapeutic issues.

Pharmaceutical companies have a fundamental role in the organization of trials for drug therapy. I have tried to give a balanced view of their activities in this area and hope that my approach to clinical trials is conducive to maintaining high standards of research in the clinical testing of new drugs. However, I wish to emphasize that randomized controlled trials should also be applied to assessing other (non-drug) aspects of therapy and patient management.

The practice of medicine poses a need to interpret wisely the published findings from clinical trials. Accordingly, the medical profession at large and others concerned with the treatment and management of patients may benefit from an increased understanding of how clinical trials are (and should be) conducted.

The proper use of statistical methods is important at the planning stage of a clinical trial as well as in the analysis and interpretation of results. I also recognize that many clinicians and others without mathematical training experience some difficulty in understanding statistical concepts. Hence, I have used a straightforward non-mathematical approach in describing those statistical issues that I consider of relevance to the practice of clinical trials. In particular,

I would like to think that the basic principles of statistical analysis described in chapter 13 may be of more general interest beyond clinical trials. Indeed, some readers who are unfamiliar with statistical terms may find it instructive to begin with this chapter.

My own experience in teaching undergraduate medical students has encouraged me to believe that the introduction of clinical trials and related statistical ideas is a useful aspect of preclinical education. Accordingly, my approach to such courses is reflected in much of this book.

As a medical statistician I believe that clinical trials require a successful collaboration of clinical, organizational and statistical skills. I feel that my profession needs to strive harder to achieve effective communication of our ideas to non-statistical colleagues and I would be delighted if this book could persuade other statisticians towards a commonsense and less theoretical approach to medical research. In this respect, students of biostatistics may find this book a useful antidote to their more mathematical courses!

Lastly, my policy has been always to introduce each concept via actual examples of clinical trials. In this way, the reader should experience the reality of clinical trials, not as an abstract collection of methods, but as a practical contribution to furthering medical knowledge.

I greatly appreciate the contributions of Sheila Gore and Austin Heady who read the book in draft and made many suggestions for improvement. I am also grateful to Tom Meade and Simon Thompson for their helpful comments on the draft. I am indebted to Peter Armitage for first stimulating the publishers to realize the need for such a book. I wish to express sincere thanks to Yvonne Ayton for typing the manuscript and to other colleagues for their invaluable support. Lastly, this whole project was made easier by the help and encouragement of my wife Faith.

CHAPTER 1

Introduction: The Rationale of Clinical Trials

The evaluation of possible improvements in the treatment of disease has historically been an inefficient and haphazard process. Only in recent years has it become widely recognized that properly conducted clinical trials, which follow the principles of scientific experimentation, provide the only reliable basis for evaluating the efficacy and safety of new treatments. The major objective of this book is therefore to explain the main scientific and statistical issues which are vital to the conduct of effective and meaningful clinical research. In addition, some of the ethical and organizational problems of clinical trials will be discussed. The historical perspective, current status and future strategy for clinical trials provide a contextual framework for these methodological aspects.

In section 1.1, I discuss what constitutes a clinical trial and how clinical trials may usefully be classified. Section 1.2 deals with the underlying rationale for randomized controlled clinical trials and their relation to the scientific method. Section 1.3 goes on to describe one particular example, a clinical trial for primary breast cancer, as an illustration of how adherence to sound scientific principles led to an important advance in treatment.

1.1 TYPES OF CLINICAL TRIAL

Firstly, we need to define exactly what is meant by a 'clinical trial': briefly the term may be applied to any form of *planned experiment* which involves patients and is designed to elucidate the most appropriate treatment of future patients with a given medical condition. Perhaps the essential characteristic of a clinical trial is that one uses results based on a limited *sample* of patients to make inferences about how treatment should be conducted in the general *population* of patients who will require treatment in the future.

Animal studies clearly do not come within this definition and experiments on healthy human volunteers are somewhat borderline in that they provide only indirect evidence of effects on patients. However, such *volunteer studies* (often termed phase I trials) are an important first step in human exposure to potential new treatments and hence are included in our definition when appropriate.

Field trials of vaccines and primary prevention trials for subjects with presymptomatic conditions (e.g. high serum cholesterol) involve many of the same scientific and ethical issues as in the treatment of patients who are clearly diseased, and hence will also be mentioned when appropriate.

An individual *case study*, whereby one patient's pattern of treatment and response is reported as an interesting occurrence, does not really constitute a clinical trial. Since biological variation is such that patients with the same condition will almost certainly show varied responses to a given treatment, experience in one individual does not adequately enable inferences to be made about the general prospects for treating future patients in the same way. Thus, clinical trials inevitably require *groups of patients*: indeed one of the main problems is to get large enough groups of patients on different treatments to make reliable treatment comparisons.

Another issue concerns *retrospective surveys* which examine the outcomes of past patients treated in a variety of ways. These unplanned observational studies contain serious potential biases (e.g. more intensive treatments given to poorer prognosis patients may appear artificially inferior) so that they can rarely make a convincing contribution to the evaluation of alternative therapies. Hence, except in chapter 4 when considering the inadequacies of non-randomized trials, such studies will not be considered as clinical trials.

It is useful at this early stage to consider various ways of classifying clinical trials. Firstly, there is the *type of treatment*: the great majority of clinical trials are concerned with the evaluation of drug therapy more often than not with pharmaceutical company interest and financial backing. However, clinical trials may also be concerned with other forms of treatment. For instance, surgical procedures, radiotherapy for cancer, different forms of medical advice (e.g. diet and exercise policy after a heart attack) and alternative approaches to patient management (e.g. home or hospital care after inguinal hernia operation) should all be considered as forms of treatment which may be evaluated by clinical trials. Unfortunately, there has generally been inadequate use of well-designed clinical trials to evaluate these other non-pharmaceutical aspects of patient treatment and care, a theme which I shall return to later.

Drug trials within the pharmaceutical industry are often classified into four main phases of experimentation. These four phases are a general guideline as to how the clinical trials research programme for a new treatment in a specific disease might develop, and should not be taken as a hard and fast rule.

Phase I Trials: Clinical Pharmacology and Toxicity

These first experiments in man are primarily concerned with drug safety, not efficacy, and hence are usually performed on human volunteers, often pharmaceutical company employees. The first objective is to determine an acceptable single drug dosage (i.e. how much drug can be given without causing serious side-effects). Such information is often obtained from dose-escalation experiments, whereby a volunteer is subjected to increasing doses of the drug according to a predetermined schedule. Phase I will also involve studies of drug metabolism and bioavailability and, later, studies of multiple doses will be undertaken to determine appropriate dose schedules for use in phase II. After studies in normal volunteers, the initial trials in patients will also be of the phase I type. Typically, phase I studies might require a total of around 20–80 subjects and patients.

Phase II Trials: Initial Clinical Investigation for Treatment Effect

These are fairly small-scale investigations into the effectiveness and safety of a drug, and require close monitoring of each patient. Phase II trials can sometimes be set up as a screening process to select out those relatively few drugs of genuine potential from the larger number of drugs which are inactive or over-toxic, so that the chosen drugs may proceed to phase III trials. Seldom will phase II go beyond 100–200 patients on a drug.

Phase III Trials: Full-scale Evaluation of Treatment

After a drug is shown to be reasonably effective, it is essential to compare it with the current standard treatment(s) for the same condition in a large trial involving a substantial number of patients. To some people the term 'clinical trial' is synonymous with such a full-scale phase III trial, which is the most rigorous and extensive type of scientific clinical investigation of a new treatment. Accordingly , much of this book is devoted to the principles of phase III trials.

Phase IV Trials: Postmarketing Surveillance

After the research programme leading to a drug being approved for marketing, there remain substantial enquiries still to be undertaken as regards monitoring for adverse effects and additional large-scale, long-term studies of morbidity and mortality. Also the term 'phase IV trials' is sometimes used to describe promotion exercises aimed at bringing a new drug to the attention of a large number of clinicians, typically in general practice. This latter type of enquiry has limited scientific value and hence should not be considered part of clinical trial research.

This categorization of pharmaceutical company sponsored drug trials is inevitably an oversimplification of the real progress of a drug's clinical research programme. However, it serves to emphasize that there are important early human studies (phases I/II), with their own particular organizational, ethical and scientific problems, which need to be completed before full-scale phase III trials are undertaken. The Food and Drug Administration (1977) have issued guidelines for drug development programmes in the United States. The guidelines include recommendations on how phase I–III trials should be structured for drugs in 15 specific disease areas.

It should be remembered that each pharmaceutical company has an equally important *preclinical research* programme, which includes the synthesis of new drugs and animal studies for evaluating drug metabolism and later for testing efficacy and especially potential toxicity of a drug. The scale and scientific quality of these *animal experiments* have increased enormously, following legislation in many countries prompted by the thalidomide disaster. In particular any drug must pass rigorous safety tests in animals before it can be approved for clinical trials.

The phase I–III classification system may also be of general guidance for clinical trials not related to the pharmaceutical industry. For instance, cancer chemotherapy and radiotherapy research programmes, which take up a sizeable portion of the U.S. National Institutes of Health funding, can be conveniently organized in terms of phases I–III. In this context, phase I trials are necessarily on patients, rather than normal volunteers, due to the highly toxic nature of the treatments.

Development of new surgical procedures will also follow broadly similar plans, with phase I considered as basic development of surgical techniques. However, there is a paucity of well-designed phase III trials in surgery.

1.2 CONTROLLED CLINICAL TRIALS AND THE SCIENTIFIC METHOD

I will now concentrate on full-scale (phase III) trials and consider the scientific rationale for their conduct. Of course, the first priority for clinical research is to come up with a good idea for improving treatment. Progress can only be achieved if clinical researchers with insight and imagination can propose therapeutic innovations which appear to have a realistic chance of patient benefit. Naturally, the proponents of any new therapy are liable to be enthusiastic about its potential: preclinical studies and early phase I/II trials may indicate considerable promise. In particular, a pharmaceutical company can be very persuasive about its product before any full-scale trial is undertaken. Unfortunately, many new treatments turn out not to be as effective as was expected: once they are subjected to the rigorous test of a properly designed phase III trial many therapies fail to live up to expectation; see Gilbert *et al.* (1977) for examples in surgery and anaesthesia.

One fundamental rule is that *phase III trials are comparative*. That is, one needs to compare the experience of a group of patients on the new treatment with a *control group* of similar patients receiving a standard treatment. If there is no standard treatment of any real value, then it is often appropriate to have a control group of untreated patients. Also, in order to obtain an unbiassed evaluation of the new treatment's value one usually needs to assign each patient randomly to either new or standard treatment (see chapters 4 and 5 for details). Hence it is now generally accepted that the *randomized controlled trial* is the most reliable method of conducting clinical research.

At this point it is of value to present a few examples of randomized controlled trials to illustrate the use of control groups. Table 1.1 lists the six trials I wish to consider.

The first trial, for bacterial meningitis, represents the straightforward situation where a new treatment (cefuroxine) was compared with a standard treatment (the combination of ampicillin and chloramphenicol) to see if the former was more effective in killing the bacterium.

The anturan trial reflects another common situation where the new treatment (anturan) is to be compared with a placebo (inactive oral tablets that the patients could not distinguish from anturan). Thus, the control group of myocardial infarction patients did not receive any active treatment. The aim was to see if anturan could reduce mortality in the first year after an infarct.

The mild hypertension trial has two active treatments which are to be compared with placebo to see if either can reduce morbidity and mortality from cardiovascular-renal causes.

The trial for advanced colorectal cancer is unusual in having three new treatments to compare with the standard drug 5-fluorouracil (5-FU). Two of the new treatments consisted of 5-FU in combination with other drugs. Most trials have just two treatment groups (new *vs.* standard) and in general one needs to be wary of including more treatments since it becomes more difficult to get sufficient patients per treatment.

The last two trials in Table 1.1 are included as reminders that clinical trials can be used to evaluate aspects of treatment other than drug therapy. The stroke trial is concerned with patient management: can one improve recovery by caring for patients in a special stroke unit rather than in general medical wards?

The breast cancer trial represents an unusual situation in that it set out to compare two treatments (radical mastectomy or simple mastectomy + radiotherapy) each of which is standard practice depending on the hospital. In a sense each treatment is a control for the other. Such trials can be extremely important in resolving long-standing therapeutic controversies which have previously never been tested by a randomized controlled trial.

I now wish to consider how a clinical trial should proceed if the principles of the scientific method are to be followed. Figure 1.1 shows the general sequence of events. From an initial idea about a possible improvement in therapy one needs to produce a more precise definition of trial aims in terms of specific hypotheses regarding treatment efficacy and safety. That is, one must define exactly the type of patient, the treatments to be compared and the methods of evaluating each patient's response to treatment.

The next step is to develop a detailed design for a randomized trial and document one's plan in a study protocol. The design needs to fulfil scientific, ethical and organizational requirements so that the trial itself may be conducted efficiently and according to plan. Two principal issues here are:

Table 1.1. Some examples of randomized controlled trials

Reference	Disease	Treatments (control group in italics)*
Swedish Study Group (1982)	Bacterial meningitis	cefuroxine v. *ampicillin + chloramphenicol*
Anturane Reinfarction Trial (1980)	Acute myocardial infarction	anturan v. *placebo*
Medical Research Council Working Party (1977)	Mild hypertension	bendrofluazide v. propranolol v. *placebo*
Douglass *et al.* (1978)	Advanced colorectal cancer	methyl-CCNU v. $\dfrac{\text{5-FU}}{\text{TG}}$ v. $\dfrac{\text{5-FU}}{\text{CTX}}$ v. *5-FU*
Garraway *et al.* (1980)	Acute stroke	special stroke unit v. *general medical ward*
Langlands *et al.* (1980)	Operable breast cancer	radical mastectomy v. *simple mastectomy + radiotherapy*

* 5-FU = 5-fluorouracil, TG = 6-thioguanine, CTX = cytoxan

(a) *Size*   The trial must recruit enough patients to obtain a reasonably precise estimate of response on each treatment.

(b) *Avoidance of bias*   The selection, ancillary care and evaluation of patients should not differ between treatments, so that the treatment comparison is not affected by factors unrelated to the treatments themselves.

Statistical methods should be applied to the results in order to test the prespecified study hypotheses. In particular, one may use significance tests to assess how strong the evidence is for a genuine difference in response to treatment. Finally, one needs to draw conclusions regarding the treatments' relative merits and publish the results so that other clinicians may apply the findings.

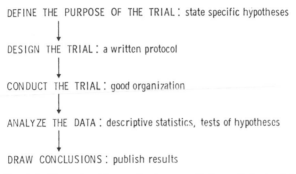

Fig. 1.1. The scientific method as applied to clinical trials

The aim of any clinical trial should be to obtain a truthful answer to a relevant medical issue. This requires that the conclusions be based on an unbiassed assessment of objective evidence rather than on a subjective compilation of clinical opinion. Historically, progress in clinical research has been greatly hindered by an inadequate appreciation of the essential methodology for clinical trials. After a brief historical review in chapter 2, the remainder of this book is concerned with a more extensive and practical account of this methodology. As a useful introduction to the main concepts, I now wish to focus on one particular trial for primary breast cancer.

1.3 AN EXAMPLE OF A CLINICAL TRIAL FOR PRIMARY BREAST CANCER

In 1972 a clinical trial was undertaken in the United States to evaluate whether the drug L-Pam (1-phenylalanine mustard) was of value in the treatment of primary breast cancer following a radical mastectomy. Fisher *et al.* (1975) presented the early findings with a subsequent update by Fisher *et al.* (1977). We now consider the development of this trial in the context of the scientific method outlined in figure 1.1.

(1) **Purpose of the Trial**

Earlier clinical trials for the treatment of patients with advanced (metastatic) breast cancer had shown that L-Pam was one of a number of drugs which could cause temporary shrinkage of tumours and increase survival in some patients. Therefore, it seemed sensible to argue that for patients with primary breast cancer who might still have an undetected small trace of tumour cells present after mastectomy, a drug such as L-Pam could be effective in killing off such cells and hence preventing subsequent disease recurrence. Such a *general concept* is an essential preliminary for a worthwhile clinical trial, but more precise *specific hypotheses* must be defined before a trial can be planned properly. There are four basic issues in this regard: the precise definition of (1) the *patients eligible* for study, (2) the *treatment*, (3) the *end-points* for evaluating each patient's response to treatment, and (4) the need for comparison with a *control group* of patients not receiving the new treatment. In this case these four issues were resolved as follows:

Eligible patients were defined as having had a radical mastectomy for primary breast cancer with histologically confirmed axillary node involvement. Patients were excluded if they had certain complications such as peau d'orange, skin ulceration, etc., or if they were aged over 75, were pregnant or lactating. Thus the trial focussed on those patients who were considered most likely to benefit from L-Pam if indeed it conferred any benefit at all.

Treatment was defined as L-Pam to be given orally at a dose of 0.15 mg/kg body weight for five consecutive days every six weeks, this dose schedule having been well established from studies in advanced breast cancer. Since haematologic toxicity will occur in some patients, *dose modifications* were defined as follows: reduce dose by half if platelet count < 100 000 or white cell count < 4000, and discontinue drug while platelet count < 75 000 or white cell count < 2500. For patients without toxicity after three consecutive courses, dosage was increased to 0.20 mg/kg. L-Pam was to be started less than four weeks after the patient's radical mastectomy and continued until treatment failure or for two years, whichever occurred first.

End-points for evaluating treatment were the disease-free interval (i.e. the time from mastectomy until first detection of tumour in local, regional or distant sites), the survival time (i.e. time from mastectomy until death) and also patient toxicity (haematologic and also nausea/vomiting). Disease-free interval would be the main criterion (that is, what percentages of patients were still alive and disease free after one year, two years, etc.), since there would not be many deaths in the first few years of follow-up and toxic effects were reasonably well known from studies in advanced disease.

A control group of patients would need to be treated in a standard way: that is, a separate group of patients just as eligible for the study would need to have a radical mastectomy but no subsequent L-Pam. They should then be followed in the same way to allow comparison of the percentages disease free in the treatment group and control group after one year, after two years, etc. Exactly how such a control group can be arranged is described in the design section to follow.

After the above clarifications, one is in a position to state the *main hypothesis* under study: Does L-Pam (as defined above) prolong the disease-free interval of primary breast cancer patients (as defined above) if given after a radical mastectomy?

Several subsidiary hypotheses concerning patient survival, toxicity and whether any increase in disease free interval is confined to particular subgroups of patients (e.g. prcmenopausal) are also to be tested if possible.

(2) Design of the Trial

As is necessary for any clinical trial, a *written protocol* was produced which documented all information concerning the purpose, design and conduct of the trial. Just a few of the salient design points will be mentioned here.

It was anticipated that the *number of patients* needed to obtain a clear answer to the main hypothesis would be of the order of several hundred. This required a *multi-centre* trial whereby, in fact, 37 American cancer hospitals agreed to enter patients into the trial. The study was coordinated by the National Surgical Adjuvant Breast Project (NSABP) and funded by the US National Cancer Institute.

The basic design was that each eligible patient was *randomly assigned* to receive either L-Pam or a *placebo* (an inert substance which looked and tasted the same as L-Pam). This randomization was by telephone to a central office in Pittsburgh. Patients were *stratified* by age (under or over 50), nodal status (1–3 or 4+ positive axillary nodes) and institution so that the randomization could be restricted to ensure the two treatment groups of patients would be comparable as regards these three factors. Each patient had a 50/50 chance of being assigned to L-Pam. The precise mechanics of such a stratified randomization will be explained in chapter 5.

The trial was *double-blind* so that neither the patient nor her attending physician nor others concerned with patient care or evaluation knew which treatment she was on, the oral drug or placebo being supplied in anonymous containers. Stratified randomization, the use of placebo and the double-blind restriction were all considered essential to ensure that the comparison of treatment and control groups could not be influenced by any extraneous factors such as the physician's personal judgement or the patient's morale. Such plans to eliminate bias are the key to any successful trial.

Each patient was to have a follow-up examination every six weeks and tests for haematologic toxicity every three weeks. Other blood tests, chest X-rays and bone scans were performed at less frequent but regular intervals. Thus, *endpoint evaluation* was performed in the same consistent and objective manner for all patients.

(3) **Conduct of the Trial**

The first patient was entered into the study in September 1972. *Patient accrual* was terminated in February 1975, by which time 370 patients had been entered from the 37 participating institutions. In each case, *informed patient consent* to take part in the trial was obtained in accordance with standard United States procedure.

In a trial of this size and complexity there were inevitably some *protocol violations*. For instance, five patients were ineligible for the study and 17 patients did not start their treatment according to protocol. These patients were excluded from further study, so that there were 348 patients for analysis, 169 on placebo and 179 on L-Pam.

There were also a few subsequent *patient withdrawals* from the study: reasons included two patients refusing further treatment (placebo, in fact), three patients developing a second cancer unrelated to their primary breast tumour, one myocardial infarction and one renal failure death. It was decided that each of these withdrawals bore no relation to treatment and hence in analysis such patients were handled as if they were lost to follow-up at the time of withdrawal.

For such a large multi-centre trial it was important to have an effective *trial committee* (including a *study chairman*) which would meet periodically to assess progress and make alterations as necessary. For instance, it became evident after a few months that there was some resistance to the initial decision to restrict patient entry to those with four or more positive axillary nodes, so that an early protocol alteration was to allow patients with one or more positive nodes to enter the trial.

In addition, day-to-day running of the trial was handled by the NSABP Headquarters Office in Pittsburgh. Besides monitoring patient entry, such a *central coordinating office* is essential for supervising *data collection* and *processing* prior to statistical analysis. In this case, it was the responsibility of *data managers* to ensure that all *forms* with patient data were received promptly, checked for errors or missing data and computer processed.

(4) **Data Analysis**

For a trial that takes over two years to recruit sufficient patients and which requires subsequent follow-up of each patient for several years, information about the relative merits of the treatments is accumulated slowly. It is therefore common practice to undertake occasional *interim analyses* of the accumulating results while the trial is in progress. In this particular trial there was considerable pressure to reveal the findings about disease-free survival at an early stage, since it was widely recognized that this trial would provide a major breakthrough in the treatment of primary breast cancer if the results were positive. The study chairman and his trial committee resisted this pressure for premature publication and maintained strict secrecy over their results until there was strong statistical evidence of improved disease-free survival on L-Pam especially in premenopausal women. Thus, such early findings were first revealed in 1975 but I will now concentrate on the more extensive results published by Fisher *et al.* (1977).

The easiest item to note first as regards disease-free survival is the number of patients on each treatment who had a recurrence of their disease and/or died. However, in such a *follow-up study* this comparison is over-simple since it fails to take into account the different lengths of time patients had been followed for: ranging from 20 months to 48 months in the 1977 analysis. Hence, a statistical technique known as life-table analysis of survival data was used to produce the results in figure 1.2, which shows for each treatment the estimated percentage of patients still alive and disease-free according to the time since mastectomy. This graph shows that 11 % of patients on L-Pam had disease recurrence within a year of mastectomy compared with 24 % of patients on placebo. After two years' follow-up the estimated percentage recurrence was 24 % and 32 % on L-Pam and placebo, respectively. Such *descriptive statistics*, clearly displayed in graphical or tabular form, are an important indication as to whether an interesting treatment difference may have arisen.

However, referring back to the main hypothesis before the trial began, one needs a formal *test of hypothesis* to assess whether the apparent improvement in disease-free survival on L-Pam can genuinely be attributed to the drug or could have arisen by chance. Conventionally this is done using a *statistical significance test*, the logic of which is as follows:

(1) Suppose L-Pam and placebo are really equally effective as regards disease-free survival (this is called the null hypothesis).
(2) Then, what is the probability P of getting such a big observed difference in disease-free survival as was found in figure 1.2, if the null hypothesis is true.

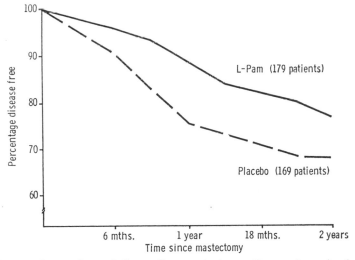

Fig. 1.2. Comparison of disease free survival on L-Pam and on placebo

(3) The answer is $P = 0.009$, i.e. such a difference is to be expected by chance 9 times in 1000. This was determined by a statistical method called the modified Wilcoxon test, the details of which need not concern us. The standard phraseology is then to declare that the treatment difference in disease-free survival is statistically significant at the 1% level (i.e. $P < 0.01$ for short).

(4) This formal procedure enables one to say that there is strong evidence that L-Pam does prolong disease-free survival. However, it should be noted that in any clinical trial one can *never* obtain absolute proof of a treatment difference, but merely assess the extent to which the evidence is indicative of a treatment difference; such is the reality of the scientific method.

In addition to this global comparison of treatments relating to all patients in the trial, it is useful to examine whether the apparent benefit of L-Pam might depend on some *prognostic factors*, i.e. clinical or personal features of a patient as recorded in the initial patient status upon entry into the trial. In this trial it was anticipated that the patient's age, menopausal state and number of positive axillary nodes might influence the effect of L-Pam. As shown in figure 1.3 it turned out that the difference between L-Pam and placebo was more marked in patients under age 50 than in those over age 50. However, one needs to be careful in interpreting such apparent subgroup differences in treatment effect.

Patient survival has also been studied, there being 84% and 90% alive after two years on placebo and L-Pam, respectively. This difference is not statistically significant, but this does not indicate that L-Pam has no effect on patient survival. One really needs to follow such patients for up to five years in order to give a clear verdict on patient survival.

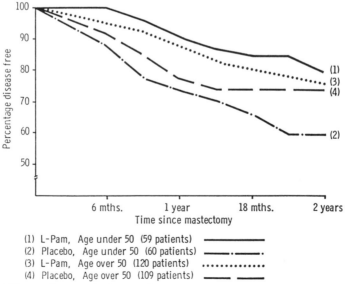

(1) L-Pam, Age under 50 (59 patients) ————————
(2) Placebo, Age under 50 (60 patients) ——.——— .
(3) L-Pam, Age over 50 (120 patients) ••••••••••••
(4) Placebo, Age over 50 (109 patients) ——— ———

Fig. 1.3. Disease-free survival according to treatment (L-Pam or placebo) and age

Assessment of the *toxic side-effects* of L-Pam is important, since one wants to avoid undue drug toxicity in treating patients who have no observable disease after mastectomy. White cell count and/or platelet counts were lowered in the majority of patients on L-Pam, sufficient to require treatment to be stopped for a while in over a quarter of patients, but no life-threatening cases were reported. Also, 40 % of L-Pam patients experienced some degree of nausea and vomiting (so did 11 % of placebo patients, an indication that all untoward events cannot automatically be attributed to drug therapy). However, in view of the serious nature of the disease and other potential benefits of L-Pam, such toxicity was generally considered acceptable.

(5) Conclusions from the Trial

The overall assessment of L-Pam treatment focusses on the main hypothesis concerning disease-free interval, with appropriate account being taken of the subsidiary hypotheses concerning survival and toxicity. Thus it appears that L-Pam after mastectomy is a useful supplement to treatment of primary breast cancer with positive axillary nodes, but the benefit is more evident for younger premenopausal women than for older postmenopausal women. However, patient follow-up continues and subsequent survival comparisons will extend the conclusions. The trial organizers felt that the benefits were sufficient to prohibit the use of placebo in their next clinical trial started in 1975 which compares L-Pam with L-Pam + 5-FU. Another trial of three-drug chemotherapy has also now been started. It is interesting to note that the new trials have accrued patients at a much faster rate: that is, it is much easier to get physicians to enter patients on a clinical trial once earlier pioneering trials have shown the general approach to be beneficial. Fisher *et al.* (1981) review subsequent progress in these trials.

The main means of bringing the outcome of a trial to the attention of a general medical audience is to *publish the results* in a medical journal. The introduction, methods, results and conclusions sections of such a paper (the standard layout of scientific articles) correspond to the purpose, design and conduct, analysis and conclusions stages of a trial as outlined in figure 1.1. All of the paper prior to the conclusions will concentrate on objective statements of factual evidence, whereas the conclusions tend to be a more subjective opinion of the authors based on their experienced interpretation of the evidence. However, in any trial, and indeed this trial of L-Pam for primary breast cancer is no exception, the ultimate conclusion rests with other practising physicians whose subsequent experience of L-Pam and similar therapies either in future trials or as part of their regular practice will determine whether such therapy is generally applicable.

I hope the above description of one specific clinical trial has given a sense of reality to the main requirements of clinical trials in general. Of course citing one such example has its limitations since each particular trial has its own unique aspects. Nevertheless, many of the principles described in chapters 3–15 have been encapsulated in this example.

CHAPTER 2

The Historical Development of Clinical Trials

Attempts to evaluate the use of therapeutic procedures can be traced back to prehistoric times, and Bull (1959) provides an extensive account of the historical development of clinical trials up until 30 years ago. However, it is largely in these last 30 years that we have seen the development and general acceptance of properly conducted clinical trials which have conformed to the scientific principles outlined in this book. Furthermore, there has been an enormous continuing expansion in clinical trial activity throughout the 20th century which will probably carry on through the 1980's. A comprehensive historical review of clinical trials would require a book all to itself. Hence only a few of the major highlights in actual trials and conceptual developments will be mentioned here.

Section 2.1 gives a brief account of some interesting landmarks in clinical trials pre-1950, culminating in the pioneering postwar trials by the Medical Research Council. Section 2.2 brings us into the modern era of properly designed clinical trials, focussing on two early randomized trials in polio vaccine and diabetes. Sections 2.3–2.5 deal with three general areas of progress: cancer chemotherapy, post-infarction trials and the pharmaceutical industry.

2.1 CLINICAL TRIALS BEFORE 1950

There are some early landmarks in clinical investigation which anticipate the current methodology. For instance, Lind (1753) planned a comparative trial of *the most promising treatments for scurvy*. He says,

I took twelve patients in the scurvy on board the Salisbury at sea. The cases were as similar as I could have them ... they lay together in one place ... and had one diet common to them all. Two of these were ordered a quart of cider a day. Two others took twenty-five gutts of elixir vitriol ... Two others took two spoonfuls of vinegar ... Two were put under a course of sea water ... Two others had each two oranges and one lemon given them each day ... Two others took the bigness of a nutmeg. The most sudden and visible good effects were perceived from the use of oranges and lemons, one of those who had taken them being at the end of six days fit for duty ... The other ... was appointed nurse to the rest of the sick.

14

Although the trial appeared conclusive, Lind continued to propose 'pure dry air' as a first priority with fruit and vegetables as a secondary recommendation. Furthermore, almost 50 years elapsed before the British navy supplied lemon juice to its ships. Unfortunately, many trials today also experience such delays before their conclusions are applied to general medical practice.

However, most pre-20th century medical experimenters had no appreciation of the scientific method. For instance, Rush (1794) had this report of his *treatment of yellow fever by bleeding*:

> I began by drawing a small quantity at a time. The appearance of the blood and its effects upon the system satisfied me of its safety and efficacy. Never before did I experience such sublime joy as I now felt in contemplating the success of my remedies . . . The reader will not wonder when I add a short extract from my notebook, dated 10th September. 'Thank God', of the one hundred patients, whom I visited, or prescribed for, this day, I have lost none.

Such totally subjective and extravagant claims were the norm for this era, though some researchers were becoming critically aware of the need for objective and statistically valid trials.

Louis (1834) lays a clear foundation for the use of the *'numerical method'* in assessing therapies:

> As to different methods of treatment, if it is possible for us to assure ourselves of the superiority of one or other among them in any disease whatever, having regard to the different circumstances of age, sex and temperament, of strength and weakness, it is doubtless to be done by enquiring if under these circumstances a greater number of individuals have been cured by one means than another. Here again it is necessary to count. And it is, in great part at least, because hitherto this method has been not at all, or rarely employed, that the science of therapeutics is still so uncertain; that when the application of the means placed in our hands is useful we do not know the bounds of this utility.

He goes on to discuss the need for: (1) the exact observation of patient outcome, (2) knowledge of the natural progress of untreated controls, (3) precise definition of disease prior to treatment, and (4) careful observation of deviations from intended treatment. He also lays stress on the difficulties to be overcome in conducting such experiments. Louis (1835) is the best illustration of his approach: he studied the value of bleeding as a treatment for pneumonia (78 cases), erysipelas (33 cases) and throat inflammation (23 cases) and found no demonstrable difference between patients bled and not bled. This finding totally contradicted current clinical practice in France and instigated the eventual decline in bleeding as a standard treatment. Louis had an immense influence on clinical practice in France, Britain and America and can be considered the founding figure who established clinical trials and epidemiology on a scientific footing.

However, in each country there continued *the arbitrary creation of ineffective therapies* whose supporters claimed dramatic success. Sutton (1865) conducted an interesting study in rheumatic fever where 20 patients received only mint water (this may have been the first use of a placebo) and demonstrated the immense natural variation in the disease process and the tendency to a natural cure in some cases. Holmes (1891) indicated the need for progress in American clinical research to counteract overmedication: he cites the major reasons for this situation as incapacity for sound observation, inability to weigh evidence, the counting of only favourable cases, the assumption that treatment was responsible for any favourable outcome, failure to learn from experience and a public which 'insists on being poisoned'.

There were many advances in surgery during the 19th century, thanks to the discovery of *general anaesthetics*. The immediate efficacy of many such procedures was considered so dramatic as to deny the need for control groups and substantial patient numbers. This informal approach to surgical research still applies today and carries the risk of falsely establishing a poor surgical procedure as being effective. Fortunately, many of the 19th century developments were so genuinely and remarkably beneficial that inadequate trials could not hinder such progress. Lister (1870) undertook a more substantial study of amputation operations comparing mortality of 43 % in 35 cases before the use of antiseptics with mortality of 15 % in 40 cases treated by the new antiseptic method. He argues cautiously that 'the numbers are doubtless too small for a satisfactory statistical comparison' though in fact the improvement in survival is statistically significant using a chi-squared test ($\chi^2 = 7.19$, $P < 0.01$ as reported nowadays). In reality, his self-criticism would have been better directed to the inadequacies of such retrospective comparison with a historical control group, since selection of cases for operation or other relevant features might have changed. Bull (1959) comments 'had it been possible a careful comparative trial of rival methods at this stage might have prevented the bitter and profitless controversy which raged for many years on the subject of the importance and technique of prevention of infection at operation'.

Fibiger (1898) in a trial of serum for diphtheria, is an early illustration of *alternate assignment* of patients to treatment and untreated control, in contrast to many other inadequately controlled studies of that period. Greenwood and Yule (1915), in a review of anticholera and antityphoid studies, appear to be the first to suggest that some form of random allocation of patients to treatment is necessary to generate truly comparable treatment groups.

Ferguson et al. (1927) in a study of vaccines for the common cold may have been the first to introduce *blinding*. Their study was single blind in that the research workers, but not the patients, knew who received saline or vaccine injections.

During the 1930's two major areas for clinical trials were *the sulphonamides and antimalarial drugs*. Colebrook and Purdie (1937) showed a mortality reduction from 22 % to 8 % for sulphonilamide treatment of puerperal fever compared with a historical control group of the previous year's patients treated at the same hospital. Evans and Gaisford (1938) achieved similar results comparing sulfapyridine with routine non-specific therapy for 200 patients with lobar pneumonia, alternate assignment of patients being used. The League of

Nations Malaria Commission (1937) describe the trials of antimalarial drugs: an extensive multidisciplinary research programme which had tremendously valuable consequences both in prevention, treatment and understanding of the disease.

The discovery of penicillin can be considered the most important therapeutic advance in the 20th century. Clinical trials, e.g. Abraham *et al.* (1941), began with very few extremely ill patients due to shortage of drug, but such dramatic results were seen that the lack of controls did not seriously impede the clear conclusions. The effects of penicillin treatment of war wound infections were investigated in North Africa: a controlled trial involving many collaborative surgeons was intended, but the wish of surgeons not to withhold penicillin from severe cases led to the penicillin group as a whole having a higher proportion of the seriously ill. Nevertheless, the superiority of penicillin was so great that its effectiveness could be demonstrated despite this bias. However, Bull (1959) observes that 'in retrospect this trial would appear to have been more successful than might have been anticipated with such indirect organisation and multiple observers. Had penicillin been less effective the biased control might have caused an inconclusive result: since the effect was so great perhaps a smaller and more precise trial would have demonstrated it with greater efficiency.'

However, the evaluation of penicillin treatment for more minor conditions such as finger pulp infections undoubtedly benefitted from properly controlled trials. After conflicting early studies with inadequate controls, Harrison *et al.* (1949) undertook a study in which patients were randomly allocated to the different treatment groups which clearly established the benefit of penicillin for finger pulp infections.

It is generally agreed that *the first clinical trial with a properly randomized control group* was for streptomycin in treatment of pulmonary tuberculosis (see Medical Research Council, 1948). This trial is remarkable for the degree of care exercised in its planning, execution and reporting, such that it represents many of the desired features of modern-day clinical trials. The trial involved patient accrual from several centres at each of which random allocation to treatment, streptomycin and bed-rest, or bed-rest alone, was made by a system of sealed envelopes. Evaluation of patient X-ray films was made independently by two radiologists and a clinician, each of whom did not know the others' evaluations or which treatment the patient was on. This blinded and replicated evaluation of a difficult disease end-point added considerably to the final agreed patient evaluation. Both patient survival and radiological improvement were significantly better on streptomycin.

The conflicting reports on antihistaminic drugs for treatment of the common cold led to another randomized controlled trial (Medical Research Council, 1950). This trial was notable for *using a placebo control in a double-blind manner*; neither the patient nor the investigator knew whether antihistamine or control tablet had been given in a particular case. This was important since patients were asked to evaluate their own improvement and over 20 % of the 1550 cases failed to comply either to treatment or evaluation. The end-results showed no benefit (e.g. 40 % on antihistamine and 39 % on placebo considered themselves cured within a week). It is hard to see how such a clear rejection of an ineffective treatment could have been achieved other than by a large multi-centre double-blind placebo-controlled randomized trial.

2.2 CLINICAL TRIALS SINCE 1950

Sir Austin Bradford Hill was the prime motivator behind these Medical Research Council trials and had much to do with the subsequent development of controlled clinical trials in Britain. In the early 1950's he produced several general articles on the conduct of clinical trials (see Hill, 1962, chapters 1–3) in which he clearly presents such fundamental concepts as concurrent controls, random allocation, definition of eligible patients, definition of treatment schedule, objective evaluation and statistical analysis. Hill (1962) also includes reports of later trials in rheumatoid arthritis, cerebrovascular disease and field trials of vaccines for tuberculosis, influenza and whooping cough, in all of which he had a major collaborative role.

One relevant question to ask at this point is why it took until 1950 to establish the ground rules for conducting clinical trials on a scientific basis. Bull (1959) lists some relevant factors: 'reverence for authority, the relationship of doctor and patient, the paucity of records, lack of facilities for investigation, polypharmacy and lack of active remedies'. Another important reason for this development of properly designed clinical trials was the *increasing concern with treatment of non-communicable disease* where (1) dramatic clear-cut advances in therapy are less likely than with communicable disease, and (2) the search for moderate, but valuable, improvements in treatment can only be resolved by randomized controlled trials.

However, one cannot say that progress in clinical trials since 1950 has been of consistent scientific quality. Therefore, the examples I now present include some problems as well as successes. The complete range of clinical trial effort since 1950 is too vast to summarize briefly. Instead, I will discuss two interesting trials (the field trial of the Salk polio virus and the University Group Diabetes Program) and then focus on three broader areas of research:

(1) clinical trials of cancer chemotherapy in the United States
(2) clinical trials for the treatment of acute myocardial infarction
(3) the development of clinical trials within the pharmaceutical industry.

The Field Trial of the Salk Polio Vaccine

In 1954 1.8 million young children in the United States participated in the largest field trial ever undertaken to assess the effectiveness of the Salk vaccine in preventing paralysis or death from poliomyelitis. Such a large experiment was needed since the annual incidence rate of polio was about 1 per 2000 and clear evidence of treatment effect, if present, was needed as soon as possible so that the vaccine could be routinely given.

One approach would have been to introduce the vaccine into certain areas and compare subsequent polio incidence with untreated areas. The problem is that polio tends to occur in epidemics which can affect some cities and not others so that geographic differences could not necessarily be attributed to treatment. Therefore, it was proposed that each area participating in the study should offer vaccination to all second-grade children and use untreated first and third graders as a control group, and over 1 million children participated in such a scheme. Difficulties in this *observed control approach*, anticipated beforehand, were that:

(1) only volunteers could be vaccinated and these tended to be from a wealthier and more highly educated background
(2) evaluating physicians would be aware which children had been vaccinated and such knowledge could in theory influence their more difficult diagnoses.

Hence, an alternative *randomized double-blind placebo-controlled trial* was undertaken simultaneously in other areas where health departments were anxious to avoid the above possibilities of bias. A further 0.8 million volunteer children were randomly assigned to placebo or vaccine in a manner such that neither the child, his or her family, nor the evaluating physicians were aware of whether the child had the vaccine. Only after a final diagnosis of whether polio had occurred was identification made as to whether the child had received vaccine or placebo. The results of this placebo-controlled part of the trial were very convincing: the overall polio incidence in the vaccinated group was half that of the placebo group, the incidence of paralytic polio was over 70% less and all four deaths occurred in the placebo group. Results from the 'observed control' areas supported these findings but there also was evidence that children who were invited but declined to volunteer for vaccination had lower incidence than the non-vaccinated controls in both parts of the study. The presence of this 'volunteer effect' means that the non-randomized 'observed control' part of the study could not by itself have provided such unequivocal evidence of the vaccine's value.

The Salk vaccine was widely used after the trial but subsequent developments revealed some problems with the vaccine, specifically that a few lots of the vaccine were inadequately prepared and actually caused polio in some children, so that within a few years the killed-virus Salk vaccine was displaced by live-virus vaccine. Thus, even though the trial was well designed and conclusive it was in reality just one step in the continuing progress of preventive medicine. More detailed descriptions of the trial are given by Francis *et al.* (1955) and Meier (1972), the latter forming the basis for this brief summary.

The University Group Diabetes Program (UGDP)

This randomized multi-centre trial in the United States began in 1961. In the original seven collaborating clinics the four treatments for adult-onset diabetics were tolbutamide (an oral hypoglycaemic agent), variable-dose insulin, standard-dose insulin and placebo. In 1962–1963 phenformin (another oral drug) was added to the trial in five new clinics plus one of the original seven. The trial was partially double-blind in that the oral drugs and placebo were considered indistinguishable. The six centres with phenformin randomized 3/7ths of patients to that drug and 1/7th to each of the others in order to achieve sufficient patients on phenformin overall. The other centres randomized equal numbers to each of the four treatments. More than a thousand patients entered the trial.

As patient follow-up continued through the 1960's it began to appear that there was an excess of cardiovascular deaths occurring in the tolbutamide group such that in 1969 a decision was taken to discontinue the drug. In 1971 phenformin was discontinued for the same reason, but here we will concentrate on developments relating to tolbutamide. Cardiovascular mortality had not originally been considered a major end-point of the study, and since tolbutamide was widely used in routine medical practice this apparent cardiovascular toxicity was a very surprising observation. Nevertheless, the trial organizers felt that such a highly significant difference in cardiovascular mortality (12.7% on tolbutamide versus 4.9% on placebo) meant that it was unethical to continue the drug. Since this conclusion was contrary to prior medical opinion, the methods and results of the trial have come under intense scrutiny and considerable criticism by some observers. Thus, a committee was set up to assess the evidence from this trial and their report (Gilbert et al., 1975), forms the basis of this description. The excess cardiovascular mortality was confirmed by this committee's reanalysis of the data, being particularly noticeable in older women.

The committee commented that the general organization and efficiency of the UGDP trial was of a high standard, indeed considerably better than most other trials. However, a few problems were noted:

(1) The decision to stop tolbutamide in 1969 meant that the body of evidence was not as great as might have been, but the trial organizers could not be faulted for their ethical concern for patients in the trial.
(2) Some patients had less advanced disease than might be considered necessary for oral agents in standard medical practice, but this could scarcely bias the evidence of drug toxicity.
(3) The randomization procedure resulted in some clinics having more men on one treatment than the others, but such accidental sex imbalances could not explain treatment differences.
(4) The mortality difference between tolbutamide and placebo for all causes of death was not statistically significant, which somewhat weakens the evidence against the drug.
(5) Many patients did not remain on their initial treatment, but such non-adherence to protocol was allowed for in a reanalysis without change of conclusion.
(6) The trial used a fixed dose of tolbutamide whereas it is customary clinical practice to use variable dosage.

Thus, the committee considered that the evidence of drug harmfulness was moderately strong. Evidently, such an opinion has not claimed universal acceptance since tolbutamide remains in common use for the treatment of diabetes. This problem illustrates that a single trial with an unexpected finding will not necessarily sway the balance of medical opinion, even though its evidence is statistically convincing, and it is therefore important that such findings be replicated in other studies. Unfortunately, the polarization of opinion evoked by the UGDP trial has prevented further randomized studies of tolbutamide.

2.3 CANCER CHEMOTHERAPY IN THE UNITED STATES

In 1948 there occurred *the first case reports* of children with acute leukemia achieving short-term responses when treated with aminopterin. There followed a whole variety of uncontrolled studies which showed evidence of patients with acute lymphocytic leukemia responding to treatment. Untreated control groups were considered unnecessary since the untreated disease had a uniformly fatal outcome. Difficulties arose in that the relative merits of different drugs and dose schedules could not be deciphered from such non-comparative small series of cases; many of these early trials had around ten patients and since only around 30% of patients responded the estimation of treatment effect was poor.

Therefore, in 1954 the National Cancer Institute began organizing *the first randomized clinical trial in acute lymphocytic leukemia* (see Frei *et al.*, 1958), in which two different schedules of 6 mercaptopurine and methotrexate were compared. Five collaborating centres were involved in order to accrue enough cases (56 patients in all). The successful organization of this particular trial quickly led to the formation of *two collaborative groups* for leukemia which are still operative today under the names Children's Cancer Study Group, and Cancer and Leukemia Group B. Also, during the early 1950's there was accumulating evidence that the nitrogen mustards were showing effect in the treatment of some adult malignancies so that in 1955 the Eastern Solid Tumor Group, a collaboration of five institutions on the US east coast, was established and supported by the National Cancer Institute to investigate the relative tumor activities of nitrogen mustard and thio-tepa.

The promise of early results from cancer chemotherapy plus the ready availability of funds for cancer research led to *a rapid expansion in the number of cooperative multi-centre groups* entering patients on cancer clinical trials such that by 1960 there were 21 such groups within the United States, mostly concerned with chemotherapy though a few were for evaluating radiotherapy and/or surgery. There was a large body of clinical cancer research being conducted in individual centres, but cooperative cancer groups were becoming established as the proper way to conduct meaningful trials on substantial numbers of patients. Nevertheless, much of this early research up until 1970 would be considered inadequate by current standards. Patients entered onto chemotherapy trials tended to have advanced disease so that short-term chemotherapy was applied to induce temporary shrinkage of tumour masses. Indeed, in much of the early research patient survival was not considered as a primary end-point and rarely were patients followed for more than a few months. Also, preliminary evaluation of drugs was not disease-specific, with non-randomized phase II studies across all disease sites which were hard to interpret. Although there was considerable progress through randomized studies in the treatment of childhood leukemia, the early promise of chemotherapy for adult solid tumours did not lead to major patient benefit for some years. However, the early cooperative experience did much to develop the basis of modern cancer clinical trials. Standards were set for the evaluation of tumour response, patient performance and drug toxicity, the detailed definition of trial protocols and the statistical analysis of results.

Over the past decade cancer chemotherapy has undergone many changes and I illustrate these by the experience of the *Eastern Cooperative Oncology Group* (ECOG). Formerly, the Eastern Solid Tumor Group, it had expanded from the original five institutions to include 15 cancer centres by 1971. Since then, this group has contributed to the development of more effective drug combinations particularly in breast cancer and the lymphomas. However, Williams and Carter (1978) remind us that 'a successful clinical trial is one that reaches the correct conclusion, not one that produces a positive result', and it is in this respect that cooperative group trials have had an important negative role to play. Uncontrolled studies usually in single institutions have frequently led to extravagant claims for the discovery of cancer cures: for instance, immunotherapy for the treatment of malignant melanoma was considered an exciting prospect in the early 1970's but carefully controlled trials by ECOG and other groups showed such treatment to be ineffective. Some notable advances in cancer have been initiated by single institutions, for example the highly effective MOPP four-drug regimen for Hodgkin's disease. However, large scale cooperative group trials have been an essential confirmation of its validity which has also enabled testing of various modifications of the regimen.

An important recent advance has been in *the development of combined modality trials* whereby chemotherapy has been tested as an adjuvant to primary surgical treatment of cancer. The most dramatic success has been in primary breast cancer and the study by Fisher *et al.* (1977) has already been described in chapter 1. This randomized double-blind trial comparing L-Pam and placebo after mastectomy for patients with axillary node involvement, showed fewer relapses on L-Pam for premenopausal women and subsequent follow-up confirms a survival advantage also. The results for postmenopausal patients showed less-convincing evidence of a treatment difference. Further trials within NSABP and ECOG have tested more complex drug combinations to see if further improvements can be obtained. Bonadonna *et al.* (1977) in Italy have compared a three-drug regimen CMF against no treatment after radical mastectomy and also show markedly improved results in premenopausal patients. These findings led to a proliferation of randomized surgical adjuvant trials in breast cancer throughout the world. Such intensive research in the primary treatment of such a common cancer is to be encouraged: however, interpretation of the large body of evidence to come over the next few years will not be an easy task.

The perspective of ECOG and other chemotherapy groups has thus broadened over the last few years, so that many trials now use drugs as a 'frontline weapon' to be combined with conventional surgery and/or radiotherapy for primary diseases, e.g. breast cancer, melanoma, colorectal cancer and brain tumours. Meanwhile, the development of new drugs and combinations for advanced cancer continues, though trials nowadays are more efficient, better organized and have a greater prospect of patient benefit and survival than in earlier years. Unfortunately, there remain some diseases, e.g. lung cancer, where the value of chemotherapy has remained very limited.

So far I have tended to look at cancer trials in terms of specific improvements in treatment. Of course, if promising treatments do not exist then no progress can be made. However, one vital element in US cancer trial cooperative groups such as ECOG has been *the consistent development of scientifically and statistically designed trials in a well-organized framework*. In 1982 ECOG has 26 member institutions (which include 164 affiliate hospitals attached to such institutions) and 44 active studies accruing around 2000 new patients per annum. This large-scale collaborative effort requires that concentrated attention be paid to the efficient handling of patients and the information derived from their response to treatment. For instance, in addition to the 1065 clinical investigators, ECOG has 18 statisticians and 237 'data managers', the latter being primarily responsible for ensuring that good quality data are being collected and computer-processed. Unlike those in earlier trials, all patients are now followed so that for each trial important survival data can eventually be added to the earlier response and remission duration data, and again this is a major administrative task.

One innovation in the last few years has been a 'cancer control' programme which is intended to improve the knowledge and implementation of current cancer treatment in local community hospitals by encouraging them to participate in the clinical trials of ECOG and other such groups (see Begg *et al.*, 1982). It is hoped that this additional educational role of cooperative groups will ensure that the high standards of cancer care given in specialized cancer centres can be extended to other hospitals for the benefit of the whole community.

In 1981, the National Cancer Institute supported 13 such collaborative multi-centre cancer clinical trial groups at a total annual cost of around $35 million. There are 450 major cancer centres involved and 386 currently active clinical trials accruing around 19 500 patients per annum. In addition, there is considerable local research, usually in smaller trials and phase I and II studies, at each individual cancer centre. Thus, in the American cancer trials programme, particularly as regards chemotherapy, the last 30 years have seen develop the greatest onslaught of randomized controlled trials that has ever occurred in a single disease area. Successes have not been easily come by and there are occasional accusations that such intensive research may sometimes lead to the overzealous recommendations of highly toxic and marginally effective regimes (see Nelson, 1979), but the clear advances in leukemia, lymphomas and breast cancer do much to justify this approach.

2.4 TREATMENT OF ACUTE MYOCARDIAL INFARCTION

In such a complex area as the treatment and management of patients after acute myocardial infarction I do not propose to give a comprehensive view of clinical trials. Instead I will focus attention on two types of drug therapy, anticoagulants and platelet-active drugs, and then make brief mention of a rather different type of trial concerned with methods of patient management (i.e. home *versus* hospital care).

The potential benefit of *anticoagulants* after myocardial infarction was first realized in the mid-1940's and although their use was endorsed by the American Heart Association as long ago as 1948 there still remains today considerable divergence of opinion regarding their value. This uncertainty has partly resulted from the doubtful quality of much early research which at the time suggested that anticoagulants could more than halve case fatality after an infarct. One problem emphasized in a review by Chalmers *et al.* (1977) is that the great majority of trials, indeed all trials in this area before 1960, were undertaken without a randomized control group on placebo or no treatment. Accordingly, Chalmers *et al.* show that from 18 trials, each of which compared a current group of patients on anticoagulants with a historical control group (i.e. earlier untreated patients), an apparent overall estimated 54% reduction in mortality was shown. This weight of evidence, based on over 9000 patients, seems overwhelming until one realizes how biassed such comparisons might be. Case selection for anticoagulant therapy was likely to be restricted to patients who were well enough to potentially benefit whereas there was no opportunity to exclude the sicker patients from the historical control groups, so that the mortality excess in the latter group could be much inflated. This hypothesis has been substantiated by three large randomized trials reported in 1969–1973 which collectively estimated a 21% reduction in mortality following anticoagulant therapy. Consequently, the extravagant claims for anticoagulant therapy have now been moderated to a more realistic but still important level of patient benefit. One would hope that today's improved standards of clinical research would prevent the recurrence of such a disorganized approach to the evaluation of a new therapy.

Over the last ten years there has developed considerable interest in the role of *platelet-active drugs* such as aspirin in the secondary prevention of coronary heart disease. Peto (1980) reviews the results of six large randomized trials comparing aspirin with placebo involving over 10 000 patients. The general quality of these trials has been high, but nevertheless their interpretation is not easy. Transferring this interesting and apparently simple idea (giving aspirin to prevent recurrent heart attacks) to actual clinical practice presents problems regarding the dosage and timing of drug administration. Thus, one trial has assessed the value of a single dose as soon as possible after infarct while two others have been concerned with daily dosage started several months after infarct. Another problem is that no single trial has shown a statistically significant mortality reduction though five of the six have lower mortality in the aspirin group. However, by combining results from all the trials (possibly a dubious mixture given the different dose patterns), Peto estimates that the overall mortality reduction from aspirin is liable to be of the order of 10 %. The corresponding overall reduction in reinfarctions (fatal and non-fatal) was found to be somewhat greater, around a 20 % risk reduction. This example indicates the considerable amount of time and effort required to evaluate a new therapy for such chronic conditions as ischaemic heart disease. In section 15.3, the collective findings of clinical trials for beta-blockers after myocardial infarction provide another illustration.

Past experience leads one to believe that new therapies are unlikely to produce really radical improvements in patient survival so that one is inevitably drawn into large-scale trials designed to detect moderate, but nevertheless important, therapeutic advances. In the United States such trials have tended to become very expensive. For instance, in 1979 the National Heart Lung and Blood Institute supported just 20 clinical trials at a cost of $57 million which amounted to over 40 % of the total NIH funds for clinical trials. Hence there appears a need to simplify these large-scale trials into a more economic form of investigation.

Over the past decade there has been considerable controversy in Britain over the value of *coronary care units* in the management of patients with myocardial infarction (see Rawles and Kenmure, 1980). In particular, consider studies to evaluate the relative merits of immediate admission to a coronary care unit versus treating the patient at home. Non-randomized studies in the United Kingdom have been contradictory since in Belfast the introduction of early coronary care seemed to reduce patient mortality while in Teesside it was found that risk of death was much less at home than in hospital. There have been two British randomized controlled trials of home versus hospital treatment both of which, taken at face value, show no difference in patient mortality. However, in both Bristol and Nottingham patients admitted to the trial were a highly selected group and the choice of home versus hospital was often not made early enough to cover the period of greatest risk. Nevertheless, these studies do sound a useful note of caution. They indicate that hospital coronary care units appear not to be of value for a substantial proportion of patients unless one can improve the speed and quality of the patient's initial care, perhaps by the provision of mobile coronary care units.

Past experience has shown that randomized controlled trials of this and other aspects of patient management (e.g. length of bed-rest or length of hospital stay after a heart attack) are very difficult to organize. However, as pointed out by Cochrane (1972), it is only by such objective evidence that one can hope to clarify what is the best course of action. Otherwise, one is left in a vacuum of uncertainty where the most enthusiastically supported policies, which may nevertheless be misguided, are likely to be adopted.

2.5 THE PHARMACEUTICAL INDUSTRY

Over the last 30 years there has been an enormous expansion in pharmaceutical company research, largely due to the great advances in pharmacology enabling new effective drugs to be synthesized. It is not my intention here to elaborate on this expansion. Instead I wish to comment briefly on how clinical research methods have changed and then discuss the current scale of clinical trials supported by pharmaceutical companies.

Before the Second World War there were no formal requirements for clinical trials before a drug could be freely marketed. Since about 1938 there was a requirement in the United States that animal research, particularly on drug toxicity, be formally documented but it was still sufficient for human data to be largely anecdotal. In the early 1960's the thalidomide disaster caused a tightening of government regulations both in Britain and in the United States. In Britain, the Committee on Safety of Medicines was established in 1968 as a more permanent successor to the Committee on Safety of Drugs temporarily set up in 1963. Thus, since 1963 it has been required that official approval be obtained (a) before drugs be included in clinical trials, and (b) before they are placed on the market. In the United States it was required since 1962 that 'adequate and well controlled trials' be conducted. It took several years before the full implications of this requirement were felt. The first randomized controlled trials were undertaken in the mid-1960's and it was not until 1969 that evidence from randomized controlled trials was mandatory for getting marketing approval from the Food and Drug Administration (FDA). Over the past decade the FDA has continually expanded and elaborated on the precise sort of clinical trial evidence needed for different types of drug. These FDA Guidelines form a sound model which is followed in principle by many other countries.

In the United Kingdom the nature of clinical trials within the pharmaceutical industry is broadly similar to that in the United States, though the regulatory conditions set by the Committee on Safety of Medicines are not so explicitly or extensively documented as in the FDA Guidelines.

It is undoubtedly true that there are more clinical trials currently taking place than ever before. The great majority of this clinical trial effort is for the evaluation of new drug treatments and is mostly supported directly by the pharmaceutical industry. A quantitative international assessment of the pharmaceutical company clinical trial effort would be difficult and therefore I will focus on the United States where many of the larger companies are based. The Pharmaceutical Manufacturers Association (PMA) reports financial data collected from its 149 member companies. In 1979, total research and development costs were estimated at $1.6 billion. The bulk of this expenditure is in preclinical research but an estimated 22 % was specifically devoted to clinical trials. Around half of this effort can be attributed to three types of product: anti-infectives, central nervous system agents and cardiovascular drugs. It is difficult to convert such financial costs into numbers of trials and numbers of patients, but certain less-precisely documented facts may help.

Although there are 149 PMA members, there are between 20 and 30 major US drug companies which are research-intensive. A typical one of these larger companies would have of the order of 20–50 pharmaceutical products currently undergoing clinical trials prior to marketing. Each product might require anything from 10 to 80 different trials, but typically for a common disease 25 trials (mostly phase III) involving around 3000 patients treated with the new drug would be needed to establish efficacy and safety before a drug could be marketed.

Of all new drugs synthesized in the laboratory only about 1 in every 10 000 actually reaches clinical testing. This explains why the greater expenditure is in preclinical research. Maybe 20 % of drugs which are subjected to clinical trials are eventually marketed. It takes from seven to ten years for the entire research programme of a new drug to be completed and roughly half of this time is spent in clinical trials. Hansen (1979) estimated that the average research and development cost per new drug successfully marketed was around $54 million in 1976.

The Food and Drug Administration, which regulates all drug company clinical trials in the United States, requires that each new drug has an IND (Investigate New Drug application) approved before clinical trials may be undertaken. As of October 1981, there were 2042 active INDs at the FDA. Many of these involve new formulations or continued monitoring of drugs already marketed, but it seems reasonable to conclude that there are over 1000 new drugs currently undergoing premarketing clinical trials.

Lastly, I can remember one British clinical researcher remarking, 'These FDA regulations take all the fun out of clinical trials.' Such is the discipline of doing good quality research with the ultimate aim of patient benefit.

CHAPTER 3

Organization and Planning

One essential aspect of planning a clinical trial is to write a *study protocol*: that is a formal document specifying how the trial is to be conducted. In section 3.1 I outline some of the main features to be included in a protocol, many of which are dealt with more extensively in later chapters.

For any trial to fulfil the protocol specification there must be adequate financial support and sufficient skilled staff. Section 3.2 discusses the resources required to undertake a trial and emphasizes the need for efficient organization.

There are three fundamental aspects of trial design which must be precisely defined at an early stage:

(a) which patients are eligible
(b) which treatments are to be evaluated
(c) how each patient's response is to be assessed.

These issues are considered in sections 3.3–3.5 respectively.

3.1 THE PROTOCOL

The design of a clinical trial, from initial rather vague ideas about treatment innovation through to an eventual detailed plan of action, is often a complicated process. Hence it is important to document one's intentions in a study protocol so that everyone involved in the proposed trial is fully informed.

The *initial draft* of a study protocol in the early stage of planning a trial may be a rather flimsy document which outlines the general scheme without detailed specifications. Indeed such a preliminary draft may usefully draw attention to some of the difficulties to be faced by the trial's proponents. In particular, any lack of clearly specified goals can often be pinpointed by the poorly defined aims in this first draft. Trial organizers should be encouraged to write down their proposals as soon as possible, so that any aspects of protocol which are unspecified, confusing or contentious may be resolved without delay. It will often require several redrafts of the study protocol until a final more extensive protocol is produced which contains full details of the trial's objectives and organization. Thus, the evolution of a study protocol from its primitive beginnings through to the final comprehensive document forms a systematic approach to the development of a clinical trial which is acceptable on scientific, organizational and ethical grounds.

The *final version* of a study protocol needs to serve two main functions. Firstly, it should provide detailed specifications of the trial procedure relating to each individual patient. Thus, the trial requirements for patient entry, treatment and evaluation plus data collection procedures need to be clearly stated so that each member of the investigating team knows what is expected of them for each patient in the trial. This aspect of the protocol may be termed an *operations manual*.

Secondly, the study protocol should include a description of the trial's motivational background, specific aims and the rationale behind the chosen study design. Inclusion of this more general overview of the trial's purpose and proposed conduct is important. Ethical committees and funding bodies need to be satisfied that the trial is well designed. Also, a clear statement of objectives ensures that the trial organizers adhere to a preplanned declaration of intent when it comes to the analysis and reporting of trial results. I do not mean to imply that the study protocol is a rigid straitjacket aimed at preventing the discovery of interesting and unexpected findings. Rather I wish to emphasize that progress in clinical trials can be best achieved by thoughtful and well-organized research geared to the examination of realistic prespecified hypotheses concerning treatment. This may be termed the *scientific design* aspect of the study protocol.

Now, for most clinical trials it is practicable to merge the operations manual and scientific design aspects into a single study protocol. However, if a trial is administratively complex (e.g. a large-scale multi-centre trial) then it may be advisable to have a separate operations manual in addition to the study protocol. For instance, the Medical Research Council Working Party (1977) are running a controlled trial for treatment of mild hypertension in which a large number of patients are being recruited from many different clinics throughout Britain. The organizers prepared an operations manual (26 pages long) and a study protocol (8 pages long). The latter described the study design and included a brief summary of the procedure for each patient, while the former document was intended for those people responsible for running the trial clinics.

I now wish to be more specific about what a study protocol should contain. Table 3.1 lists 14 main items which should usually be included. This is only a rough guideline and will need some adaptation for each trial's particular circumstances. Many of these items are discussed in the remainder of this book and table 3.1 gives the relevant chapter numbers in parentheses after each topic. The reader should refer to these chapters for more extensive explanation of each topic, but it might be useful briefly to run through these protocol items at this stage.

A description of the *background and general aims* of the trial is a useful preliminary which helps to explain why the trial is considered worthwhile and how it builds on experience gained from previous research. The *specific objectives* of the trial are a more concise and precisely worded definition of those hypotheses concerning treatment efficacy and safety which are to be examined by the trial. This summary of objectives is built on more expansive descriptions of *patient selection criteria, treatment schedules* and the *methods of patient evaluation.* Usually these three issues form the bulk of the study protocol since only by a precise and detailed explanation of these practical fundamentals can one ensure that the trial adheres to well-defined objectives. See sections 3.3–3.5 for further details.

Table 3.1. Main features of a study protocol

1. Background and general aims
2. Specific objectives
3. Patient selection criteria (section 3.3)
4. Treatment schedules (section 3.4)
5. Methods of patient evaluation (section 3.5)
6. Trial design (chapters 4, 6 and 8)
7. Registration and randomization of patients (chapter 5)
8. Patient consent (chapter 7)
9. Required size of study (chapter 9)
10. Monitoring of trial progress (chapter 10)
11. Forms and data handling (chapter 11)
12. Protocol deviations (chapter 12)
13. Plans for statistical analysis (chapters 13 and 14)
14. Administrative responsibilities (section 3.2)

Under the general heading of *trial design* I include such issues as the choice of a control group, the method of treatment allocation (see chapter 4 for the justification of randomized controlled trials), any procedures for implementing blindness (see chapter 6 on double-blind trials), and the explanation of a crossover design (see chapter 8) if it is relevant.

The procedure for *registration and randomization of patients* requires a straightforward account of the sequence of events required for each patient to enter the trial and receive their assigned treatment. Although the underlying method of preparing the randomization needs careful consideration (see chapter 5), it is often best not described in the study protocol in order to reduce the risk of investigators predicting the next patient's treatment.

Any protocol should explain the procedure for obtaining informed *patient consent* prior to commencement of treatment. Only a brief statement is necessary usually, but it is an important acknowledgement that the trial is conforming with recognized ethical standards.

The *required size of study* should be specified in the protocol together with a brief explanation of the statistical rationale behind the chosen number of patients. One of the greatest problems in clinical trials is the failure to include enough patients so that a realistic assessment of the likely recruitment rate is particularly valuable (see chapter 9). It is also useful to specify in advance how one intends to *monitor trial progress*, particularly so that prompt action can be taken if substantial treatment differences arise in interim analyses of results.

The procedure for completing *forms and handling data* needs careful attention. One of the less-exciting aspects of planning a trial is the preparation of forms for recording each patient's data. However, the quality of such forms and the reliability of subsequent data processing are major requirements for the successful conduct of a clinical trial.

If possible the protocol can refer to certain potential *protocol deviations*: it is better to anticipate problems rather than simply to wait for them to occur. For instance, in drug trials one can introduce checks on patient compliance with the treatment schedule. Also, one can specify appropriate dose modifications if side-effects are to be expected in some patients. Of course, one wants to avoid patients withdrawing prematurely from the trial or investigators deviating from protocol therapy; nevertheless one should specify how such departures from protocol get recorded.

It can be a valuable exercise to decide on *plans for statistical analysis* before the trial starts. Such plans should link closely with the specific objectives mentioned above. Of course, one should not be too inflexible about analysis methods at the planning stage, but some prior specification helps to identify one's priorities ready for when patient evaluation data arrive. A brief summary of analysis plans in the protocol ensures that the trial's eventual interpretation is not too far removed from the prespecified objectives.

Lastly, any *administrative responsibilities* should be mentioned so that the trial's organizational structure is clear to all participants.

Now how extensive a document does the study protocol need to be? This will depend on the complexity of the trial. For instance, a small phase II trial of short-term antihypertension therapy of a new drug versus placebo carried out in one centre may only require a brief study protocol, say three or four pages long. On the other hand, a multi-centre trial involving long-term follow-up of each patient may require a much more extensive protocol. For example, the UK-TIA study group aspirin trial is designed to see if daily aspirin after a transient ischaemic attack reduces the subsequent risk of stroke and myocardial infarction (see Warlow, 1979). This collaborative study requires many British neurologists to evaluate each of their patients over a period of several years. Hence, the study protocol is a weighty document over 50 pages long. In such a situation one should also provide a one- or two-page *summary protocol* to introduce participants and interested observers to the study's general outline.

3.2 ADMINISTRATION, STAFF AND FINANCE

Sources of Funding

When considering the organizational structure and administrative responsibilities in a clinical trial it is important first to recognize what is the motivation and source of funding for the trial. In this respect I find it convenient to identify three main types of clinical trial:

(1) trials with pharmaceutical company support
(2) trials funded by nationally based health organizations
(3) trials undertaken locally with no external backing.

Before tackling more general issues of trial organization, I now discuss some of the organizational problems specific to each of these types of trial:

(1) *Pharmaceutical companies* are responsible for organizing the great majority of clinical trials. The underlying purpose is for the company to obtain evidence regarding their product's safety and efficacy so that the product can be successfully marketed and make a healthy profit for the company. This 'profit motive' leads some people to suspect that such pharmaceutical company research is biassed towards exaggerated claims of drug efficacy; this view is encouraged by the persuasive advertising that doctors receive from company marketing departments. However, in reality one needs to draw a clear distinction between such marketing operations and the research and development activities of a company. On the whole, my experience of premarketing clinical trials (phases I–III) in the pharmaceutical industry leaves me of the opinion that such research is generally carried out in an objective manner. Particularly, standards have improved in the last 15 years as a direct result of stricter control by national regulatory bodies such as the US Food and Drug Administration.

Nevertheless, clinicians who collaborate in company-sponsored trials should give some thought as to how they are organized. The two extremes are:

(a) the clinician treats his patients according to protocol and completes the data sheets but all other aspects of the trial, including protocol design and reporting of results, are run by the company,
(b) the company finances the trial and provides supplies of the drug but otherwise the trial itself is run independently by the non-company organizers.

Most company trials are nearer to (a). Many clinicians do not have the resources to tackle organizational aspects and hence are only too pleased to play a superficial role. However, it can be valuable for clinicians to join in protocol design and obtain their own independent analysis and interpretation of results; otherwise there is the danger that trials run by companies lack the scientific input of experienced clinical investigators. Approach (b) above is where drug companies have no real control over the research they are supporting financially, and hence is not a routine arrangement for companies to accept. It operates best for large-scale clinical trials of an important issue (e.g. can a particular drug prolong survival after a heart attack?) when it may be vital that company interests are seen to be separated from the trial's conduct and evaluation.

(2) *National health organizations*, such as the British Medical Research Council or the American National Institutes of Health, generally devote

themselves to large-scale multi-centre clinical trials which require substantial funding and careful organization. As mentioned in chapter 2, the first clinical trials of acceptably high quality were conducted by the Medical Research Council over 30 years ago. Thus there is an established tradition that some of the best clinical research can be conducted within such a framework. Indeed, some people would argue that such collaborative trials are the only meaningful approach for evaluating therapy. However, I think this is overstating the case since the time and cost involved in planning and running large-scale research can only be justified for trials of major treatment issues. One needs a background of smaller scale more flexible research so that therapeutic innovations worthy of full-scale definitive trials can be identified. Further discussion of multi-centre trials is given in section 9.4.

(3) *Locally based trials* set up in a particular hospital, clinic or general practice can provide an important source of clinical and scientific creativity for the improvement of therapy. Trials funded by pharmaceutical companies and national organizations can sometimes fail to provide the flexibility of approach necessary for our most able clinical scientists to develop new treatments. This particularly applies to non-drug therapy, e.g. innovations in surgery or radiotherapy, studies of nutrition or exercise, evaluation of different approaches to medical care. Many such issues are best tackled, at least initially, in the context of small-scale studies in one institution.

Thus, the best of such studies provide an important source of new therapeutic ideas. However, many local studies are poorly organized and exhibit a low standard of scientific design: in particular, they often recruit too few patients to be scientifically viable. Thus, the ethics, organization and relevance of locally based trials should be carefully scrutinized both by the investigators and by external reviewers (e.g. hospital ethical committees). Having expressed this note of caution, I would still wish to encourage enthusiastic clinicians to undertake their own clinical research, provided it is recognized that their limited resources can usually only support feasibility studies or pilot trials (i.e. phase I/II trials) rather than full-scale (phase III) trials.

General practitioners could undertake clinical trials to evaluate the efficacy of many common treatment practices. For instance, Stott (1982) gives a fascinating account of his experiences in running a double-blind randomized controlled trial to answer the question 'do patients with cough and purulent sputum merit antibiotic treatment?' Unfortunately, except for trials motivated by pharmaceutical company interests there is inadequate use of controlled trials in general practice.

Coordination and Leadership

With the great diversity of research that comes under the heading of clinical trials, it is feasible only to give a general outline as to their administrative structure. Firstly, any trial benefits from clearly defined leadership, usually by an experienced *principal clinical investigator*. Although all but the simplest of trials requires collaboration of many participants, it would be misguided to undertake 'research by committee' without any definite decision on who is in charge.

Any substantial trial requires a *coordinating centre* to handle all administrative matters once patients are being entered. Such aspects as registration and randomization of patients, supplying treatments, collecting and processing patient records, checking that protocol procedure is being followed, dealing with enquiries and providing feedback to participants can all usefully come under the day-to-day duties of such a centre. Its nature depends on the trial's structure. Pharmaceutical companies tend to run their own trial coordination at company headquarters, each trial being managed by a 'clinical research associate' and his assistants. For a local trial (say in a single hospital) a junior doctor may act as day-to-day coordinator while the consultant acts as principal investigator. In large multi-centre trials the coordinating centre assumes a particularly important role in holding the trial together (see section 9.4).

In addition, major trials usually need a *monitoring committee* which meets periodically to assess the trial's overall progress. It should include the principal investigator (usually as chairman) and a coordinating centre representative. One or two experienced clinical investigators not otherwise involved in the trial and also a statistician can usefully contribute to such a committee by providing a more objective view of the trial. Early meetings of the committee will be concerned with finalizing the protocol and organization. Once the trial has begun matters such as interpretation of interim results, adequacy of patient accrual, protocol deviations and possible alterations to protocol need to be considered. The monitoring committee should operate in an advisory capacity leaving the principal investigator to implement any decisions.

Informed and Enthusiastic Participants

The successful conduct of a clinical trial relies heavily on each individual participant being fully informed and able to carry out his responsibilities. Both *clinical and nursing staff* have to understand protocol procedure as regards the treatment and evaluation of each patient. It will not be sufficient merely to supply copies of the protocol and hope everyone will read it. Prior instruction, maybe even a pilot study on a few patients, is a valuable prerequisite if there is no previous experience of trial procedure.

One needs particularly clear directions on who is responsible for completing each patient's trial records. In large trials one may have data managers specially employed for this task, but in smaller trials it may fall on the doctor, nurse or secretarial staff.

There may be other trial staff with specific responsibilities: for instance, laboratory technicians (e.g. for biochemical analyses of serum), radiologists (e.g. for chest X-rays), pharmacists (if drug preparation and packaging is required). Such people will often have only intermittent contact with the trial, so that one needs to be doubly sure that their duties are properly explained.

One important aspect in the running of a trial is to ensure that every participant has a lively interest in what is going on. Without this sense of enthusiasm, there is a real danger that the trial will deteriorate: protocol deviations, missing data or a fall in the rate of patient entry may occur. Hence, one may need to hold regular meetings of all trial participants. Such meetings should not be for decision-making, but for general communication, feedback of information on trial progress and for the airing of any problems that have arisen.

The Role of a Statistician

It is a common mistake to assume that the statistician need only be concerned with the analysis of results. Of course the statistician plays a major role as *data analyst* but he should also be involved beforehand in the study's design and conduct. I think an experienced statistician should be a *collaborating scientist* in ensuring that both protocol design and the interpretation of trial findings conform to sound principles of scientific investigation. In addition, the statistician is often in a good position to act as a 'policeman' in ensuring that satisfactory organizational standards are maintained throughout a trial.

As regards protocol design, the statistician has an obvious commitment to advising on the required number of patients (chapter 9), the method of randomization (chapter 5) and data processing (chapter 11). However, such help can be rather superficial whereas the statistician who is willing (and allowed) to get to grips with the protocol as a whole can make a valuable contribution to improving the overall design. One reason that makes him useful is his objectivity due to (a) lack of clinical involvement and (b) the nature of his mathematical training. On organizational matters, the statistician can act as a sensitive detector of problems by his overseeing of patient registration and subsequent data processing.

Unfortunately, statisticians are often used merely as a technical service for analysing data. I think this is especially true in the pharmaceutical industry. However, I hope that in the future an increasing number of trial organizers will recognize the important collaborative role of the statistician from their trial's inception to its completion.

3.3 SELECTION OF PATIENTS

Any clinical trial requires a precise definition of which patients are eligible for inclusion. The early stages of protocol development may proceed with only a rough outline of the intended type of patient, but before the trial gets underway this must be transformed into a detailed specification.

The main objective is to ensure that patients in the trial may be identified as *representative* of some future class of patients to whom the trial's findings may be applied. In addition, one wishes to focus on the type of patient considered most likely to benefit from the new treatment under investigation. However, one does not wish to be so restrictive about patient entry that the trial remains small and its findings lack generality. The principal aspects to consider are:

(a) the source of patient recruitment
(b) the disease state under investigation
(c) specific criteria for exclusion of patients.

As regards *the source of patients* the issue of representativeness needs particularly careful attention. For instance, in the study of depressive illness if one recruits hospital in-patients one ends up with an atypical group. Such patients tend to be the more serious chronic cases whereas any new antidepressant drug is usually under investigation with an eye to the larger group of depressed patients under the care of general practitioners.

One often has the problem that the primary source of patients (e.g. in general practice) is not ideal when it comes to detailed observation of progress on therapy. Hence in the early stages of research (e.g. phase I and II studies) one may be prepared to compromise and study a somewhat unrepresentative group of patients in order to achieve the patient availability and cooperation required for more intensive evaluation.

However, when conducting a full-scale (phase III) trial one must try and aim for a group of patients that truly represent the disease under investigation, even if this restricts the extent of patient evaluation, so that other clinicians can relate the trial's conclusions to future patients in their clinical practice.

In the context of hospital medicine, there is a tendency for clinical trials to focus on 'centres of excellence' since those willing to undertake research are often the most experienced clinical investigators in specialized institutions. One problem is that such institutions may treat a highly selected group of patients: the pattern of referral from other centres may tend to concentrate the more unusual or 'difficult' cases in these centres. Another issue is that new developments in treatment may be handled more skilfully in trial centres than they would be under routine circumstances so that their efficacy and safety may be overstated in trial reports. For instance, the results of clinical trials of cytotoxic drugs for cancer need careful appraisal because of the problem of side-effects. Of course, the source of patients may be dictated by the practicality of which investigators are willing to participate. It is important that each investigator contributes wholeheartedly to the trial and includes all his eligible patients. Hence in the quest for representative patient entry one should be wary of prejudicing the trial's quality in other respects.

The *disease state under investigation* must be established, and this often requires quite detailed criteria in the study protocol. In routine practice, individual clinical judgement may be used to decide how a patient should be treated. However, if the same freedom of clinical choice operated in a clinical trial it would often be impossible for others to interpret the results since there would be no clear guidelines on which patients were included. Hence *strict criteria of patient eligibility* are needed.

For instance, Douglass *et al.* (1978) defined the following selection criteria for patients in a trial of chemotherapy for advanced colorectal cancer:

(1) Patients must have histologically confirmed metastatic or locally recurrent carcinoma of the colon or rectum.
(2) Tumour must be beyond hope of surgical eradication.
(3) There must be tumour masses that can clearly be measured on physical examination or chest X-ray.
(4) No previous chemotherapy for their disease.
(5) An expected survival of at least 90 days and absence of severe malnutrition, nausea and vomiting.
(6) Patients must have recovered from effects of major surgery.
(7) Patients must have white cell count >4000 per mm^3, platelet count $>100\,000$ per mm^3, haemoglobin >10 g per 100 ml and creatinine <1.5 mg per 100 ml.
(8) Patients must be informed of the nature of their disease and their written consent must be obtained before instituting therapy.

This example illustrates the need for meticulous definition. Item 1 by itself declares in broad terms the type of patient required, while items 2–7 are various *criteria for excluding patients* who are unsuitable for the trial. For instance, item 3 regarding measurable disease is important since otherwise one includes patients whose progress is hard to assess.

It is often useful to restrict entry to *previously untreated patients* (see item 4) since otherwise the possible effects of therapy may be diminished. However, in certain chronic conditions such as obstructive airways disease it may be impractical since most patients have long-established disease.

One should aim for objective criteria, such as the contraindications to chemotherapy in item 7 above, though some criteria must involve a degree of clinical judgement, e.g. items 2, 5 and 6. However, one should beware of criteria which rely too much on opinion: 'expected survival >90 days' in item 5 cannot be assessed with reliability and could perhaps have been removed.

Item 8 is concerned with obtaining patient consent. This is primarily for ethical reasons (see chapter 7) but is also useful in ensuring good patient cooperation.

Almost every trial requires such a list of exclusion criteria to supplement the main definition of the disease. However, one should avoid making requirements too stringent since one might then have difficulty finding enough patients, causing those patients in the trial to be an unduly select group. For instance, it is common practice to exclude elderly patients, say over age 65. Such patients may be less responsive to therapy, more affected by side-effects or more difficult to evaluate properly. However, if the best of the therapies under investigation are liable to be used on future elderly patients then it may be wise to include them in the trial. In general, one needs to strike a balance between including all patients who may potentially benefit from trial therapy and aiming for a more select group of patients who are most suited to the trial's purpose.

For some diseases (e.g. cancer) it is relatively easy to define which patients have the disease and are eligible. However, other conditions (e.g. hypertension, depression) are less easily defined especially as their severity in untreated subjects may vary considerably over time. As an example, I will consider the patient entry requirements for the trial of mild hypertension run by the Medical Research Council Working Party (1977).

On first examination each subject has his blood pressure (BP) measured twice. If the mean of the two readings has systolic $BP > 200$ mm or diastolic $BP > 90$ mm, then the subject is recalled for a repeat double set of measurements at a later date, preferably one week but not exceeding four weeks after the first. All four blood pressure readings are then used to obtain each subject's mean systolic and diastolic BP. A subject is then eligible for the trial if:

$$90 \leqslant \text{mean diastolic BP} < 110 \text{ mm Hg}$$
$$\text{and mean systolic BP} < 200 \text{ mm Hg,}$$

and is randomized to antihypertensive drug or placebo. Subjects above the range are referred for active treatment not in the trial and subjects below the range remain untreated.

The use of *repeat examinations* prior to patient entry is helpful in ensuring that a trial does not include patients with only transitory signs and symptoms who can improve without treatment. It is beneficial to the trial and also to the patients themselves in avoiding unnecessary therapy. In some trials patients receive placebo between the two visits.

3.4 TREATMENT SCHEDULES

The study protocol will often need considerable space devoted to a precise definition of treatment procedure. Since the majority of clinical trials are to evaluate *drug therapy*, I will begin by concentrating on this aspect. Trials of non-drug therapy are mentioned below.

Conceptually, one's overview of a trial tends to focus primarily on the specific drug names such that the details of dose schedules, which are vital to any real understanding of treatment, are often not adequately emphasized. Therefore, in order to counteract this common tendency of oversimplifying the intricacies of trial therapy I provide the following list of features to consider when defining drug regimens in a study protocol:

(1) Drug formulation
(2) Route of administration
(3) Amount of each dose
(4) Frequency of dosage
(5) Duration of therapy
(6) Side-effects, dose modification and withdrawals
(7) Patient compliance with therapy
(8) Ancillary treatment and patient care

(9) Packaging and distribution of drugs
(10) The comparison of treatment policies

Firstly, *drug formulation* must obviously be absolutely clear. For many trials this presents no problems, since drug development is often based on several years of pharmaceutical research and one can safely rely on appropriate tablets, capsules, vials, etc., being manufactured in stable and accurately determined drug concentrations. However, it never pays to assume such pharmaceutical background without questioning: I recall one trial which was ruined upon discovery that the 'active' treatment deteriorated even after quite a short period of storage. Many trials have a control group of patients on placebo treatment (see chapter 6) and the manufacture of such placebos, carefully matched to the active treatment, may require ingenious preparation by pharmacists.

The *basic dose schedule* for each treatment, i.e. route of administration, amount and frequency of dosage, needs to be specified. The *route of administration* (oral, intravenous or intramuscular) is often self-evident, though in some conditions there can exist controversy over whether oral or intravenous therapy should be used: usually the former is more convenient while the latter provides a more reliable and immediately active route. In phase III trials the *amount and frequency of dose* is determined from experience in smaller phase I/II trials (where several different schedules of the same drug(s) have been studied).

Usually, the objective is to give the largest dose that falls safely below serious risk of side-effects, though this depends on the potential for drug efficacy and the seriousness of disease. With cytotoxic drugs for cancer, dosage is often set proportional to body surface area whereas in most other diseases dosage is fixed as the same for all patients. Such rigidity of dose schedule is not necessarily a satisfactory approach. Also, it is surprising, and perhaps alarming, how frequently the choice of dose schedule depends on arbitrary personal judgement rather than on clear-cut scientific evidence.

The *duration of therapy* may be fixed for all patients or be dependent on each patient's progress. The former is easier to interpret but sometimes fails to incorporate sufficient flexibility to handle therapy in each patient's best interests. Short, fixed periods of therapy are often satisfactory for phase II trials of short-term efficacy, e.g. for relief of hypertension, asthma, depression. For trials of more long-term effects the duration of therapy may require a more complex definition which incorporates plans for dealing with *side-effects, dose modification* and *patient withdrawals*.

As an example, let us study the protocol specifications in the trial of advanced colorectal cancer by Douglass *et al.* (1978) mentioned earlier. The trial had four treatments to which patients were randomly allocated, but here I will just give details for one of these, methyl-CCNU. The basic schedule was that every eight weeks the patient received a single oral dose of methyl-CCNU (175 mg per square metre of body surface area) after fasting. Patients whose condition deteriorated (i.e. an increase in tumour size) should be withdrawn from therapy while patients whose condition was unchanged or improved (i.e. tumours shrank) remained on therapy. Dose modification for haemotologic toxicity was specified in advance, e.g. if white cell count <2000 per mm^3 dose was delayed for at least two weeks and then reduced to 100 mg per square metre, and also delays in dosage were permitted to allow recovery from gastric or kidney toxicity. Clearly, administration of toxic drugs to patients with serious disease poses particularly difficult problems for defining protocol therapy. However, in protocols of less serious conditions it is also useful to try and lay down rules for departing from basic drug schedule when side-effects or patient deterioration occur. Otherwise, each clinical investigator may adjust therapy as he sees fit, without any prior guidelines.

One hopes that *patient compliance* with protocol therapy will remain good (see section 12.2 for a discussion of non-compliance). In general, it pays to adopt a realistic attitude: protocol therapy must remain sufficiently straight-forward to be followed without confusion or inconvenience. Hence, any 'biologically optimal' drug regimen which is unduly complex may have to be simplified to achieve adequate compliance. This is particularly applicable to out-patients on regular self-administered therapy: the fewer the pills, the better the compliance!

In many trials which are predominantly about drug therapy, there are other aspects to the management of patients that may usefully be defined in the study protocol. For instance, in trials of adjuvant chemotherapy after surgery (e.g. the breast cancer example in section 1.3) the exact form of surgery needs to be defined. Also, if a new drug is to supplement standard drug therapy, the latter must be clearly defined. In general, one should specify which non-protocol drugs (if any) are permissible and under what circumstances. Such ancillary treatment and patient care should be made as consistent as possible: one particularly wants to avoid any disparity of ancillary care between treatment groups and this is one reason for making the trial *double-blind* (see chapter 6).

On an organizational note, the *packaging and distribution* of drugs require efficient handling. This needs especially careful arrangements if the trial is multi-centre or double-blind. In general, it is advisable to supply each investigator with enough drugs for just a few patients initially and provide supplementary supplies as necessary when the investigator has entered some patients according to protocol. This approach is a useful aid to monitoring his participation in the trial.

In most full-scale trials of drug therapy, one must accept that the fundamental aim is to compare patient response to different *treatment policies* each of which defines as rigorously as possible the implementation of a particular drug schedule while making allowances for schedule adaptation to meet the needs of each individual patient. This means *one intends to evaluate treatment policies as they relate to actual clinical practice rather than as purely scientific evaluations of drug effect.* As a consequence of this pragmatic outlook I consider that all patients, including those who withdraw from therapy, need to be accounted for in any evaluation of treatment policies (see section 12.3 for details).

I now wish to draw attention to clinical trials of *non-drug therapy*. This is a very broad area to discuss: surgical procedures, radiotherapy, postoperative care, dietary intervention and other forms of patient management all present their own particular problems in defining what is meant by 'treatment'. I consider one aspect they all have in common is that the randomized controlled trial has been underutilized as a methodology for evaluating such therapies.

Trials of surgery or radiotherapy should not present any especial difficulties of treatment definition as such, except that the successful implementation of protocol treatment may depend considerably on the degree of skill and experience of each surgeon or radiotherapist. Of course, one also needs to recognize that trials comparing surgery with no surgery can sometimes present ethical and practical difficulties.

In trials for evaluating medical care, health education or dietary intervention procedures the concept of comparing general treatment policies is particularly relevant. For instance, the trial by Mather *et al.* (1976) randomized patients with myocardial infarction to home or hospital care. Those assigned to home care could subsequently be transferred to hospital if the family doctor thought it advisable, but in analysis they were retained in their original group. Thus, the trial was to evaluate the policy of not admitting patients to a hospital coronary care unit until specific problems of management (e.g. heart failure, deep vein thrombosis, persistent cardiac pain) made it necessary.

As another example, Hjermann *et al.* (1981) investigated the effect of diet and smoking intervention in preventing coronary heart disease (CHD). Over 1200 men in Oslo who were identified, using objective criteria, as being at high risk of CHD were randomized to intervention or control groups. Each man in the intervention group received antismoking advice and detailed dietary recommendations, mainly on how to reduce saturated fat intake. Thus the trial was to assess if a policy of intensive education on smoking and diet could reduce the incidence of CHD. The trial was successful in that 'at the end of the observation period the incidence of myocardial infarction (fatal and non-fatal) and sudden death was 47% lower in the intervention group than in the controls'.

I hope such interesting findings will encourage others to explore trials of non-drug intervention in the prevention and management of disease, so that we may counter the current obsession with drug therapy as the routine approach to medical practice in western society.

3.5 EVALUATION OF PATIENT RESPONSE

The evaluation of each patient's progress after the start of trial therapy needs to be done in an objective, accurate and consistent manner so that the trial as a whole provides a meaningful assessment of the treatments' relative merits. Hence, the methods for assessing and recording a patient's progress need precise definition in the study protocol. Indeed, patient evaluation in a clinical trial requires much tighter control than would normally occur in general clinical practice. In particular, routine case notes are a totally unsuitable basis for evaluation in a trial since they are usually far too vague, inconsistent and subjective.

It is convenient to classify patient evaluation into four main categories:

(1) Baseline assessment before treatment starts
(2) Principal criteria of patient response
(3) Subsidiary criteria, e.g. side-effects
(4) Other aspects of patient monitoring

All four categories require careful planning as regards *accuracy of information* (see later in this section) and *consistent recording of data* on specially designed forms (see chapter 11). However, one must first decide which features to measure or observe and hence I will now expand on what characterizes each type of data.

(1) Baseline Assessment

Here one's main aim is to measure the patient's *initial clinical condition* though in addition background information on *personal characteristics* (e.g. age, sex) and *clinical history* (e.g. duration of illness, previous therapy) may also be collected. It is sometimes tempting to collect a large and comprehensive battery of baseline data, but this can be misguided in that few of such data ever get used. Hence, it is useful to focus attention on those items which may influence the patient's response to treatment. The use of such *prognostic factors* in analysis of trial results is discussed in section 14.1.

Many trials are concerned with measuring the change in some measurable parameter while on treatment (e.g. blood pressure in hypertensives, lung function tests in asthmatics, Hamilton rating score in depressive illness). Hence, it is particularly important to measure accurately such parameters at baseline. For instance, measurement of blood pressure could be undertaken on two or more occasions prior to treatment so that the mean of all readings could provide a baseline measurement less affected by random fluctuation. Also, repeat baseline evaluation enables one to assess the stability of disease prior to treatment; some patients could be excluded from the trial if their condition improves or deteriorates sharply. Indeed, for any trial one important aspect of baseline evaluation is to check that a patient is eligible for the trial (see section 3.3).

(2) Principal Criteria of Response

The specific aims of the study protocol (see section 3.1) should give a direct indication of what constitute the principal criteria of response. A clinical trial can require an extensive list of observations on each patient and such a multiplicity of data can make results difficult to interpret (see section 14.3). Hence, before a trial commences some guidance should be given regarding the relative importance of the various measures of patient outcome. Indeed, it is extremely helpful if one particular measure of response can be singled out as the principal criterion for comparing treatments.

For instance, trials of cytotoxic drugs for advanced cancer can often involve the following criteria of response:

(a) survival time = time from start of therapy until death
(b) achievement of tumour response = partial or complete reduction in tumour size
(c) duration of tumour response
(d) change in performance status, e.g. ambulatory or non-ambulatory
(e) occurrence of haematologic toxicity
(f) occurrence of other side-effects

The picture is quite complex: (b) and (c) are concerned with observing the cancer itself, (e) monitors the risk of infection, while (d) and (f) give some indication of quality of life. All give insight into the nature of treatment effect, but it is often sensible to select (a), the survival time, as the single most important outcome measure in full-scale (phase III) trials of cancer chemotherapy.

The choice of principal response criterion will depend on whether new treatment(s) are in the early or later stages of clinical research. Thus, the phase I trials of cancer drugs are concerned with assessing toxicity, (e) and (f) above, so that satisfactory dose schedules can be determined, while phase II trials concentrate on tumour response, (b) and (c) above.

Trials for the relief of chronic conditions (e.g. hypertension, diabetes) require particularly careful consideration when deciding how best to compare treatments. Preliminary trials should concentrate on assessing *short-term effects* (e.g. reduction in diastolic blood pressure after one or two months' therapy) and it may sometimes be possible to employ a crossover design here (see chapter 8). However, one must not be deceived into thinking that such specific short-term measures truly reflect any overall benefit to the patient. Thus, any full-scale trial of continuous therapy needs to concentrate on assessment of *long-term effects*. For instance, there are many antihypertensive drugs which are successful in lowering blood pressure, but to what extent is this genuinely beneficial to the patient whose principal concern is to avoid more serious illness? Thus, for patients with mild hypertension, say diastolic BP in the range 90–114 mm Hg, one wants to know if antihypertensive drugs can reduce subsequent morbidity and mortality, especially from cardiovascular disease. The Medical Research Council Working Party (1977) are currently running a trial comparing long-term diuretic and beta-blocker therapy against placebo controls. Principal end-points are (a) stroke, whether fatal or non-fatal, (b) death from any cause and (c) any cardiovascular/renal event or death.

Another interesting example concerns a large trial of the drug clofibrate reported by the Committee of Principal Investigators (1978, 1980). Compared with placebo, the drug causes a substantial reduction in serum cholesterol in patients with initially high cholesterol levels (this was well known prior to the trial). The trial showed that the incidence of myocardial infarction, especially non-fatal heart attacks, was reduced on clofibrate, so that it might appear that the drug was a useful preventive of serious morbidity in high cholesterol subjects. However, mortality from all causes was significantly *higher* on clofibrate which indicates that overall the drug may actually be harmful.

This last example emphasizes that the evaluation of therapy needs eventually to be *patient-orientated*: short-term indications of clinical interest may encourage further investigation, but there is a potential danger of inappropriate therapy for future patients if such indirect measures are taken as adequate evidence of more long-term patient benefit.

(3) Subsidiary Criteria and Side-effects

After clear definition of the main criteria of patient evaluation there may be a substantial number of other features one wishes to observe. For instance, in any drug trial it is important to evaluate safety as well as efficacy so one will need to compare treatments for potential *side-effects*. This is straightforward when the side-effects are well known (e.g. reduced heart rate due to beta-blockers, lowered white cell count due to cytotoxic drugs) but more difficult to record in a relatively new drug. In these circumstances one needs to rely heavily on each patient's own assessment of side-effects. One conventional approach is to prepare a *check-list* of possible symptoms and ailments which each patient is asked to go through at regular intervals. For instance, in a typical trial of antidepressants the following might be listed:

headache	nausea	tingling in hands
tiredness	vomiting	trembling
unable to sleep	indigestion	excessive sweating
dizziness	dry mouth	swelling of hands and feet
fainting	itching	agitation
diarrhoea	rash	tenseness
constipation	dry skin	aggressiveness
	painful joints	

Note that such a list needs to be phrased in words the patient can understand. This approach has the advantage of consistent recording uninfluenced by investigator prompting and is easy for tabulating results. However, it does restrict enquiry to prespecified items and may elicit over-reporting of events. An alternative open-ended approach is simply to ask patients to describe any adverse events they have experienced and to keep a *record of events* for each patient on a special form for subsequent classification.

Simpson *et al.* (1980) provide a comparison of both approaches in a trial of zimelidine versus placebo in obese subjects and conclude that event recording was a practicable and convenient method. Whichever method one adopts it is important to be consistent on all treatments, including any placebo control group: since adverse effects, especially minor or common ones, will be reported even amongst untreated patients, the valid assessment of side-effects on active treatment requires comparison with controls.

(4) Other Aspects of Patient Monitoring

Although a study protocol may concentrate on those evaluation criteria most suited to comparison of treatments, one must also be careful to define other features for monitoring each patient which are required for the maintenance of sound clinical practice. For instance, one often requires blood tests at regular intervals for a patient just to check whether any unexpected developments occur sufficient to merit alteration in therapy or even removal from the trial. It is better that the study protocol specifies the frequency and extent of such routine tests rather than leaving it to the investigators' judgement.

Accuracy of Evaluation Data

I now wish to concentrate on the problem of obtaining reliable evaluation data on each patient. First, consider the following types of information:

(1) Factual information, e.g. age, date of death
(2) Measurements, e.g. blood pressure, white cell count
(3) Clinical assessments, e.g. Hamilton rating for depression
(4) Patient opinion, e.g. assessment of pain in rheumatoid arthritis.

(1) Factual Information

Baseline evaluation in particular may contain basic facts such as age, sex, previous therapy, etc. The main issue here is to ensure that data are recorded correctly on a well-designed on-study form (see section 11.1). One still needs to look out for potential errors. For instance, it may be better to record dates (e.g. date of birth, date of randomization, date of death) since they are less subject to error than the direct noting of age and survival time. Also, reliable data on previous therapy are best obtained from a well-planned sequence of specific questions rather than from an open enquiry for details.

One needs to be wary of inadequate definition of factual information since inconsistencies may arise if clinical judgement has to be used. For instance, the occurrence of myocardial infarction either before or during a clinical trial may appear to be factual information but in practice will depend heavily on clinical opinion if no clear guidelines are offered. Thus, the working definition of an infarction (based on ECG changes, chest pain, enzyme tests, etc.) should be included in the study protocol of any heart disease trial (see Heady, 1973, for an example). Even so, one has to accept that problem cases will arise (e.g. sudden death, interpretation of chest pain) which will prevent data on myocardial infarction being entirely without clinical judgement.

(2) **Measurements**

Ideally any measurement taken on a patient should be precise and reproducible. In particular, it should not depend on the observer who took the measurement. For instance, consider the measurement of blood pressure. It is undoubtedly true that in routine medical practice some clinicians and nurses record consistently higher blood pressure values than others. Such *observer variation* is unacceptable in clinical trials and steps must be taken to avoid it.

A starting point is to ensure that all blood pressure readings on a particular patient are taken by the *same observer*. Indeed, if the trial is not too large, the one observer may be used for all patients. However, it is often necessary to use several observers, especially in multi-centre trials. One should then consider arrangement of training sessions prior to the study to check that observers (and their differing equipment) can reproduce the same blood pressure in any given subject. Besides the mechanics of actual measurement (i.e. agreement on what sound changes indicate systolic and diastolic pressures) observers also need to be consistent in the way they communicate with the patient. If the trial lasts a long time then repeat training sessions may be needed. Basically, one should aim for as few observers as possible without exhausting the available staff. Any trial should be designed so that observer differences cannot bias treatment comparison, e.g. by having each observer evaluate patients on all treatments.

One should also ensure that the equipment is as precise and foolproof as possible. For instance, Rose *et al.* (1964) have developed a sphygmomanometer which avoids many errors associated with more routine equipment for taking blood pressure. It ensures a standard cuff deflation rate and records digital values unseen by the observer until after deflation, thus avoiding any bias or digit preference from observers taking readings directly off a continuous manometer scale.

Error may also be reduced by taking repeat measurements on each occasion. The mean of two consecutive blood pressure readings is often used. Also, in studies of respiratory disease, the measurement of lung function tests (e.g. forced expiratory volume) is often taken as the maximum of three consecutive readings.

Laboratory tests (e.g. blood and urine tests) are another aspect of measurement in which consistency is needed. Adequate quality control procedures can ensure satisfactory results within a given laboratory. It is more difficult to guarantee that different laboratories will agree, so that one should have all tests in a single laboratory when practicable.

(3) **Clinical Assessments**

Unfortunately, many aspects of disease cannot be evaluated in terms of quantitative measurements and hence require assessment by experienced clinical observers. For instance, evaluation of psychiatric illness is entirely based on clinical assessment. The basic problem is to impose some structure on the information being collected. For instance, in depressive illness it is no good obtaining a diffuse clinical statement on the condition of each patient: instead specific methods of assessing depression (e.g. the Hamilton rating scale) have been developed whereby a structured clinical interview leads to consistent recording of the patient's condition on specially designed forms.

Returning to the problem of diagnosing myocardial infarction, I wish to refer to an investigation by Gruer (1976) into observer variation in the interpretation of ECGs. Three consultant cardiologists were asked to interpret independently the same ECGs for 1252 patients suspected of heart disease. For 125 cases some form of infarction was agreed on by all three cardiologists, but for another 132 cases there was disagreement with only one or two declaring an infarct. Thus this important aspect of diagnosing myocardial infarction can suffer markedly from observer variation. Accordingly, it is useful to undertake more objective classification of ECGs, such as the Minnesota code. Rose et al. (1982, Annex 1) define the code and Heady (1973) illustrates its use in determining infarction and ischaemia in the clofibrate trial.

Another example is the clinical assessment of stroke. Garraway et al. (1976) discuss the setting up of standardized definition, technique and interpretation as a means of reducing observer variability in clinical examination.

Once a method of classifying a patient's disease has been devised one cannot assume that all observers are equally adept in using it. For instance, Ezdinli et al. (1976) compared the histological classification of 151 non-Hodgkins lymphoma patients as performed by local hospital pathologists and an experienced central pathology panel. There was some disagreement in 40 % of cases which was thought to indicate that (a) local pathologists could not be relied on for accurate diagnosis and (b) the method of classification is less objective than is generally recognized.

In difficult areas of clinical assessment it can be very useful to form a panel of two or three observers whose task it is to agree on a joint verdict after initial independent assessment followed by joint consultation. This is most practicable in assessments not requiring the patient's presence, e.g. interpretation of X-rays.

(4) Patient Opinion

In some diseases it is impossible to evaluate the effects of therapy other than by soliciting patient opinion, e.g. pain relief in trials of antirheumatic drugs. In other trials, patient opinion provides important subsidiary information, e.g. on side-effects. Hart and Huskisson (1972) illustrate some of the problems of using patient opinion by their discussion of pain measurement.

They consider several approaches:

(1) A percentage system whereby initial pain is graded as 100 % and the patient is coded to report relative changes; e.g. moderate relief might be scored as 80 %.

(2) A scale of pain severity conventionally graded as severe, moderate, mild or

none; though to measure slight changes a more detailed scale, say with 9 points, may be better.

(3) A continuous scale, say a 5 cm line, on which the patient marks his degree of pain: one extreme = none, the other extreme = extremely severe.

(4) Patient preference, whereby in a crossover trial (see chapter 8) no direct attempt to score pain is attempted and each patient is instead asked to compare the treatments and state a preference.

Naturally, each method has its problems since one is trying to measure a subjective sensation which is clearly immeasurable in any definitive sense, so that no approach can be declared universally correct. Incidentally, Hart and Huskisson also produce an insightful and amusing list of 'mortal sins' in clinical assessment. Those of relevance to this section are as follows:

1. Enthusiasm and scepticism	'A marvellous/useless drug this'
2. Change of assessor	'Do the measurements for me Jim/Miss Jones/Darling'
3. Change of time	'Don't worry about the assessment. Go ahead with lunch/X-rays/physiotherapy/your bath'
4. Rush	'Hurry up. I'm late for lunch'
5. Squeezing	'You're much better, aren't you, Miss B?' 'Any indigestion yet, Miss B?'
6. Anticipation	'A positive/negative result will delight/enrage the boss/the drug company'
7. Bias	'Seems better/worse. Joint size must be less/more'
8. Pride	'I'm honest. No need for placebos in my trials'
9. Impurity	'We're short of cases; she'll have to do'

Blinded Evaluation

The four types of information discussed here are generally in decreasing order of reliability. Naturally, one would like all trials to use precise measurement and factual reporting, but in reality most trials have to rely on evaluation criteria which are not entirely objective. Then in order to achieve a fair and unbiassed comparison of treatments it may be necessary to have *blinded evaluation*, whereby those responsible for measurements or clinical assessments are kept unaware of which treatment each patient is receiving. A double-blind trial (see chapter 6) is often advisable, in which neither the patient, treatment team nor evaluator are informed of therapy, since this should guarantee unbiassed evaluation. However, in some trials blinded evaluation is all that can be achieved (see section 6.3). Essentially blinded evaluation should be employed whenever possible, since although the investigators themselves may believe they are not influenced by knowledge of therapy, others wishing to interpret trial results have a right to be sceptical.

Frequency of Evaluation

Most clinical trials require the same methods of evaluation to be carried out at regular intervals on each patient. One then has to decide on an appropriate time interval between evaluations. Factors to consider are:

(1) The frequency of visits required for provision of effective medical care.
(2) The inconvenience to patients of frequent evaluations.
(3) The clinical resources available for evaluation.
(4) The number of evaluations required to obtain adequate comparison of treatments.

(1) to (3) are practical matters which may determine how often one can realistically evaluate each patient's progress. As regards (4), my experience is that investigators often generate more data from repeat examinations than is really necessary. For instance, in a trial of antihypertensive therapy lasting several months, one might record blood pressure every week (or even every day) whereas monthly readings would give sufficient detail. Indeed, a trial's results often focus attention on evaluation at the beginning and end of some fixed period of therapy, with intermediate evaluation data being scarcely used. Thus, one should beware of collecting a large quantity of evaluation data: one's resources may be more profitably used in obtaining a limited amount of high-quality information. The problem of analysing repeated measurements is discussed in section 14.3.

Follow-up Studies

Many trials of serious illness are conducted to see if a treatment can prevent or delay the occurrence of some major event (e.g. death, heart attack, recurrence of cancer). Such studies often require long-term follow-up of each patient but evaluation may be relatively infrequent and uncomplicated: one simply wants to know if and when certain major predefined events occur. The detection of morbid events may be based on patient check-ups every few months by the investigator, perhaps with additional reporting from the patient and/or his regular doctor (if not an investigator). In Britain reporting of deaths can be achieved through national mortality records. This is particularly useful for patients who have otherwise withdrawn from regular follow-up, since it guarantees that analysis of mortality can be based on complete data.

With follow-up studies patients entered early in the trial will be observed for a longer period than others entered later. It would be silly to miss the opportunity to achieve such extra follow-up by restricting all patients to the same length of observation, since methods of analysing survival data (section 14.2) can allow for differing follow-up times.

Lastly, one needs to be wary of cluttering up a follow-up study with extra evaluation data. They are often very expensive long-term projects in which it is often best to record a minimum of data (major events only) on a large number of patients. See Peto *et al.* (1976, 1977) for further discussion of follow-up studies.

CHAPTER 4

The Justification for Randomized Controlled Trials

The concept of random allocation when comparing different treatments has been an important aspect of the design of scientific experiments ever since the pioneering work of Fisher (1935). The first randomized experiments were in agriculture where the experimental units were plots of land to which the treatments, various crops and fertilizers, were assigned in a random arrangement. The purposes of such randomization were:

(1) to guard against any use of judgement or systematic arrangements leading to one treatment getting plots with poorer soil, i.e. to avoid bias
(2) to provide a basis for the standard methods of statistical analysis such as significance tests.

In most types of non-human experiment, the investigator has all his experimental units available at once and can maintain tight control over how the experiment is conducted so that randomization can usually be implemented with only minor inconvenience.

However, the situation is very different for a clinical trial, in which the experimental units are patients. The idea that patients should be randomly assigned to one or other form of treatment is not intuitively appealing either to the medical profession or the layman. Superficially, randomized comparison of treatments appears contrary to the need for the clinician to give every patient the best possible care and hence appears to imply a loss of freedom for both patient and clinician. So, why should randomization now be considered such a key issue in the conduct of clinical trials given that developments in medicine had taken place for centuries without any randomized studies? Indeed, as explained in chapter 2, randomized trials have only been in existence since the late 1940's and only in the last 10 or 15 years have they gained widespread acceptance. Therefore in this chapter I consider the deficiencies inherent in some of the alternative approaches to clinical research which have been tried in the past.

Sections 4.1–4.3 deal with the problems associated with uncontrolled studies, historical controls and non-randomized concurrent controls. Essentially, the aim is to show that *from all such non-randomized studies it is very difficult to obtain a reliable assessment of treatment efficacy.* In section 4.4 some of the ethical and practical issues associated with randomization will be discussed. The mechanical details of how randomization is actually prepared and carried out will be explained in chapter 5.

4.1 PROBLEMS WITH UNCONTROLLED TRIALS

Traditionally, medical practice entails the doctor prescribing for a patient that treatment which in his judgement, based on the past experience of himself and his colleagues, offers the best prognosis. Since there are few conditions for which treatment is 100 % effective any clinician with imagination is always on the look-out for potential improvements in therapy. When a possible new treatment first materializes, the more adventurous and enthusiastic investigators might try it out on a few patients in an *uncontrolled trial.* That is, *the new treatment is studied without any direct comparison with a similar group of patients on more standard therapy.* To give the new treatment a reasonable chance of success one might select less seriously ill patients: consequently, regardless of the treatment's real value such a selected experimental group of patients will appear to do surprisingly well compared with the general routine. Also, one might tend to place greater emphasis on successes, perhaps even exaggerate them a little, and might fail to report some failures on the basis that such patients were clearly 'too ill' to benefit from the new treatment. This critical opening paragraph serves to emphasize that *uncontrolled trials have the potential to provide a very distorted view of therapy* especially in the hands of slipshod, over-enthusiastic or unscrupulous investigators.

Pre-20th century medicine was largely based on such an uncontrolled approach to the promotion of a new therapy but more recent examples may still be found. Advanced cancer is one disease which has frequently experienced extravagant claims for therapeutic effect. For instance, in the United States the drug *Laetrile* has achieved widespread popular support for treating advanced cancer of all kinds without any formal testing in clinical trials. Ellison *et al.* (1978) reported an extensive enquiry by the National Cancer Institute to collect well-documented cases of tumour response after Laetrile therapy. Although an estimated 70 000 cancer patients have tried Laetrile only 93 cases were submitted for evaluation of which six were judged to have achieved a response. This examination of such an uncontrolled collection of cases is clearly not good scientific evidence, but did provide some preliminary objective indication that Laetrile is not a 'cancer cure' which helped to counterbalance the emotional claims by its advocates. Moertel *et al.* (1982) have since reported an uncontrolled trial of Laetrile treatment for 178 patients with advanced cancer. The results were not encouraging: the median survival time was 4.8 months and indications of cyanide toxicity occurred in several patients. Since uncontrolled trials are usually over-optimistic, this particular trial offers support to the realistic conclusion that 'Laetrile is a toxic drug that is not effective as a cancer treatment'. The American experience with Laetrile indicates the worst possible situation where a therapy gains wide acceptance by the lay public (though not the medical profession) without any proper evidence of patient benefit.

Interferon, another potential anticancer agent, provides an analogous situation where many clinicians as well as laymen are very enthusiastic about its activity before any properly controlled trials have been performed. Yanchinski (1980) describes the background whereby animal studies, knowledge of its antiviral properties and reports of tumour shrinkage in a few patients have led to the opinion that interferon could be a tremendous breakthrough in the treatment of cancer. Interferon is currently in very short supply such that it can only be tested in a few centres. Studies so far have been uncontrolled and for patients with many different types of advanced cancer. Results are encouraging, but past experience with many other cancer drugs tells one that the early promise shown in uncontrolled studies often fails to be substantiated once properly controlled trials are undertaken. In the case of interferon one must express doubts about how representative the selected cases are and how consistent patient evaluations have been. In Britain, clinical research into interferon had an unfortunate start since the treatment of two Glasgow children was widely publicized. The initial response led to extravagant press claims for 'cancer cure' but both children subsequently died. With a drug in such short supply it is scientifically and ethically inexcusable not to undertake randomized controlled trials as soon as possible. More recently, the British Imperial Cancer Research Fund have started a randomized trial of interferon for patients with locally recurrent breast cancer.

With more conventional chemotherapy for the treatment of cancer it has become standard practice to carry out *uncontrolled phase II trials* of new drugs once phase I trials have established an 'appropriate' dose schedule. A separate trial is undertaken for each cancer site in advanced cases and the idea is to see what percentage of patients achieve some objective measure of tumour shrinkage. Only those drugs with an adequate proportion of responders will be studied further in randomized phase III trials. Moertel and Reitemeier (1969) reported the results of 20 different trials of the same treatment (rapid injection of the drug 5-FU) for the same disease (advanced bowel cancer) and their findings illustrate the general difficulty in interpreting such uncontrolled phase II trials. The percentage of responders on these 20 trials ranged from 8% to 85%. Admittedly, these extremes arose from the smaller trials with fewer than 20 patients, but even the six larger trials with between 40 and 150 patients still showed tremendously variable results with response rates ranging from 11% to 55%. *Why such incompatible findings for seemingly identical trials*? Perhaps the single most important reason is *patient selection*. Although all patients had advanced colorectal cancer, different investigators will differ as regards the stage of disease progression their patients have reached prior to 5-FU therapy: some will have used 5-FU as a last resort for very advanced patients, perhaps after other drugs have failed, while others will have been more adventurous in using 5-FU as soon as advanced cancer was detected. Other contributory reasons will be variation in the criterion of objective tumour regression and different approaches to the continuance of treatment, especially if drug toxicity occurs. However, whatever the reasons, this example indicates that the response rate for a drug depends very much on who is doing the trial. Nevertheless, most early (phase II) trials to assess the potential of new cancer drugs remain uncontrolled. This undoubtedly means that some ineffective drugs may be over-optimistically reported and also some effective drugs given to very advanced patients may receive inadequate study due to initial poor results. The use of uncontrolled phase II trials for many other conditions (e.g. psychiatric illness) may be totally unjustified if either the definition of the disease or evaluation of patient outcome is less objective than in advanced cancer.

Perhaps this appalling situation illustrated by Moertel and Reitemeir (1969) has improved somewhat in the past decade. Greater attention is now paid to patient factors affecting prognosis, such as prior therapy and performance status, so that better homogeneity and more detailed reporting of patients entered in a trial can be expected. Also, criteria for tumour response and details of the treatment regimens have become more precise. However, there must remain considerable uncertainty as to the value of uncontrolled phase II trials. Williams and Carter (1978), in an article dealing with many aspects of cancer chemotherapy research, discuss several alternative designs for randomized phase II studies. One approach is to assign patients randomly to the new drug or standard drug therapy with the intention of transferring patients to the other therapy if they fail to respond. This has the advantage of encouraging investigators to try a new drug on less advanced patients, and hence giving it a better chance to show its worth, with the reassuring knowledge that all patients will have the opportunity to receive standard therapy if need be. One may adapt this approach by having a majority, say 2/3rds, of patients on the new drug (see section 5.4 for further discussion of such unequal randomization) thus enabling experience in using the new drug to be gained more quickly.

Another approach is to assign patients randomly to one of several new drugs, this being particularly suitable for cancer sites in which there is no effective standard treatment (e.g. lung cancer). Such a trial is randomized, but not controlled. Compared with having a separate uncontrolled trial for every new drug it has the advantage of ensuring a more representative group of patients for each drug, since investigator bias in selecting patients is not drug-specific.

One general finding is that *uncontrolled studies are much more likely to lead to enthusiastic recommendation of the treatment as compared with properly controlled trials.* For instance, Foulds (1958) reviewed 52 published uncontrolled trials in psychiatry and found that 85% of them reported a therapeutic success whereas in 20 published trials with a control group only 25% reported therapeutic success.

Grace *et al.* (1966) provide another useful example in a review of 53 studies of portacaval shunt operation for portal hypertension: 32 of these trials were uncontrolled and 75% of them gave a markedly enthusiastic conclusion in their publication. In contrast, there were only six well-controlled trials, none of which led to marked enthusiasm though three did lead to moderate support for the treatment.

Chalmers and Schroeder (1979) reviewed therapeutic trials published in the *New England Journal of Medicine* over the previous 25 years. In the years 1953 and 1963 over half the trials were uncontrolled whereas in 1975–1978 the proportion of uncontrolled trials fell to 30%. This encouraging reduction in uncontrolled trials in one major journal is probably reflected in other journals and in clinical research at large, and one hopes that the trend will continue. Chalmers and Schroeder conclude that 'the studies without controls are not likely to fool anybody'. I very much hope their assertion is true.

Lastly, one unfortunate use of uncontrolled studies by the pharmaceutical industry sometimes occurs after a drug has been approved for marketing. As a promotional exercise a large number of doctors, often general practitioners, are encouraged to use the newly marketed drug in an uncontrolled (phase IV) trial. Such a trial has virtually no scientific merit and is used as a vehicle to get the drug started in routine medical practice. I would not deny that the marketing of new drugs is of tremendous importance to pharmaceutical companies, but it should not be conducted under the disguise of a clinical trial.

4.2 PROBLEMS WITH HISTORICAL CONTROLS

After accepting the need for a control group receiving standard treatment, many researchers are still reluctant to assign patients randomly to new or standard treatment. Such reluctance often stems from the investigator's desire to enter all future patients on the new treatment because of his wish to gain as much experience of it as possible and his inclination to believe it is better anyway. The most common way of avoiding randomization is to compare retrospectively one's current patients on the new treatment with previous patients who had received standard treatment, this latter group of patients being commonly known as *historical controls*.

Such an approach has one major flaw: *how can one ensure that the comparison is fair*? That is, if the treatment and control groups differ with respect to any feature other than the treatment itself, how can one guarantee that any apparent improvement in patient response is actually due to the new treatment? *The potential incompatibility* can be divided into two broad areas, patient selection and the experimental environment, each of which may give rise to several sources of bias:

Patient Selection

(1) A historical control group is less likely to have clearly defined criteria for patient inclusion, since such patients on standard treatment were not known to be in the clinical trial when their treatment began.

(2) Since historical controls were recruited earlier and possibly from a different source there may be a change in the type of patient available for selection.

(3) There is the danger that the investigator may be more restrictive, either deliberately or subconsciously, in his choice of patients for a new treatment.

Experimental Environment

(1) One common issue is that the quality of the recorded data for historical controls is inferior, again since such patients were not initially intended to be in the trial. Any clinical trial requires forms designed in advance (see chapter 11) and retrospective extraction of information from routine case notes is unlikely to provide adequate data.

(2) The criteria of response may differ between the two groups of patients. Even if the criteria appear to be the same on paper, those evaluating response on the new treatment may differ in their interpretation of such rules as compared with the earlier evaluators for historical controls.

(3) Ancillary patient care may improve on the new treatment. It is very difficult to ensure that all aspects of managing the patient, other than the treatment under study, remain constant. Patients on experimental therapy in a clinical trial may well have closer observation than would occur for routine standard therapy and if patients are aware and approve of being experimented on this may affect their attitude to disease and hence their subsequent response.

(4) There is a tendency to invalidate more patients on a new treatment than in historical controls. Patients on new therapy who fare badly may be excluded after subsequent enquiry reveals some protocol violation whereas the corresponding exclusion of any historical controls is made difficult since considerable time will have elapsed since they were treated.

The nett result of all these problems is that *studies with historical controls tend to exaggerate the value of a new treatment.* For instance, Grage and Zelen (1982) report on the development of intra-arterial infusion therapy for the treatment of metastatic colorectal carcinoma to the liver. Several studies with historical controls, involving over 1000 patients, extolled the virtues of this therapy whereas the only randomized trial showed no advantage for intra-arterial infusion chemotherapy as compared with standard systemic chemotherapy. One problem was that the over-optimistic results from the earlier studies made it difficult to recruit patients on to the randomized trial since many clinicians were reluctant to randomize patients to systemic chemotherapy being already (falsely) convinced of its inferiority.

Ingelfinger (1972) refers to this same issue by quoting an example of a trial of hydrocortisone treatment after acute myocardial infarction. Mortality was 14.5% as opposed to 23.2% in a non-randomized control group. The authors believed that this study showed hydrocortisone to be beneficial but went on to say that they hoped their study would lead to large-scale randomized trials of hydrocortisone. This implies that poorly controlled trials are liable to convince some clinicians that a new treatment is better, but have too great a potential bias to be accepted as good scientific evidence. However, the dilemma is that, once the non-randomized study is completed, there may be great difficulty in undertaking subsequent randomized trials. In this case, one has no means of knowing whether the mortality difference is genuine or not and this places researchers in a quandary over whether it is ethical to undertake future trials with a randomized control group. Hence, trials with historical controls have the tendency to confuse rather than clarify clinical issues and should be avoided even as pilot studies. This has led Chalmers *et al.* (1972) to advocate that randomization should be introduced in the very earliest clinical trials of a new treatment.

As mentioned in section 2.4, the review of clinical trials for anticoagulant therapy after myocardial infarction by Chalmers *et al.* (1977) showed that use of historical controls led to the reduction in mortality being greatly exaggerated as compared with randomized trials. This indicates that even with such an objective outcome as death, there is ample scope for bias in non-randomized trials.

Similar exaggeration of treatment benefit is reported by Grace *et al.* (1966) in their review of trials for portacaval shunt operation mentioned earlier. Out of 15 trials with non-randomized controls ten reported marked enthusiasm for the operation compared with none of the six randomized trials. This indicates that poorly controlled studies are not dissimilar from uncontrolled trials as regards the tendency for over-enthusiastic conclusions.

Thus, *there has been increasing scepticism regarding the validity of historical controls* and this is reflected in the review by Chalmers and Schroeder (1979) of clinical trials published in the *New England Journal of Medicine*. Whereas in 1976–1978 only two trials (< 1 %) had historical controls, this applied to over 10 % of trials in earlier years.

Nevertheless, there are researchers who argue in support of historically controlled studies (see Gehan and Freireich, 1974, and Cranberg, 1979). Both articles advocate that historical controls can be of value if sufficient care is exercised in the study's conduct. Indeed, I would agree with their view that on some occasions the use of historical controls may give an unbiassed result. However, when presented with the findings of any particular trial with historical controls I see no way to evaluate whether one has been fortunate enough in this goal. That is, trials with historical controls can never be interpreted with the same degree of confidence as properly executed randomized controlled trials. Byar *et al.* (1976) and Doll and Peto (1980) are two interesting responses to the above articles, both of which argue in favour of randomized trials.

With the above divergence of medical opinion it seems likely that there will still be some trials with historical controls in the future. Hence it seems relevant to present guidelines as to which of these studies are liable to be the 'least unacceptable'.

Firstly, *literature controls*, whereby the control group is made up of patients treated elsewhere and previously reported in the medical literature, offer a particularly poor comparison of treatments. They allow ample opportunity for differences in all aspects of patient selection and experimental environment mentioned earlier, so such studies are essentially worthless. Another slightly different problem arises in a review of the literature when the response of several therapies tried in different centres is compared. For instance, Goldsmith and Carter (1974) compared 13 drugs for the treatment of Hodgkin's disease by tabulating all the available data from uncontrolled phase II trials. Thus, vinblastine had a 68% response rate in 682 patients compared with a 50% response rate in 149 patients on BCNU. However, since both sets of patients are derived from several different studies with differing patient selection and methods of patient evaluation, one cannot really be sure that vinblastine is more active. Such review articles are undoubtedly of interest but need to be interpreted cautiously.

Historical controls obtained from *within the same organization* might be thought to offer a more reliable comparison but this may not be so if the historical data were not part of a previous trial. For instance, I recall a colleague who wished to compare surgery with more conservative treatment of heel bone fractures. There were 30 new surgical cases and several hundred previous conservatively treated cases. His intention to match each case with a 'similar' control can only partly eliminate bias since, although it may largely account for differences in patient selection, the experimental environment including the advantage often associated with being in a trial will remain vastly different. In such instances, the investigator should recognize that he has really conducted an uncontrolled phase II trial which has very limited non-comparative conclusions. Most of the examples earlier in this section derived their historical controls in this way. It might seem the most logical approach, to compare one's new treatment with one's own past practice, and indeed it may well lead to a useful learning experience for the investigator concerned. However, it cannot provide a reliable advance in scientific knowledge.

If historical controls are obtained from *a previous trial* in the same organization one might seem to stand a better chance of reducing the potential bias. One should require that such a previous trial be recent and comparable to the current trial in such features as type of patient and methods of evaluation. However, Pocock (1977b) has shown that there may still be problems. From three cancer cooperative groups in the United States, 19 instances were identified where the same treatment had been used in two consecutive trials. If historical comparisons of this type are without bias, one would not expect any notable difference in survival for the two groups receiving the same treatment. In fact, the 19 changes in death rate ranged from -46% to $+24\%$, and in four instances the difference was statistically significant (each $P < 0.02$). Thus, even comparisons with one's previous trial need to be treated with caution.

Byar *et al.* (1976) illustrate the problem further with an example from a large US multi-centre trial in prostate cancer. This trial showed no survival difference between placebo and estrogen therapy, but if one compared placebo patients in the first $2\frac{1}{2}$ years with oestrogen patients in the second $2\frac{1}{2}$ years, the latter group had significantly better survival. Although the protocol had not changed, the earlier part of the study had a greater proportion of older patients with poor performance status, such that if the former had been used as a recent historical control for the latter an incorrect inference would have been drawn.

Gehan (1978) has suggested that such historical bias can be overcome by using more complex statistical methods (such as analysis of covariance) to allow for differences in patient characteristics for treatment and control groups. Indeed, Byar *et al.* go on to state that the above survival difference is removed after adjustment for the prognostic factors age and performance status. Such methods of analysis are described in section 14.1 and also by Armitage and Gehan (1974) in the more general context of how to identify and use prognostic factors in the design and analysis of clinical trials. However, I wish to state several reasons why such *retrospective adjustment for trials with historical controls is liable to be unsatisfactory*:

(1) Historical data are often of poorer quality so that reporting of prognostic factors may not be consistent.
(2) One may have only a sketchy idea of which patient factors are important and some essential factors may go undetected.
(3) Prognostic factors can only adjust for patient selection, whereas bias due to changes in experimental environment will remain.
(4) The analysis techniques are quite complex and involve certain assumptions, which may not be fulfilled. The methods may be clear to a skilled data analyst but their interpretation might confuse many clinicians.
(5) To propose that poor design can be corrected for by subtle analysis techniques is contrary to good scientific thinking.

Gehan illustrates his approach with a trial of adjuvant chemoimmunotherapy (FAC-BCG) in primary breast cancer. The historical controls who only had a mastectomy were not in a previous trial and had certain major differences from the treatment group: only 22% of controls were treated at M. D. Anderson hospital compared with 47% on FAC-BCG and 85% of controls had a radical mastectomy as compared with 55% on FAC-BCG. Such marked discrepancies indicate that the control group was being handled in a very different manner from the treatment group, and statistical techniques can only partially compensate for this. The apparent superiority of FAC-BCG may well be genuine but we will never know the extent to which poor design led to an exaggeration of treatment benefit. The intent of this trial is very similar to the L-Pam trial described in section 1.4, but I feel the manner of its conduct is a poor substitute for the randomized controlled trial.

Gehan and Freireich (1974) suggest that another means of overcoming historical bias is by matching each new patient with one or more control patients such that they are alike with regard to the major prognostic factors. They go on to describe a trial to evaluate a protected environment for acute leukemia patients reported by Bodey *et al.* (1971). Each of 33 patients receiving chemotherapy and antibiotics in a protected environment were matched to two control patients. The method of matching was quite complicated and involved some judgement since there were nine patient factors the investigators wished to account for. This illustrates the difficulty (indeed impossibility) of achieving a perfect match. The results showed that the protected patients had improved remission and survival and a reduction in infections. However, for reasons (1) to (3) mentioned above I would argue that historical bias may still be present in such a design.

One could argue that in some circumstances the benefit to be derived from a new treatment may be so great that use of historical controls could not seriously mislead. The trouble is that one only knows that a treatment is much superior *after* a trial has been performed. There are all too many instances where prior to a trial investigators will claim their new treatment as 'the greatest invention since sliced bread' implying that the clinical trial is only a formality, whereas if the trial is properly conducted the eventual findings may show no real benefit. Even if use of historical controls does give the right answer, i.e. a genuinely superior treatment is shown to be better, one still would like to know *how much* better and the uncertainty of historical bias makes this difficult to assess.

Another argument is that if a disease is rare then one will have difficulty in accumulating enough patients for a randomized controlled trial in which only half the patients receive the new treatment. Here the use of historical controls appears a convenient suboptimal solution leading to quicker results since all new patients receive the experimental therapy. This approach is not totally without foundation, but if sufficient collaborative effort is concentrated on gathering all patients with the rare condition from a large enough population then randomized trials are still feasible. For instance, in the treatment of Wilm's tumour, a rare childhood cancer, a randomized trial has been achieved by a national effort in the United States (see D'Angio *et al.*, 1976).

However, the case for historical controls is stronger for trials with very limited numbers of patients. The larger sampling error in a randomized trial needs to be balanced against the uncertainty of historical comparison and Meier (1975) has considered this concept in a mathematical setting as follows: Suppose historical controls have bias in response represented by a random variable with mean 0 and variance σ^2 and that sampling variation in response on each treatment is denoted by τ^2. Then if there are H historical controls and N new patients to be entered on trial the choice is between (a) all N patients on the new treatment, or (b) $N/2$ patients on each of the new and standard treatments using randomization. Meier shows that the former, i.e. historical controls, is to be preferred if $\sigma^2 < 3\tau^2/N - \tau^2/H$. In reality one has no simple means of determining σ^2, but the formula does indicate that the case for historical controls is made stronger as N decreases and/or H increases. Such favourable circumstances may exist for small phase II trials when substantial control data are available from previous trials.

This statistical argument has been extended by Pocock (1976) to consider 'unequal' randomization in which more than half the random assignments are to the new treatment. The optimal solution is then for the number of patients R on the randomized control group to be $R = \frac{1}{2}[N - H/(1 + H\sigma^2/\tau^2)]$. The intention would be to include both randomized and historical controls in the eventual analysis of results, though giving more weight to the former. Further comment on the use of unequal randomization to give a greater proportion of patients on a new treatment is given in section 5.4.

4.3 PROBLEMS WITH CONCURRENT NON-RANDOMIZED CONTROLS

Even when the investigators have agreed to a prospective clinical trial in which future patients are to be assigned to the various treatments, there may still be some reservations about whether such assignment should be based on a random mechanism. Instead, it may be decided to use some predetermined systematic method, or worse still some degree of judgement by investigator and/or patient may be adopted. This section is concerned with the problems that can arise from using such concurrent non-randomized controls.

Systematic Assignment

The most common methods used here are to assign patients according to the *date of birth* (e.g. odd/even day of birth = new/standard treatment) or *date of presentation* (e.g. odd/even days = new/standard treatment) or to use *alternate assignment* (e.g. odd/even patients = new/standard treatment). The main problem with all of these methods is that the investigator can easily know in advance which treatment a patient would receive if he entered the trial and this prior knowledge may affect the investigator's decision regarding entry or not.

For instance, Wright *et al.* (1948) report on a trial of anticoagulant therapy for myocardial infarction whereby patients admitted on odd days of the month received anticoagulant and patients admitted on even days did not. There were 589 treated and 442 control patients, a sizeable imbalance indicating a preference towards admitting patients onto anticoagulants. This finding brings into question the comparability of the treatment and control groups and hence the validity of the results.

Similarly, Grage (1981) reports a trial of preoperative radiotherapy for rectal cancer begun in 1957 in which patients were assigned according to birth date: 192 patients received preoperative radiation compared with 267 treated by operative resection alone, again an imbalance which casts doubt on the trial's validity.

In the case of alternate assignment it is somewhat more difficult to detect bias, since although the investigator's prior knowledge of the next treatment may affect patient selection the equality of treatment numbers will be preserved. However, one may find some lack of comparability in the characteristics of the treatment groups. For instance, Ehrenkranz *et al.* (1978) evaluated vitamin E for neonates with bronchopulmonary dysplasia by alternate assignment of 40 such infants to vitamin E and control groups. The vitamin E group had a higher mean 1-minute Apgar score, which raises the possibility that there might have been some selection bias so that the trial's findings in favour of vitamin E cannot be interpreted with quite the same confidence as if the trial was randomized. Of course, even if random assignment is used one can still get chance differences in treatment groups, but provided randomization is arranged so that investigators do not know which treatment is coming next no selection bias is possible (see chapter 5).

Thus, there would seem *no real justification for such systematic assignment methods* since they do contain a potential bias and can be replaced quite simply by randomization.

Another potentially more serious problem arises if a trial is conducted so that the treatment depends on the clinician, whereby some clinicians (or hospitals) give one treatment while other clinicians (or hospitals) give another. This approach has much the same deficiencies as historical controls since both patient selection and the experimental environment may differ considerably between treatments.

Cockburn *et al.* (1980) conducted a trial of vitamin D supplement versus placebo in pregnant women to see if vitamin D could reduce neonatal hypocalcaemia. Mothers assigned to one hospital ward received vitamin D while mothers admitted to another ward did not. Patients in the two groups were comparable for social class, parity and maternal age so that patient selection appeared no problem. However, the two wards were under the care of different consultants and this raises the possibility that the vitamin D group could have differed from the controls in some other aspects of medical care. The results showed marked benefits in the vitamin D group, but having such non-randomized controls leaves some doubt. In a subsequent larger trial with a higher dose of vitamin D the investigators have implemented randomized assignment to overcome such qualms.

The wish to compare different treatments given in different hospitals can arise if each hospital is committed to a certain fixed approach. For instance, clinical trials for the evaluation of radiotherapy for cancer in the United States have at times been difficult to get off the ground since many cancer centres are unwilling to deviate from their standard treatment. Schoenfeld and Gelber (1979) mention an unusual way round this problem whereby, in a trial with more than two treatment options, each centre could opt out of certain treatment(s) they disapprove of, and have each of their patients randomized to the remaining options. Of course, it would be better if all centres could agree on the treatments to be compared, but perhaps a randomized trial which allows options is better than a non-randomized trial or no trial at all.

Judgement Assignment

If the investigator and/or the patient is allowed to exercise his judgement in assigning one of several treatment options it is evident that this could introduce considerable bias: for instance, the investigator may favour one particular treatment for his more serious cases which is liable to make this treatment appear worse regardless of its actual merit. Hence, such *use of judgement is generally regarded as obviously unacceptable* in clinical trials and one will see few explicit examples of its use in the medical literature.

However, one instance reported by Smithells *et al.* (1980) is a trial of vitamin supplementation for prevention of neural tube defects (NTD) given to high-risk women planning a further pregnancy. Here the untreated control groups included some women who had declined to take vitamin supplements (i.e. patients were effectively allowed to choose whether they were in the treatment or control group) as well as women who were already pregnant. Lack of randomization in this trial has made it impossible to decipher whether the reduced number of NTD infants after vitamin supplementation is really due to the vitamins themselves or due to bias in patient selection. The ensuing controversy has hampered plans by the Medical Research Council to run a randomized controlled trial which could properly resolve this issue.

It should also be noted that the use of judgement in treatment assignment may still be present even when not explicitly mentioned. For instance, if a report of a clinical trial merely provides a comparison of two or more treatments with no indication as to how patients were assigned one should not automatically assume that judgement played no part.

Another problem is where the investigators interfere with a randomized trial. 'Student' (1931) describes one such classic example in *the Lanarkshire milk experiment*. In 1930, 10 000 children received 3/4 pint of milk a day at school while another 10 000 in the same schools did not, the objective being to see if such milk supplement led to increased height and weight. However, trouble arose in the trial's design as 'Student' explains:

> The teachers selected the two classes of pupils, those getting milk and those acting as controls in two different ways. In certain cases they selected by ballot and in others on an alphabetical system. So far so good, but after invoking the goddess of chance they unfortunately wavered in their adherence. In any particular school where there was any group to which these methods had given an undue proportion of well fed or ill nourished children, others were substituted to obtain a more level selection. This is just the sort of afterthought that is apt to spoil the best laid plans. In this case it was a fatal mistake for in consequence the controls were definitely superior both in weight and height by an amount equivalent to about 3 months' growth in weight and 4 months' growth in height. It would seem probable that the teachers swayed by the very human feeling that the poorer children need the milk ... must have unconsciously made too large a substitution of the ill-nourished among the 'feeders'.

Those children receiving milk tended to gain more height and weight, but the initial differences cast doubt on the extent to which this could be attributed to the milk itself.

In recent years the use of *data banks* on computer containing information on all previous patients in a given institution has been advocated by some enthusiasts as an exciting development in clinical research. For instance,

Starmer *et al.* (1974) describe the use of data banks in the management of chronic illness. It has been proposed that such data banks could be used in the evaluation of different treatments and might be a substitute for randomized clinical trials. However, Byar (1980) provides a firm rebuttal of such an idea. Basically, such retrospective comparisons of treatment from a data bank arise after several clinicians have used their judgement in deciding which treatment their patients should receive. Also, the lack of any precise protocol means that treatments, types of patients and methods of evaluation cannot conform to any consistent definition. Thus, although they may provide a useful insight into the general pattern of patient management and prognosis as experienced in one institution *data banks provide very poor quality information for treatment comparison,* perhaps even worse than the historical controls I criticized in section 4.2.

4.4 IS RANDOMIZATION FEASIBLE?

So far I have shown that various alternatives to randomization are liable to produce seriously biassed and often overoptimistic results regarding a new therapy. Hence on purely scientific grounds it is easy to deduce that the use of a randomized control group is to be preferred in all situations. Furthermore, in more practical terms randomized controlled trials are an efficient method for determining the optimal therapy for future patients. However, clinical trials are not solely to do with the advancement of scientific knowledge and one needs to take into account the actual circumstances regarding eligible patients before automatically proceeding with a randomized trial. In particular, *one must consider whether it is ethical to randomize patients* and also whether there are sufficient investigators (and hence patients) willing to participate in such randomization.

As regards the ethics of randomization, Hill (1963) provides a carefully reasoned argument. He begins by considering the first randomized trial, to evaluate streptomycin treatment for pulmonary tuberculosis, already mentioned in chapter 2. Streptomycin was in short supply at the time so that one could not have given it to all patients even if one wanted to. Since efficacy had not been previously established, Hill argues it would have been unethical *not* to seize the opportunity to conduct a randomized controlled trial. Such a situation of therapy in short supply (interferon mentioned in section 4.1 is another example) makes it particularly easy to randomize since in addition to scientific validity one is also exercising 'fairness' in giving each patient an equal chance of receiving the rare treatment.

However, the ethics of randomization require a more subtle argument if a new therapy is in plentiful supply and could, if one wished, be given to every new patient. First, one assumes that the wish to conduct a clinical trial is based on the idea that the new treatment has a reasonable chance of being a genuine improvement. Indeed, one must expect that some clinicians will already be inclined to believe that the new treatment is better. However, opinion should not necessarily preclude an investigator from entering patients on a randomized trial. It is important to draw a distinction between such subjective personal belief and objective scientific knowledge regarding efficacy. For instance, Gilbert *et al.* (1977) reviewed 46 randomized controlled trials in surgery and anaesthesia and found that in only half of such trials was the therapeutic innovation found to be preferable. The motivation behind each of these trials was a belief that the innovation was liable to be better, but it turns out that there is a substantial probability that such prior expectations will not be fulfilled.

Hence, before agreeing to enter patients in a randomized trial each investigator must come to terms with his personal judgement of the treatments involved. It is inevitable that he will have some preferences regarding treatment, but past experience (as in the above example) shows that randomized trials have a habit of often producing scientific evidence which contradicts such prior belief. Of course, if a clinician feels very strongly that one treatment in a randomized trial is unacceptable then he should not participate. However, it is for each clinician to decide whether he has the right to take such a dogmatic stance or needs to have his beliefs checked empirically by a randomized trial. Further consideration of ethical problems in clinical trials is given in chapter 7.

One further problem is in deciding when is the opportune moment in the development of a new therapy to start a randomized trial and let us consider this issue as regards *surgical trials*. Chalmers (1972) argues that randomization is introduced infrequently and too late to evaluate new operations. For instance, he refers to 152 trials of operative therapy for coronary artery disease: only two trials were randomized and both found internal mammmary artery ligation of no value. He argues that 'the only way to avoid the distorting influences of uncontrolled trials is to begin randomization with the first patient'. However, Bonchek (1979) and Van der Linden (1980) discuss some of the difficulties associated with randomized surgical trials. In particular, the skill of the surgeon is likely to have an impact on the patient's prognosis, more so than the clinician's impact in a drug trial. Thus, in comparing a new surgical procedure against non-surgery the former will be going through phases of development whereby refinements in technique will often mean that later results may surpass the achievements of the first experimental operations. Also, caution is needed in generalizing from the achievements of the most skilled and experienced surgeons in an experiment to the lesser expectations of routine surgical practice.

If a randomized trial is performed after a treatment has become standard practice then its results are likely to provoke controversy. The Danish Obesity Project (1979) compared a widely accepted surgical procedure (jejunoileal bypass) with medical treatment of morbid obesity and found the former to produce greater weight loss and improved quality of life, though with complications of surgery common and sometimes severe. Since the trial confirmed a *suspected* benefit of surgery, it might be considered unnecessary and unethical. But how is one to *know* such benefit if a randomized trial is never performed? Evidently, controversy would be avoided if the development of new surgery involved randomized trials at an earlier stage.

The comparison of alternative surgical procedures raises the problem that surgeons may be more experienced in one operation than the other, and such difference in pretrial routine may affect the results of a trial. For example, Van der Linden (1980) refers to two trials, one Swedish and one Finnish, which studied early versus delayed operation for acute cholecystitis and which came to completely opposite conclusions. Again, I do not think such contradiction is an argument against doing randomized surgical trials but more an indication that the relevance of their findings must be assessed relative to each hospital's circumstances. Grage and Zelen (1982) point out that randomization may be especially difficult if the treatment modalities are radically different. For instance, in the management of soft tissue sarcoma one would like to compare local excision plus radiotherapy with a more radical excision or amputation. However, it would be extremely difficult to conduct a trial in which whether the patient loses an arm or leg depends on random assignment. Here one may have to resort to some form of non-randomized comparison, though use of a randomized consent design (see section 7.2) is a possibility.

The purpose of this chapter has been to emphasize that in general *randomized controlled trials are an essential tool for testing the efficacy of therapeutic innovations*. The proper use of randomization guarantees that there is no bias in the selection of patients for the different treatments and also helps considerably to reduce the risk of differences in experimental environment. Randomized allocation is not difficult to implement and enables trial conclusions to be more believable than other forms of treatment allocation.

However, the acceptance of randomization remains only a starting point in the proper execution of a trial. In particular, if the randomization is not performed correctly then there is every danger that the trial might be just as biassed as the non-randomized trials mentioned earlier. Hence, the next chapter describes various methods of implementing random treatment assignment and discusses some of the pitfalls to be avoided.

CHAPTER 5

Methods of Randomization

The purpose of randomly assigning patients to treatments has already been discussed in chapter 4 so that in this chapter I confine attention to how one should actually implement a randomization scheme. In its crudest form one could introduce random treatment assignment into a clinical trial by repeatedly tossing a coin in order to decide which of two treatments each patient should receive. In principle, this approach should achieve the desired objective of ensuring against any bias or judgement in the selection of patients on each treatment. However, in practice it is advisable to adopt a more formal, well-defined routine for registering and randomizing patients and details are described in section 5.1. It is customary to arrange in advance the precise sequence of random treatment assignments, often using tables of random numbers, and various methods of achieving such a randomization list are explained in section 5.2. In some circumstances one may wish to restrict the randomization to ensure that the different treatment groups are comparable with regard to certain major patient characteristics and such stratified randomization is discussed in section 5.3. In certain trials it may be worth allocating a higher proportion of patients onto one treatment compared with another. The principles and implementation of such unequal randomization are considered in section 5.4.

5.1 PATIENT REGISTRATION

For each patient who might be considered suitable for inclusion in a clinical trial the following formal sequence of events should take place:

(1) Patient requires treatment
(2) Patient eligible for inclusion in the trial
(3) Clinician willing to accept randomization
(4) Patient consent is obtained
(5) Patient formally entered on the trial
(6) Treatment assignment obtained from the randomization list
(7) On-study forms are completed
(8) Treatment commences

This sequence enables the registration of patients into the trial to proceed in an efficient and ethical manner while ensuring that the rules for random treatment assignment are followed correctly.

In a multi-centre trial this whole procedure of patient registration may be carried out by the clinician being in contact with a *central registration office*, usually *by telephone*. This centralization helps the correct implementation of each step and ensures that someone has an overview of how the trial is going (see section 3.2 on trial coordination). Indeed, even for a trial in just one institution it may help to have one person, preferably not a participating clinician, who is responsible for supervising patient registration. However, if a trial has only one investigator or if one is unable to centralize operations then patient registration will have to be left to the individual clinician. I will now expand on the justification and mechanics of the above formal sequence of events, by discussing each of the eight steps in turn:

(1) Patient Recruitment

The identification of appropriate patients may seem an obvious step, but it is important to ensure that the patients entered in the trial are representative of the disease under investigation so that the trial's conclusions can be readily applied to the entire population of such patients. Thus, the manner in which patients are attracted towards a trial needs consideration: each participating clinician should see a reasonably representative group of patients and should commit himself in advance to consider seriously all relevant patients for the trial. In particular, the clinician should avoid being unduly selective in his choice of patients.

(2) Checking Eligibility

The eligibility of each possible patient should be checked right away. The clinician should go through the list of eligibility criteria in the protocol (see chapter 3) and exclude the patient automatically if any criterion is not fulfilled. In a multi-centre trial the individual clinician may be less familiar with eligibility criteria in which case it is advisable that the central registration office should run through the list when first contacted. Of course, some ineligible patients may slip through the net only to be identified later and such patients may be excluded from the results (see section 12.1). A more serious problem is the ineligible patient who goes undetected due to poor supervision.

(3) Agreement to Randomize

It is vital to ensure that the clinician should agree to accept any of the random treatment assignments *before* he formally enters the patient into the trial. Otherwise, one may have the problem that after treatment is assigned the clinician opts to use some other treatment instead; such action is totally unacceptable and could seriously invalidate the trial. It is preferable that each clinician be willing to enter and randomize all his eligible patients, but in practice one must allow a clinician to exclude the occasional patient he considers unsuitable. However, any clinician who is unwilling to randomize a substantial proportion of relevant patients should not participate in the trial at all.

(4) **Patient Consent**

In general, there is an ethical need to inform each patient about his entry into a clinical trial and obtain his agreement before proceeding further. In the United States it is a legal requirement that fully informed patient consent be obtained in writing prior to randomization whereas in some countries there is a more informal attitude to patient consent. This issue along with other ethical aspects of clinical trials is discussed more fully in chapter 7. In particular, one alternative proposal is to obtain patient consent after randomization and such 'randomized consent' designs are discussed in section 7.2.

(5) **Formal Entry on Trial**

It is essential that each patient entering the trial be formally identified *before* random treatment assignment is revealed. This can be achieved by having the patient's name, and possibly a few other details such as hospital number or date of birth (or institution if a multi-centre trial), recorded on a *log sheet* of patients in the trial. An example is shown in table 5.1. If patient registration is by telephone to a central office this log sheet will be kept at the office. At the same time the patient could be given a trial number to aid future identification. The reason for such registration before randomization is to ensure that *all* randomized patients are followed for details of treatment and evaluation. This helps to ensure that every patient is handled according to the protocol, since the clinician is aware from the start that the trial organizers know about each patient entered. In particular, it helps to guard against investigators not giving the randomized treatment: such deviant investigators, and they do exist in a poorly organized trial, should be readily identified and hence excluded. In addition, there is value in keeping a separate log of eligible patients who are *not* entered into the trial, since this provides insight into the representativeness of patients who are in the trial (see section 12.1 for further comment).

(6) **Random Treatment Assignment**

Only after steps (1) to (5) have been successfully completed does the doctor learn which treatment the patient has been assigned to. In most clinical trials, a *randomization list* of consecutive random treatment assignments has been prepared in advance and section 5.2 describes how this is done. One essential is that the clinician does not know the order of this list and is unable to predict

Table 5.1. An example of a log sheet for patient entry

Trial number	Date of entry	Name	Date of birth	Institution	Investigator's initials	Assigned treatment*
001	17.7.81	John Doe	9.3.40	Hammersmith	AFP	A
002	24.7.81	David Green	28.6.32	Royal Free	JDR	B
003	4.8.81	Henrietta Bloggs	1.8.26	Barts	MSC	B
004	5.8.81	Arbuthnot Shuttlebottom	13.7.31	Guys	PHD	B
⋮	⋮	⋮	⋮	⋮	⋮	⋮

* Treatment assignments may usually be added to the log sheet after each patient is entered, though in a multi-centre trial with telephone registration one could transfer the randomization list to the log sheet before the trial commences.

what the next assignment will be. To achieve this aim the list should be prepared by an independent person, possibly a statistician. One of several mechanisms can be adopted for revealing each patient's assigned treatment:

(a) The randomization list could be transferred to a sequence of *sealed envelopes* each containing the name of the next treatment on a card. The clinician then opens the next envelope in the sequence when the patient has formally entered the trial. This method is advisable only if each clinician is having to register his own patients, i.e. there is no central registration office and no other person he can consult when entering the patient. Even then, one needs to guard against 'dirty tricks' such as the clinician resealing the envelope or rearranging the order of envelopes if the next assignment is not to his liking. Of course, the great majority of investigators are above such dubious practices but they have been known to happen and are hard to check on. Thus, sealed envelopes are a well-tried method of randomizing but are not totally foolproof.

(b) If the trial is a *double-blind* evaluation of drug therapy (see chapter 6 for clarification) then the *pharmacist* preparing the drugs should be involved. He needs to be given the randomization list in order to produce a corresponding sequence of drug 'packages' containing the appropriate treatments but identical in appearance, etc. These packages are then presented to the clinician and treatment assignment proceeds as for sealed envelope randomization except that the clinician still does not know which treatment the patient is on even after randomization. An unsuitable alternative is to supply each clinician with sufficient supplies of each drug, suitably coded A or B so that he does not know which drug is which, and then to use one of the other methods for randomization to assign A or B to each patient. This approach is ill-advised since if the clinician 'breaks the code' for any single patient either by necessity, chance or dubious ingenuity then the actual treatment is revealed for all his patients and blindness is destroyed.

(c) For a *multi-centre trial* with a *central registration office* the treatment assignment can be read off the randomization list and given to the investigator while he is still on the phone. Such an arrangement obviously requires substantial preparation and involves a certain expenditure in terms of personnel and telephone calls. However, such effort is worthwhile in that it does provide a reasonably foolproof system of randomization. Accordingly most American cancer cooperative groups for multi-centre trials have adopted this approach. In international trials, problems of cost and communication in several languages can mean that randomization has to be performed in each centre using sealed envelopes. However, the European Organization for Research on Treatment of Cancer (EORTC) with headquarters in Brussels has successfully overcome this problem by using English as the international language in telephone randomization for many centres throughout Europe.

Even if telephone randomization is the most reliable method for multi-centre trials, it still requires strict control and agreement to 'follow the rules' for the system to work properly. For instance, I recall one multi-centre trial in which one institution deliberately avoided randomization and entered all its patients on one treatment. As a consequence other institutions received more patients on the other treatment, but the eventual publication gave no account of such interference with randomization. Hence, whatever system of randomization is used one needs to maintain close supervision and leave no loophole for such deviations.

The double-blind multi-centre trial poses an extra problem since the treatment cannot be explicitly revealed over the phone. Here, one can simply decentralize patient registration and have each hospital's pharmacist arrange drug 'packages' according to the randomization list, as described in (b) above. However, it may be possible and indeed preferable still to have central registration. For instance, the Medical Research Council Cancer Trials Unit in Cambridge has one-double blind multi-centre trial in which each hospital pharmacist obtains random treatment assignment by phone from a central office.

Of course, one needs someone manning the phone at central office at all times during which calls for patient registration might occur. Even so, there will be the occasional patient, especially in acute illness, who requires assignment outside normal hours, e.g. over the weekend. In these rare circumstances, some random method needs to be employed and at worst one can allow the clinician literally to toss a coin. However, it should be made clear that non-randomized assignment, i.e. letting the clinician choose, is not permitted.

(d) For a trial in a *single institution* the most suitable arrangement is to have an *independent person* responsible for patient registration and randomization who is not concerned with treating any of the patients. Here the system can proceed as described in (c) above, except that the clinician entering the patient can actually meet this person rather than just telephone. This should be an advantage in ensuring that eligibility checks, etc., can be more rigorously applied. For an institution where clinical research is substantial, such as the cancer trials programme at the Mayo Clinic, there may be several persons whose main responsibility is patient registration. However, where a clinical trial is a one-off effort a person otherwise employed as, say, a secretary, nurse or research assistant may need to act also as this independent person. Since errors in patient registration and randomization are perhaps most likely to occur in such small-scale single-institution research, the organizers of such trials might be advised to be extra careful in this respect.

(7) Documentation

After the treatment has been assigned, one should complete necessary documentation prior to start of treatment. Besides the log sheet already described in table 5.1 it may be appropriate to have a *confirmation of registration* form for each patient containing essentially the same information: name, date of birth, trial number and assigned treatment. In a multi-centre trial this could be mailed to the clinician from the central registration office as soon as the phone call is completed. If randomization is decentralized and by sealed envelopes, then the confirmation of registration needs to be in the reverse direction, from the clinician to a central office collecting all the trial data, and should also be mailed as soon as the sealed envelope has been opened. Such a confirmation form may seem superfluous to some but it can be a valuable aid in ensuring that the individual clinician and trial organizers are in agreement regarding patient registration and is an extra safeguard against 'losing' patients after randomization.

In addition, every trial needs an *on-study form* for each patient containing all relevant information prior to treatment such as previous therapy, personal details (e.g. age and sex), details about their clinical condition and certain tests (e.g. lung function in respiratory illness). As for all documentation, any on-study form needs careful planning as regards which items to include and which layout is appropriate, and any draft form should be tested before the trial commences. Chapter 11 gives further details on the design of such forms.

(8) Efficiency and Reliability

All the above formalities should be completed before treatment commences. Accordingly, the whole process of patient registration and randomization needs to be prompt and efficient so that there is no delay in treatment. One essential is that every patient should stay in the trial so that their treatment and evaluation can be properly recorded. In this respect, a suitably obsessive attitude to patient registration pays dividends in that it helps the clinician to appreciate the commitment to serious clinical research that he is undertaking by entering his patients in the trial.

One extra problem of correct timing for randomization concerns trials in which each patient is subjected to *more than one type of therapy*. For instance, consider the trial of adjuvant chemotherapy following mastectomy described in section 1.4. Should random assignment to L-Pam or placebo take place before or after mastectomy? In fact it is better if patients are registered and randomized after mastectomy so as to avoid any unnecessary drop-outs due to patients becoming ineligible.

Another example is a trial reported by Ezdinli *et al.* (1976) in which patients with non-Hodgkins lymphoma were initially randomized to one of two 'induction' treatments (cytoxan-prednisone or BCNU-prednisone). Those who responded after three months were then randomized to one of two 'mainten-ance' treatments (BCVP or chlorambucil). In fact, both the random induction and random maintenance treatment assignment were obtained at the same time when the patient entered the trial whereas it would have been better if the maintenance assignment was obtained separately after the patient had re-sponded at three months. Knowledge of which maintenance schedule was to follow could influence the investigators' evaluation of response on induction and the precise timing of transfer, if at all, from induction to maintenance therapy. Also, drop-outs prior to maintenance might lead to an imbalance in the numbers on each maintenance therapy. Hence, in such multi-therapy trials each randomization should be delayed until the patient is ready to receive such randomized treatment. Further discussion of patient registration, especially in multi-centre trials, is given by Herson (1980).

5.2 PREPARING THE RANDOMIZATION LIST

In this section I shall describe several ways of preparing a list of random treatment assignments which can then be used one at a time as patients are registered into the trial, as already explained in section 5.1.

First, I shall consider a simple unrestricted method of randomization which is essentially equivalent to repeated coin tossing. Then, various methods are described for restricting randomization to ensure approximately equal numbers of patients on each treatment. There are also various 'stratified' randomization methods which take into account a few patient characteristics in order to ensure that the treatment groups are not dissimilar: the merits and mechanics of such stratification are described in section 5.3.

For each method, the basic principle is followed by a brief explanation of how the list can be generated using tables of random numbers. However, in any group extensively involved in clinical trials it may be more convenient to use computer programs to produce lists based on some computer-generated sequence of random numbers.

Simple Randomization

For a randomized trial with two treatments (call them A and B) the basic concept of tossing a coin (heads = A, tails = B) over and over again is quite reasonable, but it is rather clumsy and time-consuming. Thus, people find it more convenient to use tables of random numbers instead. For instance, table 5.2 shows such a table of random digits 0 to 9. Each digit occurs on average the same number of times, there is no discernible pattern of digit values and the table presents digits in pairs merely to help the user in scanning across the page. A randomization list may be generated by using the digits, one per treatment assignment, starting with the top row and working downwards:

For *two treatments* assign A for digits 0–4 }
B for digits 5–9 }

Hence, the numbers in the top row of table 5.1

0 5 2 7 8 4 3 7 4 1 6 8 3 8 5 1 5 6 9 6 etc.

produce a list starting   A B A B B A A B A A B B A B B A B B B B etc.

For *three treatments*, say A, B and C, assign A for digits 1–3 }
B for digits 4–6 }
C for digits 7–9 }
and ignore 0

so that numbers   0 5 2 7 8 4 3 7 4 1 6 8 3 8 5 1 5 6 9 6 etc.
produce a list starting   - B A C C B A C B A B C A C B A B B C B etc.

Table 5.2. A table of random numbers

```
4 7 8 8 7 4 0 8 1 8 9 6 9 9 5 1 5 6 3 8 8 8 1 4 3 7 4 8 7 2 0 5
4 7 5 0 5 8 1 1 2 1 9 9 9 9 6 9 0 7 5 6 6 1 4 6 2 3 8 4 2 7 9 5
9 2 3 5 8 8 2 8 2 1 4 6 5 5 9 9 6 5 4 8 8 4 6 3 9 8 3 0 8 9 2 0
2 4 3 8 8 9 5 9 4 8 8 4 5 5 9 5 2 0 6 0 5 4 3 6 3 3 4 3 6 3 5 8
1 5 2 1 1 5 0 2 0 5 6 8 3 1 4 8 9 8 6 8 4 5 2 8 2 2 5 5 3 1 6 3
5 5 9 8 8 1 0 1 0 8 5 7 9 8 9 9 1 5 8 5 1 7 6 8 1 7 1 8 6 6 7 6
2 3 2 8 3 9 4 8 0 2 3 7 5 1 7 9 7 9 7 6 3 7 0 7 1 9 3 0 3 8 7 7
6 5 9 4 4 5 2 6 5 1 3 5 5 9 5 3 2 1 2 0 9 9 5 9 2 3 1 6 6 2 8 4
4 4 6 4 3 5 0 1 5 4 3 4 1 7 3 8 2 1 6 6 4 2 5 8 3 1 4 9 4 1 7 1
3 3 7 4 0 2 0 3 3 3 8 4 0 9 8 5 1 0 3 3 3 3 2 6 9 2 2 4 3 6 6 3
9 9 2 1 3 5 6 5 8 8 2 9 4 9 0 7 5 5 0 2 1 0 8 2 9 0 0 3 5 4 4 3
4 3 4 9 8 2 3 5 4 4 2 2 5 1 4 4 5 6 4 4 3 6 9 6 3 4 7 9 9 5 5 5
2 7 0 2 0 9 1 3 0 5 0 2 1 2 1 9 2 9 5 5 0 2 8 3 5 5 3 6 2 8 2 2
9 9 7 1 4 0 9 8 4 5 7 0 7 1 2 5 9 1 5 6 2 2 0 1 7 1 5 6 9 8 2 3
3 4 9 7 2 4 8 0 5 6 0 6 8 9 2 7 1 6 2 3 1 9 8 9 0 8 8 0 7 7 0 0
4 3 4 3 1 7 4 4 6 3 3 8 4 1 8 3 9 5 4 2 8 4 8 6 9 0 2 2 1 6 3 6
9 6 0 8 2 0 4 0 3 1 2 8 5 3 0 7 5 0 6 3 8 1 8 6 3 6 9 6 5 7 4 2
3 5 3 6 3 4 4 1 4 4 9 2 4 4 0 5 7 1 0 5 2 3 1 7 3 7 4 9 8 1 5 4
4 1 4 7 8 0 2 0 6 3 2 8 5 5 7 3 5 5 1 5 4 0 3 1 7 1 1 7 9 7 7 0
5 0 9 1 9 5 0 5 4 2 2 6 7 2 5 8 6 0 0 9 4 1 5 9 7 8 7 9 5 8 6 4
9 8 6 2 8 9 9 2 6 9 4 9 8 1 1 7 9 0 9 8 1 2 6 3 9 6 7 8 5 6 2 8
6 2 6 2 9 8 9 0 2 0 5 6 6 9 1 7 3 8 3 6 5 1 3 9 6 6 6 5 7 3 4 4
0 9 8 8 4 7 1 9 8 5 8 9 5 6 2 8 5 6 4 6 0 7 4 9 0 0 1 5 6 7 8 0
9 8 6 9 9 4 3 8 5 7 6 1 2 8 6 0 2 0 8 8 8 1 5 5 9 6 5 3 1 8 5 0
```

Table 5.2. A table of random numbers

For *four treatments*, say A, B, C and D, assign   A for digits 1–2 ⎫
                                            B for digits 3–4 ⎪
                                            C for digits 5–6 ⎬
                                            D for digits 7–8 ⎭
and ignore 0 and 9

so that numbers   0 5 2 7 8 4 3 7 4 1 6 8 3 8 5 1 5 6 9 6 etc.

produce a list starting - C A D D B B D B A C D B D C A C C - C etc.

Such randomization lists can be made as long as necessary and since the process is so easy one should make the list before the trial starts and make it long enough to complete the whole trial. One should consider starting the list at some arbitrary point in table 5.2, rather than the top left, just in case anyone should know how to refer to this actual table to 'break the code'. (What a suspicious mind I have!)

The advantage of such a simple method is that *each treatment assignment is completely unpredictable*, and probability theory guarantees that in the long run the numbers of patients on each treatment will not be radically different. However, clinical trials are of finite size and one should consider the possibility that the treatment numbers may end up unequal. For instance, using the above list for two treatments and 20 patients one ends up with eight patients on A compared with 12 on B: not a huge difference but somewhat inconvenient and inefficient especially if A happens to be the new treatment and B the standard. Furthermore, table 5.3 illustrates what sort of difference in treatment numbers may occur with probability at least 0.05 or at least 0.01. Clearly, it would be catastrophic if a trial with 20 patients had four on one treatment and 16 on the other. The fact that such an event should occur with probability slightly greater than 0.01 is no consolation to the unlucky investigator. With 100 patients an inequality of 40:60 or worse is to be expected with probability slightly above 0.05. This would not be a major fault if it occurred, but would best be avoided if possible. Only in large trials, say with over 200 patients does the chance of severe imbalance become so remote that simple randomization may be

Table 5.3. Possible imbalance in simple randomization with two treatments. This table shows the difference in treatment numbers (or more extreme) liable to occur with probability at least 0.05 or at least 0.01 for various trial sizes

Total number of patients	Difference in numbers Probability $\geqslant 0.05$	Probability $\geqslant 0.01$
10	2:8	1:9
20	6:14	4:16
50	18:32	16:34
100	40:60	37:63
200	86:114	82:118
500	228:272	221:279
1000	469:531	459:541

recommended, but a problem could still arise if one intends to analyse early results while the trial is in progress.

Thus, *it is often desirable to restrict randomization to ensure similar treatment numbers throughout a trial* and here I will describe three possible approaches:

Replacement Randomization

After preparing a randomization list as described above one can check if there is any serious inequality in treatment numbers. If it is unsatisfactory then one can generate an entirely new simple randomization to replace the first one. It is unlikely that one will need to repeat this more than once to achieve reasonably equal-sized treatment groups throughout a trial. The decision to replace a randomization list should be based on objective criteria: for instance, for a trial with two treatments and around 100 patients one could specify that a simple randomization with inequality of 10 or more at any point should be replaced. Such replacement of randomization lists might seem a little odd to some people, but provided it is all carried out before the trial starts there should be no problem. It has the advantage of ensuring reasonable balance, being simple to do and gives investigators little scope for guessing future patient assignments, especially if they are not aware of the rules for replacement.

Random Permuted Blocks

A more conventional method of restricted randomization is to ensure exactly equal treatment numbers at certain equally spaced points in the sequence of patient assignments. Suppose we have T treatments, then for each block of say kT patients we produce a different random ordering of k assignments to each treatment. Firstly, for blocks of relatively small size one can use a table of random numbers as in table 5.2 to produce the randomization list:

For two treatments, blocks of two patients assign AB for digits 0–4
BA for digits 5–9

Then, the numbers   0   5   2   7   8   4   3   7 etc. produce a list
starting   AB BA AB BA BA AB AB BA etc.

For three treatments, blocks of three patients assign ABC for digit 1
ACB   2
BAC   3
BCA   4
CAB   5
CBA   6
and ignore 0 and 7–9

so that numbers 0   5   2 7 8 4   3 7 etc. produce a list
starting   - CAB ACB - - BCA BAC - etc.

For two treatments, blocks of four patients assign AABB for digit 1
ABAB   2
ABBA   3
BBAA   4
BABA   5
BAAB   6

and ignore 0 and 7–9

so that numbers 0   5   2   7 8   4   3   7   etc. produce a list
starting   - BABA ABAB - - BBAA ABBA -   etc.

One problem here is that at the end of each block a clinician who keeps track of previous assignments could predict what the next treatment would be, though in double-blind or multi-centre trials this would not normally be possible. Evidently the smaller the choice of block size the greater is the risk of randomization becoming predictable so that one should particularly avoid a block size of two. However, note that in stratified randomization (see section 5.3) one may use random permuted blocks for patients classified separately into several types (or strata) and in these circumstances the block size needs to be quite small, so that the above description of how to generate small blocks is not without purpose.

Thus, in general *a trial without stratification should have a reasonably large block size* so as to reduce predictability but, if interim analysis is intended, not so large that serious mid-block inequality might occur. For example, a trial with say 100 or more patients could have a block size of 20. Table 5.4 gives a list of random permutations of numbers 0 to 19 to be used as follows.

For two treatments, blocks of 20 patients assign A for 0– 9
and B for 10–19

Then, starting with the top left-hand permutation and working downwards numbers 11 19 15 5 9 0 6 13 7 2 16 1 12 18 4 17 10 8 3 14 produce a list B   B   B A A A A B A A   B A B   B A   B   B A A   B

block 1

14 12 0 1 19 8 7 17 11 18 2 15 5 9 4 16 10 6 13 3
B   B A A   B A A B   B   B A   B A A A   B   B A   B A

block 2, etc.

For three treatments, blocks of 15 patients assign A for   1– 5
B   6–10
C   11–15

and ignore 0 and 16–19

Table 5.4 Random permutations of 20 numbers (each row represents a random ordering of the numbers 0 to 19)

11	19	15	5	9	0	6	13	7	2	16	1	12	18	4	17	10	8	3	14
14	12	0	1	19	8	7	17	11	18	2	15	5	9	4	16	10	6	13	3
5	17	2	4	16	19	10	11	14	7	12	15	1	18	6	9	0	3	13	8
8	13	3	12	10	5	17	2	6	7	16	19	0	1	4	11	14	15	18	9
11	6	8	0	1	10	13	18	12	14	17	7	4	5	3	9	19	16	2	15
17	18	3	6	9	15	14	5	4	19	2	1	0	8	11	13	7	12	10	16
14	19	13	16	1	9	18	0	5	15	4	12	10	11	2	3	8	6	7	17
0	3	2	13	7	8	19	12	5	9	16	6	4	17	15	14	1	11	18	10
11	19	2	6	12	15	17	0	10	3	4	14	7	5	16	13	1	8	9	18
13	18	9	6	5	17	19	0	8	10	15	7	11	3	12	4	16	1	2	14
9	3	4	17	18	2	13	14	15	11	0	8	1	7	6	19	16	12	10	5
2	9	17	12	6	19	14	4	1	7	5	3	10	13	0	18	8	15	11	16
14	8	11	2	13	6	5	0	10	12	19	4	16	15	9	17	7	18	1	3
5	9	11	3	7	14	19	15	0	17	2	12	18	4	13	16	10	1	6	8
3	19	11	17	18	10	6	4	14	2	1	16	9	5	7	8	12	13	0	15
13	3	9	11	2	7	0	15	19	4	14	10	12	6	5	1	17	16	18	8
0	5	18	12	3	11	8	15	6	16	9	4	7	2	19	17	14	10	1	13
10	15	0	16	7	5	4	13	12	1	17	3	9	14	11	8	6	18	2	19
2	16	13	19	8	6	17	9	14	4	12	3	1	11	5	15	0	10	7	18
18	15	5	11	6	3	14	13	7	0	9	17	2	1	8	10	12	19	4	16
9	14	3	6	16	1	0	11	4	2	10	12	19	13	7	15	18	8	17	5
15	18	4	12	1	7	11	10	5	17	14	8	2	0	3	6	9	19	13	16
12	1	7	13	19	8	6	4	10	14	0	18	15	9	17	16	11	2	5	3
15	11	3	10	14	9	16	2	5	17	18	19	4	6	13	1	8	0	7	12
1	17	16	10	15	18	0	7	11	9	2	14	3	5	13	12	6	4	19	8
5	9	16	12	6	17	19	15	2	14	11	0	3	10	8	18	1	4	7	13
9	8	0	7	4	17	19	3	5	6	13	15	16	10	11	12	1	14	2	18
9	2	17	7	16	14	5	15	19	8	13	6	0	4	18	3	10	11	1	12
9	4	14	1	5	0	6	10	15	17	8	16	19	18	7	2	11	13	3	12
6	4	17	14	16	2	1	8	15	11	3	0	10	18	5	13	19	7	12	9
11	6	14	13	10	4	7	18	19	12	15	2	8	5	17	3	1	16	9	0
17	2	14	8	4	11	9	12	3	18	6	13	1	19	7	0	16	5	10	15
1	11	5	9	4	17	14	7	6	12	0	10	19	15	8	16	3	13	2	18
8	19	5	15	9	14	4	1	18	16	11	0	3	12	17	13	7	10	2	6
12	11	6	18	7	13	3	2	14	19	10	9	16	0	4	15	5	8	17	1
17	7	11	4	3	15	16	9	8	0	5	18	10	19	2	13	12	14	1	6
7	11	18	0	17	19	15	12	10	5	8	3	9	13	4	14	1	2	16	6
5	8	0	2	3	13	15	19	6	18	1	10	9	12	14	16	4	7	17	11
15	11	1	12	7	14	13	19	2	16	10	6	18	8	3	17	0	5	4	9
8	1	9	10	6	15	4	19	0	18	2	7	16	13	5	3	11	14	17	12
13	1	17	14	11	16	3	5	7	9	0	15	19	6	18	12	4	10	8	2
3	12	9	4	6	15	5	16	17	18	7	2	19	11	14	8	1	13	10	0
10	3	8	15	2	16	19	4	1	5	13	14	6	7	11	0	17	12	18	9
16	5	9	1	15	18	17	12	10	19	8	13	6	11	4	14	7	3	0	2
19	1	9	16	3	11	8	15	4	13	12	18	0	10	7	6	2	14	5	17
0	10	3	5	13	17	19	8	7	16	14	9	11	12	4	6	2	18	15	1
3	16	15	13	7	9	0	2	18	14	5	10	17	4	19	11	12	1	8	6
14	16	15	7	4	17	2	10	3	1	8	11	18	0	19	12	6	13	5	9
3	1	17	18	19	0	5	9	14	10	8	2	15	4	12	6	16	7	13	11
11	17	13	19	16	18	2	15	1	8	7	10	14	6	0	9	4	5	3	12

so that permutations

      11 19 15 5 9 0 6 13 7 2 16 1 12 18 4 17 10 8 3 14

produce a list starting

     C - C A B - B C B A   - A C   - A   - B B A C

block 1

    14 12 0 1 19 8 7 17 11 18 2 15 5 9 4 16 10 6 13 3

    C C - A   - B B   - C   - A C A B A   - B B C A

block 2, etc.

Again, one could consider starting at an arbitrary point in table 5.3 rather than at the top left.

If one prefers to use random permuted blocks of size 10 or less, one can still use table 5.4 by simply ignoring numbers 10–19 in each block. Alternatively, Fisher and Yates (1974) contains a table of random permutations of length 10.

To help reduce the predictability of random permuted blocks one could vary the block size at random from one block to the next. Also, it is advisable not to inform clinicians that blocking is being used and especially they should not know the block size.

The Biassed Coin Method

Even though the above 'blocking' is widely accepted one should consider whether such strict equality is necessary. One really needs to avoid major inequalities in treatment numbers and Efron (1971) has proposed the biassed coin method which is as follows for the two-treatment case. At each point in the trial one observes which treatment has the least patients so far: that treatment is then assigned with probability $p > 1/2$ to the next patient. If the two treatments have equal numbers then simple randomization is used for the next patient.

One has to choose an appropriate value for p and here some probability theory is helpful. It turns out that for $p = 3/4$ ⎫ a difference in treatment
                                           2/3 ⎬
                                         3/5 ⎬
                                or 5/9 ⎭

numbers of 4 ⎫ or more has less than a 1 in 20 chance of occurring at any
             6 ⎬
          10 ⎬
          16 ⎭

particular point in the trial. Hence, $p = 3/4$ maintains very strict control on treatment numbers but as a consequence is somewhat predictable once any inequality exists. $p = 2/3$ may be an appropriate choice for a relatively small trial whereas $p = 3/5$ is satisfactory for larger trials of say 100 patients. The randomization list for such a method can be generated using table 5.2 as follows:

For $p = 3/5$ assign the treatment with least patients for digits 0–5 ⎫
the treatment with most patients for digits 6–9 ⎬
When treatment numbers are equal assign A for digits 0–4 ⎫
B for digits 5–9 ⎬

Hence, numbers 0 5 2 7 8 4 3 7 4 1 6 8 3 8 5 1 5 6 9 6 etc.
produce the list A B A A A B B A B B B B A B A A B B B B
       ↑ ↑   ↑   ↑

↑ indicates those points where treatment numbers were equal and simple randomization was used.

One possible extension would be to use simple randomization as long as the difference in treatment numbers remains below some prespecified limit but introduce the biassed coin method to correct imbalances beyond that limit. For instance, with a trial of size 100 patients one could set a limit of 6 (say) beyond which the treatment with least patients is assigned with probability $p = 2/3$. With three or more treatments the biassed coin method becomes a little more complex to follow and Pocock (1979) provides further details.

Other authors have produced further, more elaborate methods for restricted randomization with suitable theoretical justification. However, I feel that one should try and keep a basically simple approach as illustrated above.

5.3 STRATIFIED RANDOMIZATION

In this section, I will describe two main methods of stratified randomization, *random permuted blocks within strata* and *minimization*, but wish to begin by considering the basic rationale behind stratification.

In any randomized trial it is desirable that the treatment groups should be similar as regards certain relevant patient characteristics. For instance, in a breast cancer trial, such as in section 1.3, it would be unfortunate if the proportion of premenopausal patients was very different between treatments. Firstly, it would cast doubt on whether the randomization had been correctly performed. Also, it would affect the credibility of any treatment comparisons: although there exist methods of statistical analysis to allow for such lack of comparability (see section 14.1), readers are more likely to be convinced when valid conclusions can be achieved from a simple presentation of results for comparable treatment groups. Lastly, there would be some loss of statistical efficiency no matter what methods of analysis are used.

The larger a trial becomes the less likelihood there is of any serious non-comparability of treatment groups and this property has led some authors, e.g. Peto *et al.* (1976) and British Medical Journal (1977), to suggest that stratification is an unnecessary elaboration of randomization. I have some sympathy with this attitude to the extent that I would consider *three main reasons for not using stratification* and sticking to the unstratified methods in section 5.2:

(1) If the trial is very large, say several hundred patients, and interim analysis of early results is either not feasible or of minor interest, then stratification has little point.
(2) If the organizational resources for supervising randomization are somewhat limited then the increased complexity of stratification may carry a certain risk of errors creeping in, so that simpler methods may prove more reliable.
(3) If there is uncertainty about which patient characteristics might influence response to treatment, or the relevant information is not easily or reliably obtained, then one clearly has inadequate knowledge on which to carry out stratification. For instance, in a multi-centre trial for non-Hodgkins lymphoma the pathological diagnosis is of major significance but cannot be reliably confirmed until histological specimens have been evaluated by a central pathologist, by which time the patient will have already been randomized.

However, there remain many clinical trials which are not very large, which are well organized and for which there are patient factors well known to influence response. In these circumstances stratification based on such patient factors would seem worthwhile. Of course, even if randomization makes no allowance for such patient factors one will usually be fortunate enough to get a well-balanced trial. Thus, stratified randomization is rather like an insurance policy in that its primary aim is to guard against the unlikely event of the treatment groups ending up with some major difference in patient characteristics.

The first issue is to *decide which patient factors one should stratify by*. This is best achieved by studying the outcome of previous patients, preferably in earlier trials. For instance, Stanley (1980) carried out an extensive study of prognostic factors for survival in patients with inoperable lung cancer based on 50 such factors recorded for over 5000 patients in seven trials for the Veterans Administration Lung Group. He showed that performance status, a simple assessment of the patient's ability to get around, was the best indicator of survival. Weight loss in the last six months and extent of disease (confined to one hemithorax or not) also affected survival. Hence, one could say with confidence that these would be the three factors to account for in any future randomization. In my experience trial organizers will often propose factors for stratification which although of clinical and technical interest (e.g. histology in this example) may be of little relevance to patient outcome, whereas one or two simple observations on the patient's current and previous physical status (e.g. performance status and weight loss) may be much more relevant.

In most situations evidence about which are the relevant patient factors will be less rigorously determined. However, I feel one should be quite convinced about a factor's potential for making an impact on outcome before it is included in stratification. If investigators have only a vague idea about which factors may affect the outcome, then they may be wise to proceed with unstratified randomization.

Random Permuted Blocks within Strata

In my description of this most common form of stratification I will begin by returning to the breast cancer example of section 1.3. There were two patient factors considered to be of major prognostic importance in primary breast cancer: nodal status (i.e. the number of positive axillary nodes) and age. As regards the former, one expects a poorer prognosis for patients with a larger number of positive nodes. The importance of age is not only that older patients tend to have shorter survival, a fact not directly due to disease, but that the potential benefits of adjuvant chemotherapy such as L-Pam may depend on the patient's age.

After choosing the relevant patient factors, the next step is to categorize each one into two or more levels. Accordingly age was split into under or over 50 while nodal status was split into 1–3 or ≥ 4 positive nodes. The choice of split is inevitably somewhat arbitrary but should take into account the numbers of patients likely to be in each category. Also, in this case age 50 provides an approximate division into pre- and postmenopausal.

The purpose of categorizing each factor is to end up with several patient types or *strata*. In this case the four ($=2 \times 2$) strata are:

$$\text{age} < 50 \text{ and } 1\text{--}3 +\text{ve nodes}$$
$$\text{age} \geq 50 \text{ and } 1\text{--}3 +\text{ve nodes}$$
$$\text{age} < 50 \text{ and } \geq 4 +\text{ve nodes}$$
$$\text{age} \geq 50 \text{ and } \geq 4 +\text{ve nodes.}$$

Then before the trial begins *a separate restricted randomization list is prepared for each of the patient strata* using the methods described in section 5.2, random permuted blocks being the usual approach. Generally one adopts a relatively small block size when several strata are involved, the rationale being that stratified randomization needs to be more tightly restricted to be effective while the chances of any investigator predicting the last assignment in any block is considerably reduced given the greater complexity.

Hence, in this example blocks of 4 could be used in which case the method already described in section 5.2 produces four entirely separate randomization lists (one for each stratum) as shown in table 5.5. If there is no chance of investigators predicting treatment assignments (e.g. if there are many strata, the trial is multi-centre and/or double-blind) then one could restrict further and use blocks of two rather than four.

In practice, as each patient enters the clinical trial the process is as previously described in section 5.1 except that one has to identify which stratum that patient is in and obtain the next random treatment assignment from the corresponding randomization list.

The above example includes two patient factors each at two levels (hence four

Table 5.5. An example of random permuted blocks within strata for a
trial in primary breast cancer (A = L-Pam, B = placebo)

Age:	<50	≥50	<50	≥50
No. of positive axillary nodes:	1–3	1–3	≥4	≥4
	B	B	A	B
	A	B	A	A
	B	A	B	A
	A	A	B	B
	A	A	B	A
	B	A	A	B
	A	B	B	B
	B	B	A	A
	A	B	B	B
	B	A	A	B
	B	A	B	A
	A	B	A	A
	B	A	B	A
	B	B	A	B
	A	B	A	A
	A	A	B	B
	⋮	⋮	⋮	⋮

strata) and in a great many trials there will be no need to have more strata than
this. Indeed, it will often suffice to have just one major patient factor for
stratified randomization. However, there are situations where it may be
considered important to stratify by more than two factors. For instance, in a
clinical trial comparing two forms of chemotherapy in advanced breast cancer it
was decided that randomization should be stratified according to four patient
factors:

> performance status (ambulatory or non-ambulatory)
> age (<50 or ≥50)
> disease-free interval (<2 years or ≥2 years)
> dominant metastatic lesion (visceral, osseous or soft tissue)

This means that there were $2 \times 2 \times 2 \times 3 = 24$ different strata each requiring
a separate randomization list. Evidently, this extends the pre-trial documentation and also increases the amount of information required each time a
patient is registered in the trial so that one should really consider whether this
extra burden is justified, particularly if one has doubts about the efficiency of
the trial organization. In this case, all four factors were well known to influence
prognosis and the trial was well organized through a central registration office.

However, another problem is whether random permuted blocks for so many
strata will achieve the desired end of getting comparable treatment groups. For

example, table 5.6 shows how the first 80 patients were actually distributed across the 24 strata. One stratum has 13 patients while there are seven strata still empty and five with only one patient. Such an uneven distribution across strata is quite typical of clinical trials and may possibly result in substantial imbalance. For instance, here there are 12 strata with an odd number of patients so that even with blocks of two within each stratum one could have a difference in treatment numbers as large as 34:46. Furthermore, the percentage of non-ambulatory patients on the two treatments could differ by as much as 17%: 31%. This example illustrates that over-stratification can be self-defeating since a large number of strata with incomplete randomized blocks can lead to substantial imbalance between treatment groups.

Table 5.6. Distribution of patients across strata in an advanced breast cancer trial

Performance status:	Ambulatory				Non-ambulatory			
Age:	<50		$\geqslant 50$		<50		$\geqslant 50$	
Disease-free interval (years):	<2	$\geqslant 2$	<2	$\geqslant 2$	<2	$\geqslant 2$	<2	$\geqslant 2$
Dominant metastatic lesion:								
Visceral	13	1	9	5	3	1	7	1
Osseous	6	0	4	0	0	0	4	1
Soft tissue	8	1	7	7	2	0	0	0

This *problem of overstratification* is particularly evident in small clinical trials but at the same time the chance of serious imbalance is greater in small trials without stratification. Hence one may need an alternative approach as follows.

The Minimization Method

The rationale behind 'random permuted blocks within strata' is to aim at approximate equality of treatment numbers for every type of patient. However, as the number of strata (or types) increases this becomes rather irrelevant: for instance, no one is especially interested in ambulatory patients aged less than 50 with visceral metastases and disease-free interval over two years since this is a very small subgroup of patients with advanced breast cancer. In reality, one is more interested in ensuring that the different treatment groups are similar as regards the percentage ambulatory, percentage under age 50, etc., and the 'minimization' method attempts to achieve this in a more direct manner than does random permuted blocks within strata. In statistical jargon, the purpose is to balance the marginal treatment totals for each level of each patient factor.

The method is best described with the aid of an example. Consider the situation reached in the advanced breast cancer trial after 80 patients have already entered and the next patient is ready to receive treatment assignment.

Table 5.7 shows the numbers of patients on each of the two treatments, A and B, according to each of the four patient factors. Thus, each one of the 80 patients appears four times in this table, once for each factor. Suppose the next patient is ambulatory, age < 50, has disease-free interval ≥ 2 years and visceral metastasis (as indicated by the arrows in table 5.7). Then for each treatment one adds together the number of patients in the corresponding four rows of the table.

Thus, for A this sum $= 30 + 18 + 9 + 19 = 76$
while for B this sum $= 31 + 17 + 8 + 21 = 77$

Table 5.7. Treatment assignments by the four patient factors for 80 patients in an advanced breast cancer trial

Factor	Level	No. on each treatment		Next patient
		A	B	
Performance status	Ambulatory	30	31	←
	Non-ambulatory	10	9	
Age	< 50	18	17	←
	≥ 50	22	23	
Disease-free interval	< 2 years	31	32	
	≥ 2 years	9	8	←
Dominant metastatic lesion	Visceral	19	21	←
	Osseous	8	7	
	Soft tissue	13	12	

In its simplest form, minimization requires one to give the treatment with the smallest such sum of marginal totals to the next patient. In this case, the 81st patient is therefore assigned to treatment A. If the sums for A and B were equal then one would use simple randomization to assign the treatment.

Having explained the principle behind minimization I will now consider some of the practical details for its actual implementation. Unlike the other methods of treatment assignment one does not simply prepare a randomization list in advance. Instead one needs to keep continually an up-to-date record of treatment assignments by patient factors such as is shown in table 5.7. Such information might best be recorded on a set of index cards, one for each level of each factor. In our example, this would require $2 + 2 + 2 + 3 = 9$ cards. As each patient enters the trial one would need to pull out the four relevant cards to produce the treatment sums as above, make the treatment assignment and then add one onto that treatment's number on each of the four cards. This small amount of clerical effort and addition required for each assignment is not a problem and even if randomization is by telephone to a central registration office the assignment should be accomplished within a minute while the investigator is on the phone.

One possible problem with minimization as described so far is that treatment assignment is determined solely by the arrangement to date of previous patients and involves no random process except when the treatment sums are equal. This may not be a serious deficiency since investigators are unlikely to keep track of past assignments and hence advance predictions of a next assignment should prove infeasible. Furthermore, the claim that lack of true randomization makes standard statistical analysis inappropriate has no foundation in practice. Nevertheless, it may be useful to introduce an element of chance into minimization by assigning the treatment of choice (i.e. that with the smallest sum of marginal totals) with probability $p < 1$. $p = 3/4$ or $2/3$ might be a suitable choice. This random element is perhaps more important in single-institution trials where investigator prediction is more likely than in multi-centre trials.

Hence, before the trial starts one could prepare two randomization lists. The first is a simple randomization list where A and B occur equally often (as described in section 5.2) for use only when the two treatments have equal sums of marginal totals, e.g. A B B A B B A B A A B A A B etc. The second is a list in which the treatment with smaller sum of marginal totals (call it S) occurs with probability $3/4$ while the other treatment (L, say) occurs with probability $1/4$. Using table 5.2 this is prepared by assigning S for digits 1 to 6, L for digits 7 or 8 and ignoring 9 and 0; e.g. S S L S S S S S L S L S etc. In a larger trial this second list could be used initially, say for the first 50 patients, and then S could be assigned automatically thereafter once advance prediction by investigators clearly becomes impossible. Note that the very first patient is assigned by simple randomization. The extension of minimization to trials with more than two treatments should be obvious and presents no real difficulty.

Further details of minimization can be found in White and Freedman (1978) and Miller et al. (1980) with more theoretical background in Pocock and Simon (1975) and Freedman and White (1976). Begg and Iglewicz (1980) have proposed an alternative method which, though more complicated, provides even better balance between treatments. These more complex approaches become more feasible if one uses a computer to assist in patient registration and randomization (as is done by the Northern California Oncology Group) but this is beyond the resources of most trials. In general minimization is of greatest value in relatively small trials (say with < 100 patients) where several patient factors are known to be of prognostic importance, though it may still be of use in larger trials provided the administrative effort does not over tax the available resources.

Balancing for Institution

In multi-centre trials, one must consider whether the institution entering a patient should also be a factor worth including in stratification. Different institutions can show very different response rates for their patients for reasons of patient selection and experimental environment already mentioned in chapter

4. Also, it seems desirable that each institution should have a fair opportunity to try all treatments.

If there are no other factors in stratification then such balancing for institutions can simply be achieved by having a separate randomization list for each institution using some form of restricted randomization, e.g. random permuted blocks. However, if there are other stratifying factors as well as institution then use of random permuted blocks within strata can sometimes lead to a ridiculous situation. For instance, if there were ten institutions in the above advanced breast cancer this would increase the number of strata from 24 to $24 \times 10 = 240$. Indeed, I have come across one trial with more strata than patients!

Zelen (1974) has proposed a way round this problem as follows. One uses random permuted blocks within strata to balance for patient factors other than institution, so that as each patient enters the trial a provisional assignment is made. One then checks if the institution entering this patient would then have its range of treatment totals increased beyond some prespecified value d ($d = 3$ might be suitable). If so, one replaces this provisional assignment by the next acceptable one down the list for the patient's stratum. The rejected assignment is used later for the next suitable patient in that stratum. One possible problem could be a certain predictability of assignments within institution but this could be overcome by only using such replacement with some prespecified probability (say 2/3).

If the minimization method is employed then it is a simple matter to include institution as another patient factor to be used in the same way as the others.

In this section, I have tried to present both the pitfalls and advantages of stratification. Although stratification is theoretically efficient, the practical circumstances must dictate whether its use is desirable in any specific trial. A recent survey by Pocock and Lagakos (1982) has shown that in multi-centre trials for cancer both in Europe and America most groups do use stratification whereas in my experience most trials run by the pharmaceutical industry tend not to. Further useful discussion on stratification has been made by Simon (1979) and Brown (1980).

5.4 UNEQUAL RANDOMIZATION

In a clinical trial with two treatments it is standard practice to randomize roughly equal numbers of patients to each treatment and the methods of sections 5.2–5.3 have been based on this premise. Equal-sized treatment groups provide the most efficient means of treatment comparison for any form of response. Although such comparison is the essence of randomized trials, it is not the only purpose. If the trial is comparing a new treatment against a standard, one is also interested in gaining greater experience and insight into the new treatment's general profile whereas such background information is often well known for any standard treatment. Also the trial is usually motivated by some enthusiasm for the new therapy. These influences make it worth considering whether one should put more than half the patients on the new treatment, even though it would involve some loss of statistical efficiency. Peto (1978) has argued that the benefits of such unequal randomization might be especially useful in randomized phase II trials which are often quite small and generally have no prior information on efficacy for a new treatment.

I will now demonstrate the statistical consequences of unequal randomization. One commonly assesses the evidence for a treatment difference by using statistical significance tests and the 5% level of significance (i.e. $P < 0.05$) is widely regarded as a useful indication. Then, as is described more fully in chapter 9, one standard approach to determining the required size of a trial is as follows. One calculates how many patients are needed such that a certain prespecified true underlying treatment difference would be detected as significant at the 5% level with some high degree of assurance, say with probability 0.95. This latter probability is called the *power* of the trial.

Now, the question is what happens to this power to detect a certain treatment difference as significant at the 5% level if one decides to put a greater proportion on the new treatment. Figure 5.1 shows that, if the overall size of trial is kept constant, this power decreases relatively slowly as one begins to move away from equal sized groups. For instance, the power decreases from 0.95 to 0.925 if one has 2/3 patients on the new treatment. However, the loss of power becomes more marked as one reaches grosser inequalities in size. For instance, power is down to 0.82 if one has 4/5 patients on the new treatment. More theoretical results and other examples are given by Pocock (1979).

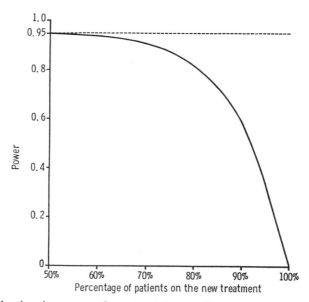

Fig. 5.1. Reduction in power of a trial as the proportion on the new treatment is increased

Thus *randomization in a 2:1 or 3:2 ratio for new:standard treatment is a realistic proposition* but a randomization ratio of 3:1 or more extreme may be undesirable in view of the considerable loss of statistical power. Setting up such an unequal randomization list involves a simple adaptation of the various methods in sections 5.2–5.3 so details will not be given here.

Unequal randomization is relatively uncommon but one or two examples may be useful. Epstein *et al.* (1981) describe a trial comparing D-penicillamine and placebo in the treatment of primary biliary cirrhosis. Since this was a relatively uncommon trial in a rare disease and a substantial proportion of patients on D-penicillamine had to withdraw due to side-effects, it was decided that the best use of resources could be achieved by randomizing a higher proportion of patients on the active drug. The trial accrued 32 patients on placebo versus 55 (including withdrawals) on D-penicillamine and produced evidence of substantial survival benefit on active therapy.

Starting in 1973, the Eastern Cooperative Oncology Group ran a trial of cyclophosphamide versus adriamycin in advanced lung cancer. Since adriamycin was the new treatment it was decided that it should be given to 2/3 patients. Also, there was some uncertainty about the best dosage so that half the adriamycin patients had a lower dose. In one sense, the end-result was three equal sized groups: cyclophosphamide, low-dose adriamycin and high-dose adriamycin. However, there remained the possibility of combining these two adriamycin groups if they produced similar results for a single overall comparison with cyclophosphamide.

Another example in advanced breast cancer emanates from the same organization. Adriamycin and vincristine was compared with the more standard three-drug regimen CMF. As a subsidiary question it was decided to add prednisone treatment for half the CMF patients so that the resultant three treatments were randomized in a ratio of 2:1:1. This illustrates that unequal randomization can also apply to trials with more than two treatments.

In conclusion, I consider *there is a reasonable case for more widespread use of unequal randomization* in clinical trials provided that the inequality is not so great as to seriously impair the statistical efficiency of treatment comparison.

CHAPTER 6

Blinding and Placebos

In any randomized trial the comparison of treatments may be distorted if the patient himself and those responsible for treatment and evaluation know which treatment is being used. This problem can sometimes be avoided by making the trial *double-blind*, whereby neither patient, physician nor evaluator is aware of which treatment the patient is receiving. The reasons for introducing blinding are discussed in section 6.1. In particular, the role of placebos for control patients not on active treatment is discussed. Section 6.2 describes how double-blind studies are actually carried out. It is often infeasible to conduct a double-blind trial so that in section 6.3 I consider some guidelines as to when blinding is practicable. The role of partially blinded studies (e.g. blinded evaluators only) is also discussed.

6.1 THE JUSTIFICATION FOR DOUBLE-BLIND TRIALS

In chapter 4 I emphasized the need for a randomized control group when evaluating a new therapy. One might think that the correct use of randomization guarantees an unbiassed clinical trial, but in fact there remain many possible sources of bias to be mentioned in this and subsequent chapters. Here we consider *the potential bias that can occur if everyone involved in a trial is aware of which treatment each patient is receiving.* In this respect there are three main participants to consider: the patient, the treatment team and the evaluator.

(1) *The patient*   If the patient knows he is receiving a new treatment this may be of psychological benefit. In contrast, the patient knowing he is on standard treatment (or no treatment if there is no effective standard) may react unfavourably especially if he is aware that other patients are 'privileged' to receive a new therapy. The reverse psychological effect could apply to some patients who feel more assured when on standard therapy. Such a patient's attitude towards his therapy may affect his cooperation in the study (e.g. compliance with intended therapy, attendance for evaluation) and may also influence how the patient responds.

The impact that full therapy information can make on patient response will depend on the type of disease and nature of the treatments. Clearly, in psychiatric illness such information could make a huge psychological difference to response: patients who knew they were receiving a new antidepressant drug could be expected to respond better than untreated controls, even if the drug was really ineffective. However, one should not underestimate the importance of psychology in other non-psychiatric diseases: whether it be asthma, cancer or heart disease the manner in which patients are informed of therapy can have a sizeable effect on subsequent performance.

(2) *The treatment team*   By the term 'treatment team' I mean everyone who participates in the treatment and management of the patient. The principal (and sometimes only) member of such a team is the patient's attending physician who can obviously affect the course of therapy in a number of ways. Decisions on dose modification, intensity of patient examination, continuance of trial therapy and need for other additional treatment are all his responsibility. How these decisions are made may be influenced by the physician's knowledge of a patient's treatment. For instance, if a patient is known to be receiving a new treatment, the physician may observe his progress more closely than the progress of others on standard therapy. Such differences in ancillary patient care, which nursing staff can also determine, may affect the eventual response. In addition, their enthusiasm for a new treatment may be conveyed to the patient and consequently affect patient attitude.

(3) *The evaluator*   The importance of a reliable evaluation of patient response was discussed in section 3.5. One key issue is to ensure that those responsible for assessing patient outcome are as objective as possible. In this respect, problems may arise if such evaluators are informed of each patient's treatment. There is potential danger that evaluators will err towards recording more favourable responses on the new treatment: after all, most trials are conducted in the hope that a new treatment will appear superior and it is only human nature to anticipate such superiority.

Assessment bias is particularly inviting if response evaluation requires clinical judgement. For instance, in psychiatric disease patient evaluation is usually based on a structured clinical interview so that there is enormous scope for knowledge of treatment to bias assessment no matter how hard the evaluator tries to remain objective. However, other apparently more objective measurements can also be influenced by knowledge of therapy. For instance, the recording of blood pressure can be affected by the evaluator's attitude to the patient and by his interpretation of what he hears. If a patient is on a new antihypertensive drug the evaluator may tend to anticipate and hence record readings lower than is really the case. Even with apparently 'hard' end-points such as myocardial infarction there is still a need for clinical judgement in the more borderline cases such that awareness of treatment could bias evaluators for or against diagnosing an infarct. Basically, knowledge of patient's therapy puts considerable pressure on the evaluator's ability to be objective. In any one trial evaluators may be successful in avoiding such bias, but for those interpreting results there will remain some doubt of this which can jeopardize a trial's credibility.

The above three aspects of bias will vary in their importance depending on the type of trial. For instance, bias is minimal if the treatments under comparison are quite similar to one another and patient evaluation is clear-cut (e.g. the effect of two cytotoxic drugs for advanced lung cancer on patient survival). At the other extreme are trials in which a new treatment is compared with an untreated control group. In this context lack of blindness, i.e. knowledge of who is being treated, can make a marked impact on patient, treatment team and evaluator. Use of placebos can then make a major difference.

The Value of Placebo Controls

In many diseases there exists no effective standard treatment so that it is appropriate for the control group in a randomized trial of new therapy to remain untreated. Also, even if alternative therapies do exist the early (phase II) trials of a new treatment may require short-term evaluation for the existence of some therapeutic effect by comparison with untreated controls. Now, one great danger in having control patients who are completely without treatment is that one cannot decipher whether any response improvement in the treated group is genuinely due to therapy or due to the act of being treated in some way. Even if therapy is irrelevant to the patient's condition the patient's attitude to his illness, and indeed the illness itself, may be improved by a feeling that something is being done about it.

This problem has been given particular emphasis in oral drug therapy. Gribbin (1981) argues that *many patients could be effectively treated by placebos*, inert and preferably attractive pills, especially if the doctor was persuasive as to their value. The argument applies most convincingly in minor psychiatric illness but can also extend to more physical ailments, e.g. hypertension.

The power of suggestion by a caring physician should not be underestimated in a whole variety of symptomatic conditions. For instance, British Medical Journal (1970) reports an appreciable reduction in frequency of angina attacks in untreated patients and also quotes examples of response on placebo for relief of postoperative pain and inhibition of cough reflex.

Hence, in any randomized trial of an oral drug versus untreated controls it is worth considering giving the latter a placebo. As a consequence one is able to eliminate the so-called 'placebo effect' from one's therapeutic comparison. The use of placebo controls has become commonplace in many diseases. For instance, trials in hypertension, rheumatoid arthritis, asthma or depression would virtually always include placebo rather than untreated control patients.

Note that it is an entirely separate issue to decide whether placebo or some standard active drug therapy should be a control. One basic principle is that patients cannot ethically be assigned to only a placebo if there exists an alternative standard therapy of established efficacy. The difficulty comes in deciding what constitutes 'established efficacy'. Ideally, one would like support- ive evidence from previous controlled trials but often a standard therapy has been around for so long without such formal testing. In such instances, one has to rely on clinical experience and opinion in deciding whether it is unethical to withhold what has become accepted as standard therapy. However, I suspect there exist some widely accepted therapies which would appear to lack efficacy if subjected to placebo-controlled trials, e.g. the UGDP trial mentioned in section 2.2.

Suppose a previous trial on the same type of patient has reported that a certain therapy improved response. Does this automatically mean that it is unethical to conduct a placebo-controlled trial hereafter? I think not, since there is a tendency for the medical literature to contain some 'false-positive' results, as discussed in section 15.2. Any single trial is on a limited number of patients, and is liable to encounter some methodological difficulties so that one would usually require replication in different circumstances before claims of 'established efficacy' can be justified.

The prime reason for introducing placebo controls is often to make patient attitudes to the trial as similar as possible in treatment and control groups. However, it can also give the opportunity to make the trial double-blind as defined below.

The Double-Blind Trial

The potential source of bias so far mentioned in this chapter can sometimes be eliminated by ensuring that *neither the patient nor those responsible for his care and evaluation know which treatment he is receiving.* This is called a double-blind trial, perhaps a slightly misleading term since in fact there are three types of blinded participants: patients, the treatment team and evaluators. But often the same clinicians handle both therapy and patient evaluation in which case double-blind refers quite accurately to patient and clinician.

The importance and feasibility of making a trial double-blind depends on the disease, the type of therapy, method of evaluation and available resources. We return to these issues and the possibility of partial blinding in section 6.3. First, let us consider the practical aspects of how to run a double-blind trial.

6.2 THE CONDUCT OF DOUBLE-BLIND TRIALS

The great majority of double-blind trials are for oral drug therapy and most of these have one treatment group compared with a control group on oral placebo. Though 'double-blind' is not synonymous with 'oral placebos' it makes sense to deal first with this large subgroup of double-blind trials.

Matched Placebos

One first needs to arrange the manufacture of an oral placebo which is identical in all respects to the active oral drug except that the active ingredient is absent. Particular features requiring matching are the colour, taste, texture, shape and size of placebo and pharmaceutical skills have enabled 'perfect' placebos to exist for a wide range of active drugs. One needs to decide on the mode of oral therapy: capsule, liquid or tablet. Since many active drugs have a distinctive taste which is hard to match, the use of capsules is often the most feasible. Even if a perfect match is not achieved the double-blind procedure may still be worthwhile. For instance, differences in taste are often not as readily identified as one might think. One example concerns medical students whom we randomized to alcohol, barbiturate or placebo as a teaching exercise. All three liquid treatments were flavoured with lime juice, orange squash and chalk but to us teachers the distinctive taste of alcohol (vodka) seemed to remain. Nevertheless many students failed initially to identify their 'treatment' though subsequent side-effects made their classification easier!

Coding and Randomization

The aspect of double-blind trials requiring most careful organization is the allocation of treatments. Standard procedure is for a randomization list to be prepared first as described in chapter 5. To preserve blinding it is then important that this list should not be shown to the therapists or evaluators. Thus the randomization list must be prepared by someone else, perhaps a statistician. The list is then needed by the pharmacist, either at the drug company or in the hospital, so that he may make up identical drug 'packages' containing either active drug or placebo for each patient.

If the pharmacist is readily accessible, say in the same hospital, then each time a patient enters the trial the investigator contacts the pharmacist to have the next unidentifiable drug package on the randomization list sent up. If the pharmacist is less accessible then a whole batch of unidentifiable assigned treatments may be sent in advance to the investigator, so that the next assignment is available immediately the patient is entered. The latter approach will usually be required for trials in general practice.

In either case it is essential to have a simple coding system linking the drug packages to the randomization list. Each package must have a unique trial *code number* which is also written on the randomization list. The code number is then clearly noted on the patient's trial forms. Usually the code numbers can simply correspond to the order of patients entering the trial, though a slightly more elaborate code may be needed for stratified randomization or multi-centre trials.

Breaking the Code

Before analysing the trial results one needs to 'break the code' and identify which treatment each patient was on. However, rather than waiting until analysis, it may be more reliable for the pharmacist and/or data centre to keep an up-to-date log sheet of randomized treatment assignments with patients identified. Remember it is essential that other trial participants remain unaware of such a list. Perhaps it is obvious to state that one should be careful to ensure that one breaks the code correctly. Nevertheless, I recall with embarrassment one occasion when I mistakenly showed a highly effective placebo in an initial analysis with the treatments the wrong way round.

One must also decide whether the interpretation of trial results should also be undertaken blind initially, in the sense that treatments be unidentified. This applies particularly to interim analyses while a trial is still in progress, where decisions on the trial's future are to be made by a monitoring committee. Friedman *et al.* (1981) refer to this as a 'triple-blind' study. The advantage is that it enables more objective interpretation of response data whereby the uncertainty over which treatment is which prevents individual opinion and prejudice affecting a committee's judgement. For instance, Cochrane (1972) reports an occasion where the treatment names were deliberately reversed in the first interim analysis of a trial comparing home and hospital care after myocardial infarction. One enthusiast for coronary care units declared that the trial was unethical and should be stopped since hospital care appeared to have a slightly lower mortality. However, once the treatments were correctly ordered 'he could not be persuaded to declare coronary care units unethical'. The issue of confidentiality of interim results is discussed further in section 10.2.

One particular advantage of double-blind studies is that they allow *more objective evaluation of side-effects*, both by the patient and his physician. For instance, one invariably gets side-effects reported by some patients on placebo (usually minor features such as headache, fatigue, nausea). This enables one to correct for the over-reporting of side-effects on active therapy and get an unbiassed estimate of adverse reactions attributable to the treatment itself.

On the other hand, if the clinician feels that the blinded treatment is harmful to the patient either because of side-effects or clear failure to respond then *he must be allowed to break the code for that particular patient* if he so wishes. This clinical freedom is ethically important in order that full information be available for planning future therapy for that patient. For such circumstances, one needs effective communication between the clinician and the pharmacist (or data centre) so that the code may be broken as soon as possible. Indeed, it may sometimes be necessary for each clinician to have on hand some means of immediately identifying each patient's treatment, say in a sealed envelope. However, one wants to ensure that investigators' code-breaking for individual patients is kept to a minimum justified on ethical grounds otherwise the reason for blinding, avoidance of biassed evaluation, may be jeopardised.

If a drug frequently gives rise to side-effects then the attending physicians may be able to guess which treatment many patients are on without needing formally to break the code. For instance, the drug L-Pam in the double-blind breast cancer trial described in section 1.3 tended to produce lowered white cell and platelet counts and also some nausea and vomiting. Clearly, such adverse reactions, rather unlikely to occur on placebo, give the physician a strong indication that L-Pam is being given, so that blinding will not be maintained in some patients. However, it was still considered worthwhile to start off each patient in a double-blind manner since one is consequently liable to get a closer consistency of therapeutic care and evaluation in both treatment and control groups.

When the whole trial is completed and results interpreted it is then desirable that investigators be informed of each patient's treatment, both for patient records and to aid each investigator's experience and understanding of the treatments.

Other Types of Double-blind Study

So far I have concentrated on trials of oral drug therapy versus matched oral placebos. However, one can sometimes make double-blind a trial comparing two active drugs by arranging for both to be in an identical form, except for differing active ingredients.

The situation becomes more complex if the two drugs have different dose schedules. For instance, an antihypertensive trial was conducted double-blind to evaluate once-daily (slow release) versus twice-daily oral beta-blocker. Each patient was given two bottles of tablets, marked A and B, and instructed to take one tablet from bottle A each morning and one tablet from bottle B each evening. The bottles actually contained the following:

Once-daily treatment	Twice-daily treatment
A = slow-release tablet (200 mg)	A = conventional tablet (100 mg)
B = placebo	B = conventional tablet (100 mg)

All three tablets were identical except for active ingredient. Patients were randomized to one or other combination of A and B, and the trial was successfully carried out double-blind.

Sometimes two active drugs cannot be matched satisfactorily in which case one can produce two different matched placebos, one for each drug. Then patients may be randomized to receive drug A + placebo B or drug B + placebo A. Blinding can then be preserved though at the expense of involving more 'pill taking' which could possibly affect patient compliance.

It is occasionally possible to run even more complex double-blind trials. For instance, Willey et al. (1976) report a crossover trial involving ten different dose schedules of two oral drugs, pirbuterol and salbutamol, for asthma. To preserve blinding each patient was required to take four green capsules on each day's therapy, the ten different schedules being as follows:

4 placebo capsules	3 placebo + 1 pirbuterol (5 mg)
3 placebo + 1 salbutamol (2 mg)	3 placebo + 1 pirbuterol (7.5 mg)
2 placebo + 2 salbutamol (2 mg each)	2 placebo + 2 pirbuterol (5 mg each)
1 placebo + 3 salbutamol (2 mg each)	1 placebo + 3 pirbuterol (5 mg each)
4 salbutamol (2 mg each)	4 pirbuterol (5 mg each)

All capsules were identical except for active ingredients so that the trial was double-blind. Four capsules were required since capsules containing more than 2 mg salbutamol or 7.5 mg pributerol were not available. Other aspects of this trial's design are described in section 8.3. Evidently, this degree of complexity requires very careful organization and a high degree of patient cooperation which is most likely to occur in such short-term phase II studies.

The use of placebos for trials of therapy other than oral drugs is much less common. Placebo injections present a greater practical and ethical problem but can be used in some circumstances. For instance, Hjalmarson *et al.* (1981) in a trial of metoprolol for myocardial infarction patients gave control patients placebo (saline) injections followed by oral placebo tablets so that their course of inert treatment was comparable to the metoprolol group.

Double-blind trials in other modes of therapy (e.g. surgery) are extremely rare if not impossible. Johnstone *et al.* (1980) report an unusual example concerning electroconvulsive therapy (ECT). Seventy depressed patients were randomly assigned to receive real ECT or simulated ECT. To preserve blindness, each control patient was given the same anaesthetic and handled in an identical manner except that no electricity was passed. Treatment allocation was known only to the psychiatrist administering ECT and the anaesthetist. Neither the doctors involved in patient care or assessment, nor the patients themselves, knew the assigned treatment. The trial showed strong evidence that ECT was beneficial, a result that could not have been reliably demonstrated without the double-blind procedure.

6.3 WHEN IS BLINDING FEASIBLE?

I wish to begin this section by drawing a clear distinction between blinding and randomization. Many randomized controlled trials have been successfully conducted without blinding and hence the argument over randomized versus non-randomized studies (see chapter 4) is a separate (possibly more important) issue not directly related to blinding. However, the use of blinding techniques is largely confined to randomized trials.

The individual circumstances of each clinical trial make it impossible to give any general rule on blindness (yes or no) which could be applied to all trials. Instead, one's decision for each trial requires careful consideration of the following aspects:

(1) *Ethics*   The double-blind procedure should not result in any harm or undue risk to a patient.
(2) *Practicality*   For some treatments it would be totally impossible to arrange a double-blind trial.
(3) *Avoidance of bias*   One needs to assess just how serious the bias might be without blinding.
(4) *Compromise*   Sometimes partial blinding (e.g. independent blinded evaluators) can be sufficient to reduce bias in treatment comparison.

Ethical problems can often immediately rule out a double-blind trial. For instance, in surgical trials it would clearly be unethical to subject a control group to an incision under anaesthetic to mimic genuine surgery. Van der Linden (1980) suggests that lack of blindness in surgical trials means that we will usually have to restrict our interest to objectively measurable results. Other modes of treatment may require more careful ethical considerations. For instance, use of placebo injections has been possible (an example was given in section 6.2) but they may be ethically unacceptable if frequent repeat injections are required. Hill (1963) points out that the Medical Research Council's trial of streptomycin for tuberculosis (already mentioned in section 2.1) could not be made double-blind for this reason so that the control group received bed-rest alone.

The double-blind approach is only practicable when comparing treatments of a similar nature. Suitable use of placebos can sometimes contrive to achieve such similarity but this is not always ethical or practicable. For instance, cancer trials of cytotoxic drugs are usually not double-blind, though section 1.3 describes an exception. Reasons are that complicated dose schedules, the likelihood of serious side-effects and dose modifications to suit each patient all make it necessary for the treating physician to know a patient's therapy.

For other less-toxic therapies the double-blind technique may also require unduly rigid adherence to fixed dose schedules (see Ritter, 1980). Such lack of flexibility may mean that therapy cannot be adjusted finely enough to suit each patient's needs. However, many treatments have fixed schedules anyway so that this will often not be a problem.

Another ethical argument against double-blind trials is that 'the patient is being deceived' (see Lancet, 1979a). The whole issue of informed patient consent is discussed in section 7.2, though I should mention here that such ethical debate becomes particularly important in placebo-controlled double-blind trials. Essentially, if the patient is informed of the trial's nature, including the possibility of his receiving a placebo, and there is no clear evidence that placebo is inferior, then it should be ethical to continue. The Lancet (1979a) goes on to suggest that 'mutual trust between doctor and patient is maintained by a trial being double blind. Both are in the same boat of ignorance and this ... brings otherwise inherently unequal parties into a joint adventure or partnership.' Perhaps the truth lies somewhere between this view and the alternative of 'planned deception'.

One obvious practical point is that *double-blind trials require considerable time and effort to ensure they work properly*. Indeed, blinding may adversely affect participation by some investigators in an otherwise acceptable trial, their reason being inconvenience rather than ethical concern. Therefore, such practical problems need to be set against the benefits of blinding.

In studies without blinding, the manner in which bias can materialize has already been discussed in section 6.1. Briefly, it depends on the extent to which treatments differ in nature, the liability of patients and their clinicians to influence the course of disease by attitude and suggestion and the degree of subjectivity in evaluation. For each trial one must try to assess where the main sources of potential bias arise and how important they will be. In some cases, a trial needs to be double-blind since all the above factors could affect response, e.g. depression, hypertension. However, one can sometimes isolate the main source of bias and eliminate it by partial blinding. One approach is the *single-blind study*, where only the patient is not informed of his treatment. This will be of particular use in trials where the patients evaluate their own response (e.g., pain relief studies). One then has to guard carefully against clinical influence of the patient, and suitable training of investigators to avoid suggestion may help. The problem here is that, even if such influences are avoided, the trial's credibility could still be questioned since one cannot prove that clinical bias was absent. Thus, a study may need to be double-blind in order to convince others that its findings are reputable.

Sometimes it is most important to ensure *blinded evaluation*, even if the patient and his treating clinician know the treatment. For instance, the Medical Research Council (1948) in the trial of streptomycin for tuberculosis had X-ray evaluation by two independent observers who were unaware of each patient's therapy. Hill (1963) expresses the belief that blinded evaluation was sufficient in this instance. He goes on to say that 'in a controlled trial, as in all experimental work there is no need in the search for precision to throw common sense out of the window'.

Blinded evaluation is not quite so straightforward if it requires the patient's presence for results to be assessed. For instance, the Diabetic Retinopathy Study Research Group (1976) required patients to be trained not to inform the evaluator which eye had been treated with photocoagulation so that visual tests were carried out in the same way on both eyes. The value of blinded evaluation, which is perhaps underutilized in some diseases, is also mentioned in section 3.5.

In summary, there is no single answer regarding the value of the double-blind technique in clinical trials. In some diseases (e.g. psychiatric disorders) it would otherwise be impossible to get objective evidence, whereas in other situations (e.g. surgery, radiotherapy) it is generally impossible to do a double-blind trial. Most other trials lie somewhere between these extremes and trial organizers must weigh up the pros and cons for themselves.

CHAPTER 7

Ethical Issues

Every clinical trial requires careful assessment of whether it is ethically acceptable for patients to participate in the proposed manner. Of paramount importance is the avoidance of unnecessary patient suffering, inconvenience or loss of freedom as a consequence of participation in a trial. However, can one carry out a scientifically designed and well-organized trial in order to clarify which treatment is most appropriate for future patients, while still looking after the best interests of each current patient in the trial? The balance between achieving medical progress and ensuring individual patient care is the essence of the ethical dilemma and forms the basis of section 7.1.

One particular ethical issue is whether each patient should be informed and his consent be sought for inclusion in a clinical trial and this is discussed in section 7.2. Ethical problems also relate to several aspects of trial conduct mentioned in other chapters (e.g. randomization in chapter 4, blinding and placebos in chapter 6, and interim analyses in chapter 10). Such specific comments should complement this chapter's more general discussion on ethics.

7.1 MEDICAL PROGRESS AND INDIVIDUAL PATIENT CARE

Guidelines and Ethical Committees

Ethical considerations should be of continuing concern throughout the design and conduct of a clinical trial. The general ethical requirements of clinical research world wide are outlined in the *Declaration of Helsinki* issued by the World Medical Association in 1960 and revised in 1975. This brief document has been accepted internationally as the basis for ethical research. The sections most relevant to clinical trials are as follows:

I. Basic Principles

1. Biomedical research involving human subjects must conform to generally accepted scientific principles and should be based on adequately performed laboratory and animal experimentation and on a thorough knowledge of the scientific literature.
2. The design and performance of each experimental procedure involving human subjects should be clearly formulated in an experimental protocol which should be

transmitted to a specially appointed independent committee for consideration, comment and guidance.

3. Biomedical research involving human subjects should be conducted only by scientifically qualified persons and under the supervision of a clinically competent medical person. The responsibility for the human subject must always rest with the medically qualified person and never rest on the subject of the research, even though the subject has given his or her consent.

4. Biomedical research involving human subjects cannot legitimately be carried out unless the importance of the objective is in proportion to the inherent risk to the subject.

5. Every biomedical research project involving human subjects should be preceded by careful assessment of predictable risks in comparison with foreseeable benefits to the subject or to others. Concern for the interests of the subject must always prevail over the interests of science and society.

6. The right of the research subject to safeguard his or her integrity must always be respected. Every precaution should be taken to respect the privacy of the subject and to minimize the impact of the study on the subject's physical and mental integrity and on the personality of the subject.

7. Doctors should abstain from engaging in research projects involving human subjects unless they are satisfied that the hazards involved are believed to be predictable. Doctors should cease any investigation if the hazards are found to outweigh the potential benefits.

8. In publication of the results of his or her research, the doctor is obliged to preserve the accuracy of the results. Reports of experimentation not in accordance with the principles laid down in this Declaration should not be accepted for publication.

9. In any research on human beings, each potential subject must be adequately informed of the aims, methods, anticipated benefits and potential hazards of the study and the discomfort it may entail. He or she should be informed that he or she is at liberty to abstain from participation in the study and that he or she is free to withdraw his or her consent to participation at any time. The doctor should then obtain the subject's freely-given informed consent, preferably in writing.

10. When obtaining informed consent for the research project the doctor should be particularly cautious if the subject is in a dependent relationship to him or her or may consent under duress. In that case the informed consent should be obtained by a doctor who is not engaged in the investigation and who is completely independent of this official relationship.

11. In case of legal incompetence, informed consent should be obtained from the legal guardian in accordance with national legislation. Where physical or mental incapacity makes it impossible to obtain informed consent, or when the subject is a minor, permission from the responsible relative replaces that of the subject in accordance with national legislation.

12. The research protocol should always contain a statement of the ethical considerations involved and should indicate that the principles enunciated in the present Declaration are complied with.

II. Medical Research Combined with Professional Care
(Clinical Research)

1. In the treatment of the sick person, the doctor must be free to use a new diagnostic and therapeutic measure, if in his or her judgement it offers hope of saving life, re-establishing health or alleviating suffering.

2. The potential benefits, hazards and discomfort of a new method should be weighed against the advantages of the best current diagnostic and therapeutic methods.

3. In any medical study, every patient—including those of a control group, if any—should be assured of the best proven diagnostic and therapeutic method.
4. The refusal of the patient to participate in a study must never interfere with the doctor–patient relationship.
5. If the doctor considers it essential not to obtain informed consent, the specific reasons for the proposal should be stated in the experimental protocol for transmission to the independent committee.
6. The doctor can combine medical research with professional care, the objective being the acquisition of new medical knowledge, only to the extent that medical research is justified by its potential diagnostic or therapeutic value for the patient.

Each country has to decide on its own approach to implementing such guidelines. For instance, in the United Kingdom a system of *local ethical committees* exists so that all clinical trials (and other types of clinical research project) need to have their protocol approved by such a committee beforehand. In multi-centre trials each separate collaborating institution must seek approval from its local ethical committee. These committees are made up of both clinicians and lay people. This has the advantage that proposals for clinical trials are subjected to broader social standards than might be achieved by the medical profession alone but has the problem that all the clinical implications and technicalities of each proposal may not be fully appreciated by committee members. Allen and Waters (1982) provide a useful discussion of one such committee's activities. In addition, any clinical trial of a new drug cannot proceed without permission from the Committee on Safety of Medicines. The British Medical Association (1980) provides guidelines on medical research involving human subjects in its *Handbook of Medical Ethics* and also the General Medical Council maintains a national overview of ethical matters.

The real difficulty is how to relate the Declaration of Helsinki and other ethical guidelines to the specifics of each clinical trial. Obvious unethical practices (e.g. withholding treatment from some patients when therapy of known efficacy exists) are easy to identify, but in general there is no simple, objective way in which one can decide whether a trial is ethical or not. Indeed, it is possible for different local ethical committees evaluating the same proposal for a multi-centre trial to disagree on its ethical acceptability. For instance, a proposed trial of multi-vitamin therapy for prevention of neural tube defects (previously mentioned in section 4.3) has met both approval and rejection from different ethical committees depending on whether prior evidence from poorly controlled trials was deemed sufficient to prohibit the use of control subjects not receiving multi-vitamins.

A society's attitude towards the medical profession and clinical research will largely determine what constitutes ethical research. For instance, national differences in approach to informed patient consent are particularly striking (see section 7.2). Although guidelines and ethical committees are a helpful safeguard against unethical practices, the main responsibility for ensuring a trial remains ethical rests with the trial organizers themselves. Furthermore, it is not only the trial's design as specified in the protocol that needs to be satisfactory but also the actual conduct of the trial as it affects each individual patient.

Hence, the maintenance of high ethical standards cannot be achieved by a purely administrative exercise based on the independent assessment of trial protocols. It is also up to each individual clinical investigator to ensure that his patients do not suffer as a result of clinical research.

High Scientific and Organizational Standards

One basic premise is that *it is unethical to conduct research which is badly planned or poorly executed.* That is, if a trial is of sufficiently poor quality that it cannot make a meaningful contribution to medical knowledge then it should be declared unethical. These statements reflect what I think is the major ethical failing of many clinical trials. It seems unreasonable that any patient should be subjected to the potential risks and inconvenience of experimentation in a clinical trial if that trial is either lacking scientific quality or efficient organization. However, I fear that this aspect of medical ethics goes largely unrecognized by the medical profession and society at large.

In considering this problem I wish to define three main outcomes that a trial should avoid:

(a) *Bias* If a trial's conclusions exaggerate the benefits of a new therapy, then the trial is clearly doing a disservice to medicine and to mankind. The avoidance of bias is a recurring theme throughout this book and I see it as an ethical as well as a scientific issue.

(b) *Too few patients* The inadequacy of small trials is referred to in section 9.3. If a trial has too few patients one cannot reach a reliable conclusion on treatment efficacy, in which case the whole trial is worthless and should not have taken place.

(c) *No published findings* It often happens that the results of a trial never get published in the medical literature, either because the investigators lost interest or the trial had serious deficiencies. Now, the whole purpose of a trial is to further medical knowledge. Hence, if findings do not get published the whole trial is pointless except perhaps as an experience for the investigator himself.

Of course, one cannot always anticipate these problems before a trial commences. If a trial unexpectedly runs into difficulties then it is perhaps reasonable to assume the investigators acted in good faith so that it would be unjust to attach the label 'unethical' to such a trial in retrospect. However, if the trial's inadequacies can be seen beforehand or become recognized while it is still in progress then I think there is a strong case for a trial being discontinued on ethical grounds. Also, I think an investigator's ignorance of the scientific and organizational needs for a clinical trial should not be seen as an excuse. It should be a moral obligation for investigators to acquire the appropriate knowledge or seek advice to ensure a trial of high quality. On a similar note, Altman (1980a) argues that the misuse of statistics in medical research is unethical.

This *strong connection between ethics and good science* suggests that the function of an ethical committee should not necessarily be confined to the ethics of what happens to each individual patient. Perhaps ethical committees should also assess the scientific merit of each trial. This would require that committees include more members with the skills to undertake such scientific evaluation. In this respect the Queen's University of Belfast is one ethical committee in the United Kingdom that has made notable efforts in combining ethical and scientific evaluation.

Poor organization in a clinical trial can have a more immediate deleterious effect on a particular patient. For instance, Brahams (1982) reports a case where a patient with rectal cancer receiving 5-FU and heparin in a controlled trial died after a failure to monitor the patient's blood in accordance with the trial protocol. The problem arose because a junior doctor had not been adequately informed of the trial protocol and the need to monitor blood samples for bone marrow toxicity. This unfortunate incident, more dramatic than most erroneous departures from protocol, illustrates the need for effective organization as previously mentioned in section 3.2.

Individual versus Collective Ethics

Lellouch and Schwartz (1971) introduced the idea that in any clinical trial there is competition between the ethics of individual benefit and the ethics of collective benefit. '*Individual ethics*' means that each patient should receive that treatment which is thought to be most beneficial for his condition. This is the clear aim of good clinical practice in which the patient and his doctor decide together on what is the best course of action. Usually, it is the clinician who is the individual determining therapy on the basis of his knowledge, experience and opinion with appropriate acknowledgement of the patient's wishes.

'*Collective ethics*' is concerned with achieving medical progress as efficiently as possible so that all patients may subsequently benefit from superior therapy. One could argue that collective ethics is aimed at future patients while individual ethics is about that patient who requires treatment now. Exclusive adherence to collective ethics is a totally unacceptable stance to adopt. It implies that clinical trials can be conducted in the same way as any other scientific experiment, the needs of each individual patient being abandoned in order to conduct that trial which best conforms to scientific and statistical principles. As pointed out by Lebacqz (1980), such an approach 'might permit the use of humans against their will, as happened in Nazi Germany. Such use is forbidden by the principle of respect for persons, which requires that we honor the free choice of a moral agent.'

In contrast, most people instinctively feel that we should pay exclusive attention to individual ethics. However, I feel if this were to be the case then properly designed clinical trials could no longer exist and there would be no constructive framework for meaningful progress in therapy. In particular, a total commitment to individual ethics would appear contradictory to the use of randomization (see section 4.4), blinding and placebos (see chapter 6).

For instance, consider a clinician whose next patient is ready for inclusion in a randomized trial with two treatments. It is quite likely that the clinician has a personal preference, say for treatment A, though this is not backed up by actual evidence of superiority. Suppose the first two patients' results are known: a good response on A and a poor response on B. Now, individual ethics would demand that the next patient be given treatment A. Evidence on two patients and clinical opinion are both favouring A so that the odds are slightly in favour of A being the better treatment. I would argue that such logic would be a recipe for chaos in clinical research and practice. Randomization would be untenable and there would be a tremendous risk that all kinds of ineffective therapies could become available after grossly inadequate testing (see chapter 4 for details).

Hence, individual ethics must be compromised to some extent since otherwise patients would be exposed to *ad hoc* therapy based on the whims of clinical opinion and insubstantive evidence. Thus, *each clinical trial requires a balance between individual ethics and collective ethics.* The prime motivation for conducting a trial is the latter: one wants to find out which therapy is better for future patients. One then has to give individual ethics as much attention as possible without destroying the trial's validity. Randomized double-blind trials do require that patients are not fully aware of their therapy, but in some conditions progress can only be achieved by such trials. Thus, ethical adjudication on any particular trial requires an assessment of whether the loss of individual freedom, which I see as being inevitable, is sufficiently serious to mean that the trial should not take place. Account should be taken of the trial's importance in resolving a therapeutic choice, prior knowledge and opinion regarding the therapies and the extent of each patient's risk, inconvenience and loss of freedom as a consequence of participation.

I feel that society as a whole and the laws on medical ethics have not fully appreciated the reality of clinical trials. For instance, in Germany it appeared for a while that randomized controlled trials would be declared illegal (see Burkhardt and Kienle, 1978), and there is continuing controversy on the ethics of clinical trials. I now wish to discuss the issue of informed patient consent where the ethical conflict becomes particularly marked.

7.2 INFORMED PATIENT CONSENT

The Declaration of Helsinki states that in clinical research 'the doctor should obtain the subject's freely-given informed consent, preferably in writing' but then goes on to declare that 'if the doctor considers it essential not to obtain informed consent, the specific reasons for this proposal should be stated in the experimental protocol . . .' These contradictory statements imply that while seeking informed consent is highly desirable there may be circumstances where it is best not to.

Different countries have adopted widely divergent attitudes to informed consent. In the United States it is a legal requirement to obtain written informed consent for every patient entering a clinical trial. This requires that the patient should be fully aware of his disease and the essentials of the trial protocol. In particular, the treatment options should be explained together with the fact that his therapy is to be determined by randomization. In general, consent is to be obtained prior to randomization though a possible alternative—the 'randomized consent design'—is discussed below.

In the United Kingdom the situation is not so clear-cut. While the British Medical Association recommends that consent to alternative therapies should be obtained from individual subjects, in practice the decision over whether informed consent be obtained is made by local ethical committees. In some trials consent is obtained in writing, in others it is verbal approval and in others consent is not sought at all. I think this diversity of approach in Britain is partly due to different clinical attitudes regarding whether patients in general should be informed of their disease. For instance, it remains a matter of some controversy whether telling a patient he has cancer is ethically desirable or 'not in the patient's best interests'. Nevertheless, a more consistent approach to informed consent would seem desirable.

In France it is customary not to obtain informed consent, particularly in cancer clinical trials. Again this reflects the pattern that patients are not usually told that they have cancer.

In the Federal Republic of Germany, the present ethical and legal debate makes it difficult to provide a clear picture. It is current practice that every trial protocol be examined by a lawyer who decides on the trial's legal and ethical status. One lawyer is said to have required that every patient be fully informed even to the extent that the trial's interim results so far (e.g. response rates on each treatment) be explained prior to consent. This is complete adherence to individual ethics (see section 7.1) and would destroy the viability of clinical trials since presumably many patients would choose that therapy which was currently ahead, no matter how non-significant the difference.

Hence, can one really expect international conformity on patient consent to be achieved? For instance, should all countries be encouraged to adopt the American approach that written informed consent is legally required? I am inclined to think not, since this would be an unrealistic and undesirable uniformity of practice. Also, such an approach is partly motivated by the need to protect doctors from subsequent litigation if trial therapy is not successful. While obviously seeking respect for human rights in all countries, I think one must accept that there are national differences as regards society's attitude to medical ethics. I suspect that by and large patients in Britain and France do not wish automatically to be informed of the full clinical implications of their disease. Certainly the medical profession in these countries tend to adopt such a view. This issue is discussed more fully by Kennedy (1981) in a wide-ranging critical appraisal of medical ethics in general.

Thus, any definite ruling on informed consent for all trials would be contrary to current medical practice. However, can one produce sensible guidelines which could help to determine which trials (and patients) should or should not have informed consent? Hill (1963) presents the following argument:

> The situation implicit in the controlled trial is that one has two (or more) possible treatments and that one is wholly, or to a very large extent, ignorant of their relative values (and dangers). Can you describe that situation to a patient so that he does not lose confidence in you—the essence of the doctor/patient relationship—and in such a way that he fully understands and can therefore give an *understanding* consent to his inclusion in the trial? In my opinion nothing less is of value. Just to ask the patient does he mind if you try some new tablets on him does nothing, I suggest, to meet the problem. That is merely paying lip-service to it. If the patient cannot really grasp the whole situation, or without upsetting his faith in your judgement cannot be made to grasp it, then in my opinion the ethical decision still lies with the doctor, whether or no it is proper to exhibit, or withhold, a treatment. He cannot divest himself of it simply by means of an illusory consent.

Similarly, Brewin (1982) reaches the following conclusion: 'The best policy—not perfect, but better than any alternative—is for a responsible caring doctor to be flexible, considerate, and discreet, never imposing unnecessary "informed consent", yet always ready to discuss anything with patients who wish it. Far from being patronising or arrogant, such a policy enhances the dignity of the patient as a unique individual, with changing moods and a changing ability to cope with fear, doubt and uncertainty. At the end of the day it shows more respect for him, or her, than any measure designed to standardize consent and treat everybody alike.'

For instance, consider a trial for acute myocardial infarction in which patients are to be randomized to beta-blocker or placebo as soon as possible after admission. The patient here is in acute distress and clearly cannot be expected to benefit from the full procedure of informed consent. An alternative approach is to seek consent from a close relative, though this may also present some practical difficulties.

At the other extreme, there are patients with chronic symptomatic conditions such as asthma and rheumatoid arthritis who are in a much better position to cope with and benefit from informed consent. Such patients are liable to have a good prior understanding of their disease and are in a suitable mental state to comprehend the nature of the clinical trial. Even so, patients' intellectual and social circumstances vary enormously, so that the manner and extent of explanation by a caring physician should depend somewhat on his perception of that patient's needs.

The situation becomes more difficult in cancer clinical trials. Is a full explanation of his disease and the trial liable to cause emotional distress in the patient? On the other hand, is it ethical to subject patients to highly toxic experimental therapies without their consent? I see no simple general solution to this problem, as long as cancer patients are not routinely informed of their true condition. Brahams (1982) emphasized the dilemma in a discussion of one patient's death from side-effects of drug therapy. Brahams argues that some 'halfway house' in consent procedure may be desirable and it is in this context that I introduce the randomized consent design below.

Another issue concerns the extent to which the alternative therapies in the trial differ from one another. If therapies are similar in nature (e.g. two drug regimes for hypertension), then patient consent is not of such great import. However, if therapies are radically different (e.g. surgical versus non-surgical therapy), then patient consent seems more desirable but is also more difficult to obtain. For example, the Danish Obesity Project (1979) did not seek patient consent in a trial of jejunoileal bypass versus medical treatment in morbid obesity. The consequent ethical controversy (*Lancet*, 1979b) emphasizes just how difficult it is to conduct such a trial. Again, the following compromise to consent may be of value in this context.

The Randomized Consent Design

It is conventional practice to seek patient consent immediately before randomization takes place, as already described in the sequence of events for patient registration in section 5.1. Such timing poses something of a dilemma in the doctor–patient relationship since

(a) the doctor has to reveal the state of ignorance which has led to a randomized trial and
(b) the patient is asked to agree to trial entry without knowing which treatment he will receive.

Zelen (1979) has proposed a new design for randomized trials which might make informed consent more practicable and acceptable to both patient and doctor. The principle of this design is best explained for the simplest trial comparing a new treatment B against a standard treatment A. Figure 7.1 illustrates the proposed sequence of events. Each eligible patient is randomly assigned to either

(1) a *do not seek consent group* (G_1) who all receive standard treatment A *or*
(2) a *seek consent group* (G_2) who are asked whether they are willing to receive the new treatment B. Some patients in G_2 may decline the offer of B, in which case they receive the standard treatment A. Evidently, such a design cannot be used in a double-blind trial.

The crux of this plan is that *the analysis of results must compare all patients in G_2 (including those on A) with all patients in G_1.* At first sight this might seem a little odd, but the logic is that one is comparing the policy of offering patients the opportunity of receiving treatment B with the policy of giving all patients treatment A. Any alternative analyses comparing patients receiving B against patients receiving A are likely to introduce bias, since patients who accept B may well differ from patients who refuse B. The successful implementation of such a 'randomized consent design' depends on the percentage of patients in the seek consent group who accept the new treatment being close to 100%. A loss of

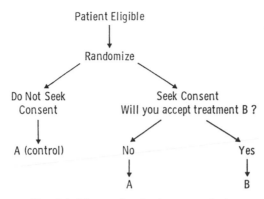

Fig. 7.1. The randomized consent design

statistical efficiency is incurred by patients refusing treatment B, but this may be compensated for by the fact that the randomized consent design may attract more patients into the trial than would be the case with conventional consent procedure. Zelen (1979) gives a more precise mathematical formulation of this aspect.

The philosophy behind this approach is that a patient's consent need only be sought after randomization has provisionally assigned him to a new experimental treatment. Patients assigned to the control group G_1 are due to receive the therapy A that they would have received anyway if they were not in the trial, so that there is no apparent need to seek their consent.

I think that the randomized consent procedure is an attractive proposition for coping with patient consent in such a way that the ethical need is fulfilled without disturbing the doctor–patient relationship. Some clinicians, e.g. Armstrong (1979), have already conducted trials along such lines but further experience is required to reveal whether randomized consent is widely applicable in the legal and ethical circumstances of trials conducted in different countries.

This chapter has explored some of the ethical issues encountered in the conduct of randomized controlled trials. Further discussion is provided by Brewin (1982), Hill (1963), Lebacqz (1980) and Smith (1977).

CHAPTER 8

Crossover Trials

Most of this book is concerned with 'between-patient' comparisons whereby each patient receives only one treatment. In some situations a more precise treatment comparison is possible by a 'within-patient' study in which each patient receives more than one treatment. The advantages and limitations of such studies are considered in section 8.1.

The most common type of within-patient study is when each patient receives two treatments one after the other, the order of treatments being decided randomly. Design and analysis of such two-period crossover trials are dealt with in sections 8.2 and 8.3, respectively.

Occasionally it is possible to give each patient more than two treatments, and such multi-period crossover designs are considered in section 8.4.

8.1 WITHIN-PATIENT COMPARISONS

One major problem with conventional 'parallel group' randomized trials is that patients vary so much in their initial disease state and in their response to therapy. This means that one needs substantial groups of patients on each treatment in order to estimate reliably the magnitude of any treatment difference (see chapter 9 on size of trials). In many diseases, clinical trials must be conducted with only one treatment per patient. For instance, when comparing different surgical procedures (e.g. radical versus simple mastectomy) or evaluating the effects of long-term drug therapy there is no scope for more than one treatment per patient and one needs to undertake large randomized trials.

However, some trials have the more limited objective of studying the patient's response to relatively short periods of therapy. This is particularly so in chronic conditions (e.g. hypertension, asthma, rheumatoid arthritis) where one's first evaluation of treatment efficacy is concerned with *measuring short-term relief of signs or symptoms*. There then arises the possibility of giving each patient a series of two or more treatments over separate equal periods of time. *For each patient one has an evaluation of both treatments*, and hence a measure of treatment difference for each individual or an individual patient preference. Statistical analysis is then based on such within-patient comparisons.

In principle, such within-patient studies allow a more precise comparison of treatments and hence need smaller numbers of patients than between-patient studies. For instance, asthmatic patients vary enormously in their lung function as measured by standard tests like forced expiratory volume (FEV_1). Some will only be marginally below normal while others may have FEV_1 well below 50% of normal. However, the variability of FEV_1 for an individual measured on different days will not be anywhere near as great. Hence, the comparison of FEV_1 after two different treatment periods on the same patient will be less affected by fluctuations unrelated to therapy than the equivalent comparison of two different patients receiving different treatments. This advantage can be expressed more precisely in terms of the statistical method called analysis of variance by assessing the relative magnitude of within patient and between patient components of variance; see Armitage (1971, section 7.2) for details.

Now, *to cross-over patients from one therapy to another* may seem at first sight to be a simple, straightforward idea but in practice one needs to consider carefully whether it is feasible and reliable. For instance, is the disease sufficiently stable and is patient cooperation good enough to ensure that all patients will complete the full course of treatments? Clearly the nature of the condition and treatment must be such that only short-term relief, not long-term cure, can be achieved in any treatment period.

A second issue is the avoidance of bias in the treatment comparison and this can be achieved by giving treatments in a random order determined separately for each patient. Problems of interpretation arise if the order of treatments is the same for all patients. For instance, Christiansen *et al* (1974) describe a trial of vitamin D treatment of epilepsy in which patients first received a placebo for 28 days followed by low-dose and then high-dose vitamin D for 28 days each. For most patients the number of epileptic seizures on vitamin D was less than on placebo. However, one cannot claim this as evidence that vitamin D caused the improvement since it might be that patients would have improved anyway over the six-month period. This is not just a theoretical issue; patients are more likely to enter a trial when their disease is most noticeable, and hence more severe than usual, so that there is a very realistic chance of a trend towards improvement while on trial regardless of therapy. Further discussion on the design of crossover trials is given in sections 8.2 and 8.4.

In ophthalmology, another type of within-patient study is the *simultaneous comparison* of different treatments applied to each of the two eyes, both being affected by the same condition. For instance, the Diabetic Retinopathy Study Research Group (1976) describe a trial which demonstrated the efficacy of photocoagulation treatment for diabetic retinopathy. For each patient one eye was randomly chosen to receive photocoagulation while the other eye remained untreated. Besides being useful scientifically, this design was also favoured ethically since it gave every patient the opportunity to receive the treatment in one eye rather than leaving some patients untreated. Such simultaneous within-patient trials may also be possible in other specialties, e.g. dermatology.

One very misleading type of within-patient trial is the simple *before and after study*. Here all patients receive the same treatment and their condition is assessed before and at various times after start of treatment. One will often see an improvement in such a treated group (indeed improvement is almost inevitable in some conditions) but one cannot attribute this to the treatment concerned. Such trials are uncontrolled and their shortcomings are mentioned in section 4.1.

8.2 THE TWO-PERIOD CROSSOVER DESIGN

I will illustrate the main features of two-period crossover trials by means of three examples. First, James *et al.* (1977) studied the effect of oxprenolol on stage-fright in musicians using the design shown in figure 8.1.

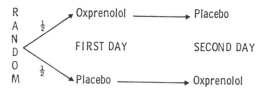

Fig. 8.1. An example of the two-period crossover design

On two separate days, 24 string musicians gave concert performances at which they were assessed for nervousness and quality of performance. Half the musicians were randomly assigned to oxprenolol on the first day and a placebo on the second, tablets being taken about 90 minutes before each performance, while the other 12 musicians had the reverse order. The trial was double-blind (see chapter 6) as is usually the case in crossover trials, in that neither the musician nor his assessors knew his order of treatments. The trial showed that oxprenolol was associated with an improved overall musical performance, especially when given on the first day.

This particular trial was simple in structure in that only one dose of drug was given and evaluation was over in a couple of hours. In other crossover trials the *duration of each therapy* needs to be longer in order to compare their effects. For instance, a trial of two steroid inhalers for the treatment of asthma randomized half the patients to receive inhaler A for four weeks followed by inhaler B for four weeks. The other half received B for four weeks followed by A for four weeks. Each patient measured his own peak flow rate every morning and evening and other lung function tests were carried out in hospital at the end of each treatment period. Here, *too short a period* on each treatment could mean that:

(1) treatment has too little time to take effect
(2) one has too few peak flow recordings to obtain an accurate mean measurement of response on each patient, or
(3) there may be some carry-over effect, whereby the effect of the treatment given first may still be present well into the second period.

Conversely, *too long a period* on each treatment may lead to:

(1) inadequate compliance with the protocol and a substantial number of patient withdrawals
(2) the disease condition not remaining sufficiently stable for some patients. For instance, in a trial for treatment of hypertension in the elderly two treatment periods of four months proved too long for some patients.

Hence, some compromise solution must be reached and four weeks per treatment was considered appropriate in this asthma trial. Also good patient cooperation is particularly important in crossover trials to ensure correct medication and evaluation in each treatment period.

In crossover trials, one is only concerned with short-term response as measured during and at the end of each treatment period. Any more long-term *carry-over effect* of the first treatment into the second period is undesirable. If such carry-over is possible one should consider introducing a *wash-out period* after the first treatment during which patients receive no treatment or a placebo. However, in the above asthma trial it was considered unethical to withhold therapy so that no wash-out was possible. Hence, daily peak flow measurement in the first week or so of the second treatment period may be influenced by the first treatment, so that one should concentrate more on comparing the last two weeks on each treatment.

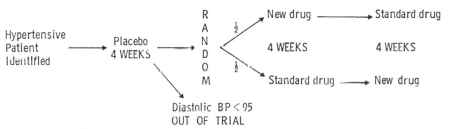

Fig. 8.2. An example of a crossover trial with a run-in period

Another problem is to ensure that patients have sufficiently *stable disease* and hence a *run-in period* for premonitoring of relevant signs and symptoms is often desirable. For instance, a trial of antihypertensive agents had the design shown in figure 8.2. Patients first received a placebo for four weeks, this being given single-blind (i.e. the patient did not know it was a placebo). Only those patients who still had hypertension (i.e. diastolic BP $\geq$ 95 mm Hg) were then considered eligible to enter the trial proper. In this way one could exclude patients who had transitory hypertension, and concentrate the trial on patients who might really benefit from therapy and hence get a more reliable therapeutic comparison.

Randomization is an important feature of any crossover trial. One has two treatment sequences:

$$C = \text{treatment A followed by treatment B}$$
$$D = \text{treatment B followed by treatment A}$$

One can then use the methods described in chapter 5 to assign patients randomly to sequence C or D.

Turpeinen *et al.* (1979) describe an unusual crossover trial in that it was non-randomized and had a very long treatment period. Patients in one Finnish mental hospital were given a diet low in saturated fats while those in another mental hospital received a normal diet. After six years the diets were reversed. The study showed a reduction in serum cholesterol and a lower incidence of coronary heart disease when the low fat diet was given. The interpretation of this trial is very difficult and lack of randomization makes comparison of the two diets in the first six years of questionable value. Also, the changing hospital population, plus a potential carry-over effect of the initial diet into the second period may bias any within-hospital comparison.

When considering the use of a crossover design, one needs to recognize the above limitations as well as the advantages. At first sight, it may seem an attractive proposition to have each patient acting 'as his own control' in this way, but the problems of patient withdrawals, unstable disease, period effects or carry-over effects can sometimes destroy the whole purpose of a crossover trial. Such problems have led some people, including the US Food and Drug Administration, to question whether crossover trials can ever be a reliable method. Indeed, in the past they probably have been used to excess in inappropriate situations. However, in the early evaluation of new drugs in phase II trials they can be of value where past experience indicates that the above problems are not too severe. Of course, one must recognize that such trials of short-term therapy are only one step in understanding a new therapy and will usually need to be followed by larger randomized phase III trials of longer-term therapy. Brown (1980) provides further discussion of crossover designs and their potential misuse.

Another very different type of crossover design is when patients who fail to respond on one treatment are crossed over to the alternative therapy. For instance, Ezdinli *et al.* (1976) describe a trial in lymphocytic lymphoma with two initial treatments (cytoxan-prednisone and BCNU-prednisone). Patients who failed to achieve adequate tumour shrinkage on one treatment could be crossed over to the other treatment in the hope that a second chance may produce a response. These optional crossovers are primarily for ethical reasons whereby each patient will get a chance to receive the 'better' treatment if necessary. Consequently, such crossover data are usually only of secondary interest, the main analysis of results being a comparison of initial treatment only.

8.3 THE ANALYSIS AND INTERPRETATION OF CROSSOVER TRIALS

The statistical analysis of results from two-period crossover trials is often incorrectly performed or misunderstood. Hence, I will describe two examples which deal with the main issues and problems. Certain statistical terms used in this section (e.g. significance tests, confidence limits) are described more fully in chapter 13.

Example 1: A Hypertension Trial

The design of this trial has already been outlined in figure 8.2. One hundred and nine patients were randomized such that 55 received new anti-hypertensive drug A for four weeks followed by standard anti-hypertensive drug B for four weeks and 54 had B followed by A. Each patient had several blood pressure readings taken at the end of each treatment period. Here, let us analyse the results of systolic blood pressure measured at the end of a standard 5-minute exercise test.

First, one can perform a *crude overall within-patient comparison* of treatments. That is, for each patient calculate the difference = systolic BP after A − systolic BP after B. For example, the first patient had BP = 174 mm Hg after A and 180 mm Hg after B so that the difference = −6 mm Hg.

The mean of these 109 differences was +3.94 mm Hg, indicating that post-exercise systolic BP tended to be somewhat higher on the new drug A. Now, one should test whether this mean is significantly different from 0 by performing a *t test for paired differences*. That is, one needs to assess whether a mean difference as big as 3.94 based on 109 patients had a reasonable chance of occurring even if treatments A and B were really equally effective. The calculation is as follows:

$$\text{Standard deviation of differences} = 17.48 \text{ mm Hg}$$

$$\text{Standard error of mean difference} = \frac{\text{standard deviation}}{\sqrt{\text{no. of patients}}}$$

$$= \frac{17.48}{\sqrt{109}} = 1.67 \text{ mm Hg}$$

$$t = \frac{\text{mean difference}}{\text{standard error of mean difference}} = \frac{3.94}{1.67} = 2.36$$

$$\text{Degrees of freedom} = \text{no. of patients} - 1 = 108.$$

This value of t is converted to a P-value using table 13.6. In fact, $t = 2.36$ implies $P = 0.02$, indicating that the treatment difference is significant at the 2% level. This means that under the null hypothesis that there is no real difference in treatments, one could expect such a large observed mean difference to occur only with probability 0.02. Hence, we appear to have fairly strong evidence that post-exercise systolic BP really does tend to stay higher on treatment A. Note that for trials with fewer patients (say <20) a more detailed table allowing for degrees of freedom should be used to determine the P-value; see Armitage (1971, table A3).

In addition it is useful to calculate the 95% confidence limits = mean difference $\pm 2 \times$ standard error = $+3.94 \pm 2 \times 1.67 = +0.60$ and $+7.28$ mm Hg. This means that one is 95% sure that the true mean difference in post-exercise systolic BP for the population of all such hypertensive patients lies between these limits.

This relatively straightforward analysis makes two main assumptions, no period effect and no treatment–period interaction, which should be checked as follows:

(1) **Period Effect**

Ideally one would prefer that the patient's underlying condition and ability to respond remain unchanged from the first to the second treatment period. However, it is often the case that patients will on average improve (or sometimes deteriorate) by the second period. This period effect can be examined by comparing the mean differences for the two treatment orders:

	A followed by B	B followed by A
Mean of differences		
BP after A − BP after B	+5.04	+2.81
Standard deviation of differences	15.32	19.52
No. of patients	55	54

In this instance, those receiving A first had higher mean BP in the first period (i.e. after A) and those receiving B first had higher mean BP in the second period (i.e. also after A). The estimated overall mean period effect $= (5.04 - 2.81)/2 = 1.12$ mm Hg higher in the first period. One can test whether this is significantly different from 0 by a *t test for period effect* as follows:

$$t = \frac{5.04 - 2.81}{\sqrt{\dfrac{15.32^2}{55} + \dfrac{19.52^2}{54}}} = 0.66$$

This is non-significant, i.e. there is no evidence of a period effect. If there were evidence of a period effect, or one does not wish to rule out the possibility of one, then the crude overall treatment comparison given at the start of this section may be slightly modified. The estimated mean difference then becomes $\dfrac{5.04 + 2.81}{2} = 3.93$ mm Hg, virtually unchanged here since the numbers on each treatment order were almost equal. The *t test for treatment effect* is modified so that

$$t = \frac{5.04 + 2.81}{\sqrt{\dfrac{15.32^2}{55} + \dfrac{19.52^2}{54}}} = 2.33, \ P = 0.02$$

In practice, I prefer to use this modification only when there is some suggestion of a genuine period effect, but some people always use it.

If a marked period effect is found, one feels somewhat uneasy about interpreting any overall treatment difference within patients, since the observed treatment difference in any patient depends so much on which treatment was given first. See the second example below.

(2) **Carry-over Effects and Other Interactions between Treatment and Period**

The above statistical analysis assumes that the effects on blood pressure of treatment and period (if present) operate independently of one another. This is not always the case: sometimes response on one treatment may be different in period 1 as compared with period 2, whereas response on the other treatment shows no such difference between periods. It is difficult to interpret such a 'treatment-period interaction' but one common reason is the carry-over effect mentioned in section 8.2.

The statistical test for interaction proceeds as follows in the hypertension trial. For each patient calculate the mean blood pressure

$$= \frac{\text{BP after A} + \text{BP after B}}{2}$$

	A followed by B	B followed by A
No. of patients	55	54
Mean of patient means	180.17	176.28 mm Hg
Standard deviation of patient means	26.27	26.56

The required two-sample t test has

$$t = \frac{180.17 - 176.28}{\sqrt{\dfrac{26.27^2}{55} + \dfrac{26.56^2}{54}}} = 0.77$$

This is not significant, there is no evidence of interaction and hence the original simple analysis remains valid.

Unfortunately, this test for interaction is not very sensitive since it is based on between-patient comparisons, so that particularly in small crossover trials one may fail to detect an interaction when it is present. If a significant interaction is found, one's best policy is to abandon the above within-patient analysis and resort to a between-patient comparison of treatments using the first period only.

Example 2: An Asthma Trial

This crossover trial of two *steroid inhalers* for treatment of asthma has already been mentioned in section 8.2. Here, we shall analyse the results of peak flow rate (PEFR) as measured every evening during the latter two weeks on each inhaler. Each patient's PEFR on each inhaler is taken as the mean of the daily readings. The analysis for treatment and period effects is as follows:

	Inhaler A followed by B	Inhaler B followed by A
No. of patients	14	13
Mean difference (PEFR on A − PEFR on B)	− 32.86 litres/min	− 3.92 litres/min
Standard deviation of differences	37.56	31.71

Estimated mean period effect $= \dfrac{32.86 - 3.92}{2} = 14.5$ litres/min higher in the second period. The test of period effect has $t = 2.17$, which is significant at the 5% level, so that this must be taken into account when assessing the treatment effects.

The estimated mean treatment difference $= \dfrac{32.86 + 3.92}{2} = 18.4$ litres/min higher on inhaler B. The test for treatment effect has $t = 2.76$, $P < 0.01$. However, given the strong period effect I would not be entirely happy with this overall comparison and prefer to see the results for the two orders presented separately as above. Then one can observe the marked (and highly significant) increase in PEFR when B follows A, and the negligible change in PEFR when A follows B.

The test for interaction was not significant, but given its lack of sensitivity this does not rule out the possibility of a carry-over effect. For instance, the mean PEFR by treatment for each order was as follows:

	Period 1	Period 2
A → B (14 patients)	310.1	343.1
	A	B
B → A (13 patients)	335.8	339.7
	B	A

There is a suggestion that A fared badly when given first, but not when given second. In fact, B is the standard inhaler that many patients had used beforehand. It could be that A was not so good to begin with because it was a change from usual therapy, but when A was introduced after B the patient improvement in PEFR (either in technique or actual lung function) over time compensated for this.

This example illustrates the difficulty that can arise in crossover trials for a chronic condition such as asthma where virtually all patients are permanently on treatment. One should consider the alternative of a conventional 'between-patient' randomized study with a longer single treatment period, though since asthmatics vary so much in their lung function this would require many more patients.

The analysis methods so far have been in terms of mean treatment differences in outcome. However, *it is also informative to display individual data* in some table or diagram. For instance, in the hypertension trial (example 1) a frequency distribution was produced as in table 8.1. This table enables one to observe that 55 patients had higher BP on A compared with 36 on B. This difference becomes more marked (33 versus 12) when A was given first and slightly reversed (22 versus 24) when B was given first. However, the variation in treatment difference was greater when B was given first.

One sometimes sees the results of a crossover trial displayed in terms of means and standard deviations separately for each treatment. For instance, in the hypertension trial the post-exercise systolic blood pressure results were

	Treatment A	Treatment B
Mean	180.21 mm Hg	176.27 mm Hg
Standard deviation	28.44 mm Hg	27.02 mm Hg
No. of patients	109	109

To present these treatment means is often a useful extra since it gives a better feel for what the mean treatment difference, 3.94 higher on A, actually relates to. Standard deviations also give an idea of patient variation provided the distribution is not very skew. However, note that the treatment comparison is not based on such data but on the treatment *differences* for individual patients and *their* mean and standard deviation. In particular, the above table should not include the standard errors of each mean which could mislead one into the erroneous use of a two-sample t test rather than the t test for paired differences; see Armitage (1971, section 4.6) for clarification.

Table 8.1. Frequency distributions for the treatment difference in post-exercise systolic blood pressure

BP after A − BP after B	All patients	A given first	B given first
Over 30 mm Hg	7	1	6
21 to 30	12	5	7
11 to 20	13	11	2
1 to 10	23	16	7
0	18	10	8
− 1 to −10	17	6	11
−11 to −20	13	4	9
−21 to −30	4	1	3
Over −30	2	1	1
Total No. of patients	109	55	54

Here I have only dealt with the analysis of trials with a quantitative measurement for response. Other crossover trials may have response in terms of more qualitative assessments, ordinal scores or patient preferences. Also, if the trial is small and measurements have a skew distribution Wilcoxon tests should be used rather than t tests. Thirdly, for some crossover trials, baseline data recorded at the start of each treatment period may be incorporated in analysis. For further details Hills and Armitage (1979), and Armitage and Hills (1982) provide more comprehensive accounts of the analysis of two-period crossover trials.

Lastly, *patient withdrawals* from the trial may seriously affect analysis and interpretation. As mentioned in section 12.3, such patients must be included in any trial report, but clearly in the absence of any evaluation for one (or both) treatments they cannot be included in the above-mentioned analyses. A large number of drop-outs after the first treatment period makes the crossover design of questionable value and it then may be advisable to use a between-patient analysis of the results in period 1 only.

8.4 MULTI-PERIOD CROSSOVER DESIGNS

Sometimes the crossover design can be extended to include more than two treatments per subject in consecutive periods. This will usually be when the intervals between treatments are very short (one day each, say) and may be particularly useful in phase I studies of healthy volunteers. My first example is not a clinical trial as such, but an experiment by Douglas (1975) into the short-term effects of various air pollutants on the lung function of volunteers. For each pollutant (e.g. sulphur dioxide) there were four dose levels (none, low, medium, high) which each subject received in a random order on four consecutive days. To ensure a balanced experiment, subjects were entered in blocks of 4 and the following *latin square design* was used to determine their order of dosage:

		Day number			
		1	2	3	4
	1	A	B	C	D
Sequence number	2	B	D	A	C
	3	C	A	D	B
	4	D	C	B	A

As each block of four subjects was ready for the experiment they were randomly assigned to sequence numbers 1 to 4, the four doses (none, low, medium, high) having already been randomly allocated as letters A, B, C, or D. This latin square ensures that (1) each subject has all four treatments, (2) each treatment occurs once on each day and (3) each treatment pair (e.g. A followed by C) occurs once only. The whole procedure can be repeated for each block of four patients.

Studies of observer variation (see section 3.5) may also employ such a latin square design. For instance, Garraway *et al.* (1976) assessed the variation in clinical assessment of stroke by having 12 patients assessed by four clinicians. Using a similar design to the above, patients arranged in blocks of 4 were randomly assigned to sequences 1 to 4, the four clinicians being randomly allocated letters A, B, C, or D. In this way, the *order* in which clinicians examined patients was balanced over the 12 patients.

Some early phase I/II trials may be concerned with the effects of different single-drug dosages over just a few hours. In this situation there may be scope for quite a large number of treatment periods on each patient. For instance, Willey *et al.* (1976) carried out a trial to assess the bronchodilatory effects of oral pirbuterol and salbutamol in patients with bronchial asthma. There were 10 different treatments in all:

Pirbuterol 5 mg	Salbutamol 2 mg
Pirbuterol 7.5 mg	Salbutamol 4 mg
Pirbuterol 10 mg	Salbutamol 6 mg
Pirbuterol 15 mg	Salbutamol 8 mg
Pirbuterol 20 mg	and placebo.

Over two weeks (five days in each week) ten patients were each given all ten treatments. On a given day, one of the treatments was given in the morning and patient's lung function monitored for 6 hours. The sequence of treatments over the ten days was determined using a latin square as follows:

		1	2	3	4	5	6	7	8	9	10
					Day number						
	1	A	B	C	D	E	F	G	H	I	J
	2	B	G	A	E	H	C	F	I	J	D
	3	C	H	J	G	F	B	E	A	D	I
Patient	4	D	A	G	I	J	E	C	B	F	H
number	5	E	F	H	J	I	G	A	D	B	C
	6	F	E	B	C	D	I	J	G	H	A
	7	G	I	F	B	A	D	H	J	C	E
	8	H	C	I	F	G	J	D	E	A	B
	9	I	J	D	A	C	H	B	F	E	G
	10	J	D	E	H	B	A	I	C	G	F

The ten treatments were randomly allocated to letters A to J and each patient in turn received one of the above ten treatment sequences.

Theoretically one could suggest various elaborations on this sort of design. For instance, if each patient could not receive all treatments, say one had four treatments but only three periods per patient was feasible, then some form of 'balanced incomplete block design' could be used. Cox (1958) provides further details on such methods.

Another quite different type of crossover design is to have more treatment periods than there are treatments, i.e. to have some treatment repetition in each patient's random sequence of treatment periods. Ebbutt (1983) discusses the use of three period crossover designs for two treatments and explains how this enables carryover effects to be allowed for.

Note that all the above studies were randomized and balanced in order to guard against any 'period effect' biassing the treatment comparisons. However, *dose-escalation studies*, in which all subjects are given the same sequence of increasing drug doses, are open to such bias. Such studies are commonly carried out in phase I trials on human volunteers or patients, but may be exceedingly difficult to interpret. For instance, a new bronchodilator was studied in ten subjects as follows. Each subject received a sequence of six doses at 30-minute intervals. The first dose was zero (a placebo) and the following five doses were of increasing magnitude. Lung function, blood pressure and heart rate were then monitored over the 3 hours of observation. The trial produced dose response curves for forced expiratory volume, peak flow rate, etc., but these are hard to interpret because of the cumulative dosage given. For instance, the increase in peak flow rate after the highest dose may be partly due to that dose itself, partly due to the carry-over effect of previous doses and partly due to natural improvements over time when under experimental conditions. Hence, dose-escalation studies are of limited value.

In principle a better design would be (1) to have longer gaps between doses to minimize any carry-over effect and (2) to arrange dose sequences using some form of balanced randomization (e.g. latin square design as above). However, the latter may not be possible in early phase I/II trials because of the ethical need to plan for a set pattern of dose escalation in case any side-effects occur at intermediate dosage.

CHAPTER 9

The Size of a Clinical Trial

One fundamental question facing the organizers of any clinical trial at the planning stage is '*How many patients do we need?*' Statistical methods can be used to determine the required number of patients to meet the trial's principal scientific objectives, and in section 9.1 these power calculation techniques will be explained with examples. However, such an approach can only be used as a guideline since practical matters such as the availability of patients and resources and the ethical need to prevent any patient receiving an inferior treatment must be taken into account. Section 9.2 considers this need to reach a compromise between scientific objectives and the 'real world'. Section 9.3 deals with the inadequacies of trials which are too small. The pros and cons of multi-centre trials are discussed in section 9.4. Another issue concerns the number of treatments that one can sensibly include in a randomized trial and this is considered in section 9.5 together with an explanation of factorial designs.

9.1 STATISTICAL METHODS FOR DETERMINING TRIAL SIZE

Although practical and ethical issues need to be considered, one's initial reasoning when determining trial size should focus on the *scientific requirements*. To this end *there is one standard statistical approach, often called power calculations*, which can be applied to a wide range of clinical trials. I will introduce the line of reasoning by using one example. This is followed by a more general description of the statistical formulae.

The Anturane Reinfarction Trial Research Group (1978) describe the design of a randomized double-blind trial comparing anturan and placebo in patients after a myocardial infarction. Before the trial began there were *five key questions regarding the trial's size*:

(1) *What is the main purpose of the trial?*
To see if anturan is of value in preventing mortality after a myocardial infarction. Prevention of further non-fatal infarction was also relevant but not the prime purpose.

(2) *What is the principal measure of patient outcome?*
Death from any cause within one year of first treatment was considered the primary indicator of treatment failure. Sudden death, especially in the first few months, ended up showing some interesting differences but when the trial was designed this was rated of secondary importance.

(3) *How will the data be analysed to detect a treatment difference?*
The simplest analysis is a comparison of the percentages of patients dying within a year on anturan and placebo. A χ^2 test will be used (see section 13.2) and the 5% level of significance will be accpeted as showing evidence of a treatment difference. Life-table methods of analysing survival data will also be used but these are more difficult to employ as a basis for determining trial size.

(4) *What type of results does one anticipate with standard treatment?*
Placebo is the standard in this case and one would expect about 10% of patients to die within a year.

(5) *How small a treatment difference is it important to detect and with what degree of certainty?*
The logic here is that very large treatment differences such as a ten-fold reduction in mortality on anturan, could be shown with quite small numbers of patients. What matters is to identify what is the smallest difference that is of such clinical value that it would be very undesirable to fail to detect it. Of course, one could argue that *any* treatment benefit is relevant and must be detected but this is unrealistic since the trial would then have to be infinitely large. In this case, it was decided that if anturan was able to halve the mortality (i.e. 5% die in one year), then one would like to be 90% sure that this was detected as statistically significant.

Given all the above information one is then able to determine that the anturan trial required around 1200 patients (half on anturan, half on placebo). I will now explain in a more general, technical manner how this number was obtained.

Statistical Method for a Qualitative Outcome

The most common statistical approach is to focus on a single outcome of patient response which is dichotomous: that is, each patient's outcome on treatment can be classified either as a 'success' or 'failure' (e.g. death in a year = failure, survival = success).

As in the above example, one then has to choose four items:

p_1 = percentage of successes expected on one treatment (usually the standard).

p_2 = percentage of successes on the other treatment which one desires to detect as being different from p_1.

α = the level of the χ^2 significance test used for detecting a treatment difference (often set $\alpha = 0.05$).

$1 - \beta$ = the degree of certainty that the difference $p_1 - p_2$, if present, would be detected (often set $1 - \beta = 0.90$).

α, commonly called the *type I error*, is the probability of detecting a 'significant difference' when the treatments are really equally effective (i.e. it represents *the risk of a false-positive result*).

β, commonly called the *type II error*, is the probability of *not* detecting a significant difference when there really is a difference of magnitude $p_1 - p_2$ (i.e. it represents *the risk of a false-negative result*).

$1 - \beta$ is called the *power* to detect a difference of magnitude $p_1 - p_2$.

Here, p_1 and p_2 are the hypothetical percentage successes on the two treatments that might be achieved if each were given to a large population of patients. They merely reflect the realistic expectations or goals which one wishes to aim for when planning the trial and do not relate directly to the eventual results.

In the anturan example above, they chose

$$p_1 = 90\% \text{ on placebo expected to survive one year}$$
$$p_2 = 95\%$$
$$\alpha = 0.05$$
$$\beta = 0.1.$$

Now, *the required number of patients on each treatment n* is given by the following formula

$$n = \frac{p_1 \times (100 - p_1) + p_2 \times (100 - p_2)}{(p_2 - p_1)^2} \times f(\alpha, \beta)$$

where $f(\alpha, \beta)$ is a function of α and β, the values of which are given in table 9.1. In fact, $f(\alpha, \beta) = [\Phi^{-1}(\alpha/2) + \Phi^{-1}(\beta)]^2$ where Φ is the cumulative distribution function of a standardized normal deviate. Numerical values for Φ^{-1} may be obtained from statistical tables such as Geigy (1970, p. 28).

Hence, for the anturan trial,

$$n = \frac{90 \times 10 + 95 \times 5}{(95 - 90)^2} \times 10.5 = 578 \text{ patients required on each treatment.}$$

Table 9.1. Values of $f(\alpha, \beta)$ to be used in formula for required number of patients

		β (type II error)		
		0.05	0.1	0.2	0.5
	0.1	10.8	8.6	6.2	2.7
α (type I	0.05	13.0	10.5	7.9	3.8
error)	0.02	15.8	13.0	10.0	5.4
	0.01	17.8	14.9	11.7	6.6

As will be discussed further in section 9.2, this statistical method is only a guideline as to how many patients are needed. However, it is important now to realize that if the trial had fewer patients than this one would automatically decrease the chances of finding a statistically significant reduction in mortality: that is, if the trial is made smaller than these calculations indicate, the power to detect important treatment differences is decreased and so the risk of a false-negative conclusion is increased.

I will now describe a couple of other examples to illustrate this method. *The clofibrate trial*, described in a report of the Committee of Principal Investigators (1978), was to compare clofibrate with placebo for the prevention of ischaemic heart disease in men with raised serum cholesterol. The annual incidence of ischaemic heart disease on placebo was postulated as 1 % per annum, i.e. 5 % in five years, and the study was designed to detect a reduction in incidence of 1/3 in the clofibrate group with type I and type II errors set at $\alpha = 0.01$ and $\beta = 0.1$. Since this was a unique trial unlikely to be replicated elsewhere it was felt that a more stringent level of significance (i.e. $P < 0.01$) would be necessary for any positive findings to be of lasting conviction.

Thus, $p_1 = 5\%$, $p_2 = 3\frac{1}{3}\%$, $\alpha = 0.01$ and $\beta = 0.1$ so that

$$n = \frac{5 \times 95 + 3\frac{1}{3} \times 96\frac{2}{3}}{(5 - 3\frac{1}{3})^2} \times 14.9 = 4276 \text{ patients are required on each treatment}$$

In practice, this was increased to 5000 per treatment. Note that here p_1 and p_2 refer to the percentage 'failures' on each treatment but the identical n is obtained if instead we set $p_1 = 95\%$ and $p_2 = 96\frac{2}{3}$ as the 'success rates'.

My next example concerns *a trial with more than two treatments*. In 1974, the Eastern Cooperative Oncology Group began a randomized trial of chemo-therapy for unfavourable histologic types of malignant lymphoma. There were four multi-drug regimens, BCVP, COPA, COPB and CPOB, the main objective being to see if any of the other three treatments could produce a higher response rate than the standard BCVP that had previously been used by the group. Response was defined as complete disapppearance of demonstrable disease. On past experience, it was considered realistic to hope for increasing response from an anticipated 30% on BCVP to 50% on one of the other regimens with type I error = 0.05 and type II error = 0.1.

Thus, $p_1 = 30\%$, $p_2 = 50\%$, $\alpha = 0.05$, $\beta = 0.1$ so that $n = 121$ patients on each treatment. Since there are four treatments in all, the trial needed an overall size of around 500 patients to meet these criteria.

It may be useful to make some general observations about the above formula. Firstly, n is roughly inversely proportional to $(p_1 - p_2)^2$, which means that for fixed type I and type II errors if one halves the difference in response rates requiring detection one needs about a fourfold increase in trial size. Also, n depends very much on the choice of type II error such that increase in power from 0.5 to 0.95 requires around three times the number of patients. Reduction in type I error α from 0.05 to 0.01 also involves an increase in trial size of around

40% when β is around 0.1. Further clarification of some of the concepts involved in this statistical approach can be found in articles by Altman (1980b) and Gore (1981a).

Much statistical work has been done in this area, such that I feel compelled to justify the relative simplicity of my approach. The non-statistical reader may wish to skip over such details. The method here is based on the normal approximation to the binomial without continuity correction, whereas there are more elaborate methods. Fleiss (1973) gives formulae and extensive tables for the same approach except *with* continuity correction. I have found these tables useful but they are correct only if one intends to use chi-squared with Yates correction. Since Grizzle (1967) has shown this test to be conservative, I prefer to recommend the use of uncorrected chi-squared in which case Fleiss's tables provide an overestimate for n. Casagrande *et al.* (1978) have produced tables based on Fisher's exact test which will be of use to those who prefer a table to a formula. In particular, for trials with a small intended size, say <50, these tables will give different results from the formula given here. For instance, for $p_1 = 5\%$, $p_2 = 50\%$, $\alpha = 0.05$, $\beta = 0.1$, their table gives $n = 21$ compared with $n = 15$ using the formula. However, this does not necessarily mean that our approach here is inferior since Berkson (1978) has argued that the exact test is too conservative. Yet another approach, using the angular transform approximation, is given by Cochran and Cox (1957). The practical value of using the above formula to calculate n is that one has an unrestricted choice of p_1, p_2, α and β. Also, one danger in using a table instead is that one scans the page in search of values to provide *post hoc* justification for one's preconceived ideas on trial size.

Another statistical issue is the choice between using one-sided and two-sided significance levels both in determining trial size and in analysis of results. This issue will be raised again at the end of section 13.2. Here I have presented all results in terms of two-sided tests which in most circumstances I think is a justifiable safeguard against prejudging the direction of treatment differences. However, for those who prefer one-sided testing, which incidentally reduces the required sample size, one needs to replace $\Phi^{-1}(\alpha/2)$ by $\Phi^{-1}(\alpha)$ in the formula for $f(\alpha, \beta)$. Alternatively, use of the above method with $\alpha = 0.05$ is effectively giving a one-sided type I error of 0.025.

In practice, the determination of trial size does not usually take account of patient factors which might influence prognosis. However, Gail (1973) describes an extension of the above approach based on the comparison of percentage successes for patients classified into several separate categories. The method is more complex and hence will not be described.

Statistical Method for a Quantitative Outcome

In some trials the main criterion of patient response is a quantitative measurement and it would seem sensible to utilize this information in determining trial size. For instance, consider a clinical trial to evaluate supplementary vitamin D given to pregnant women for the prevention of neonatal hypocalcaemia. Then, one could randomize pregnant women to vitamin D or placebo and use the infant's serum calcium level one week after birth as the principal measure of response to treatment. Cockburn *et al.* (1980) describe such a trial in an Edinburgh maternity hospital, though the estimations given below were not specifically applied to that actual trial.

The statistical method bears a close resemblance to that for a qualitative response already described. First one needs to specify for one of the treatments the anticipated mean response μ_1, and standard deviation σ. In this case, routine evaluation of previous untreated women could provide such information for serum calcium: in fact suppose we choose $\mu_1 = 9.0$ and $\sigma = 1.8$ mg per 100 ml for serum calcium.

One has to decide on what change in mean response, $\delta = \mu_2 - \mu_1$ achieved by the other treatment it would be important to detect using a two-sample t test at some prespecified significance level α (say $P < 0.05$). One also needs to decide on the power $1 - \beta$, i.e. the degree of certainty to detect such a difference if it exists. In this example, suppose we consider an increase in mean serum calcium to 9.5 mg per 100 ml of clinical relevance so that

$$\delta = \mu_2 - \mu_1 = 9.5 - 9.0 = 0.5 \text{ mg per 100 ml.}$$

Also let us choose $\alpha = 0.05$ and $1 - \beta = 0.95$.

Then, the required number of patients on each treatment is

$$n = \frac{2\sigma^2}{(\mu_2 - \mu_1)^2} \times f(\alpha, \beta)$$

where f is exactly the same as before (see table 9.1). In this case $n = \dfrac{2 \times 1.8^2}{0.5^2} \times 13.0 = 337$ patients on each treatment so that the trial requires around 700 patients in all. Altman (1980b) provides further details of this approach and also presents a useful nomogram which some might prefer to the formula given here. Again this method is an approximation which will tend to give a slight underestimate especially when the calculated n appears small and the data have a skew distribution. It also assumes that the standard deviation of response is the same on both treatments so that if one suspects that the standard deviation may also be greater on the new treatment one should accordingly increase σ in the calculation.

One major problem in using this approach is in choosing appropriate values for μ_1, μ_2 and σ. If one has no past data on patient variation on standard treatment it may be impossible to choose a realistic value for σ. Also, it is very difficult to choose an appropriate value for $\delta = \mu_2 - \mu_1$, since the clinical relevance of a treatment is not intuitively summarized by a change in mean response. Clinical thinking is more likely to focus on the need to increase the chances of a good response in each individual patient.

For instance, it may be easier to redefine the above example in terms of reducing the chances of hypocalcaemia. Serum calcium < 7.4 mg per 100 ml has been used as a criterion of infant hypocalcaemia. Suppose a reduction in percentage hypocalcaemic from 20% on placebo to 10% on vitamin D was considered of clinical relevance. Then the previous method for qualitative data may be used: $p_1 = 20\%$, $p_2 = 10\%$, $\alpha = 0.05$, $\beta = 0.05$ appears an appropriate choice so that $n = 325$ patients are required on each treatment.

Methods for Follow-up Studies

In many trials the main end-point is some time-related event such as death or relapse. Patients will be followed for different lengths of time and usually some patients will not have died or relapsed. Such survival data require appropriate methods of statistical analysis such as the logrank test (see section 14.2).

When determining trial size one can simplify the situation by focussing on a specific follow-up time (e.g. success = survival for one year) and both the anturan and clofibrate trials already mentioned illustrate this approach. There is some loss of information since clearly one is not taking account of the actual death times, so that one may end up with a slightly larger sample size than by using more complex methods. However, this will not be crucial since statistical estimation is intended only as a general guideline and also some patients may withdraw from follow-up. Freedman (1982) explains more elaborate power calculations based on logrank tests for survival data.

A Method for 'Negative' Trials

The motivation behind most randomized trials is to hope for a 'positive' result whereby one treatment is significantly better than another and the above methods have been based on that premise. However, *there are trials in which one is more interested in showing the 'negative' result that two treatments are equally effective*. This usually arises in comparing a conservative treatment with a more intensive standard therapy. For instance, in breast cancer there is some controversy about whether simple mastectomy may be as effective as radical mastectomy. Also, in the treatment of depression it would be of value to demonstrate that a new drug with fewer side-effects produces as good a response as amitriptyline.

Makuch and Simon (1978) describe a suitable method for such trials based on a qualitative measure of patient response, which works as follows. One first specifies p, the overall percentage of successes that one anticipates will occur. Then one chooses a value d such that if the two treatments really are equally effective the upper $100 (1 - \alpha)\%$ confidence limit for the difference in percentage successes on the two treatments should not exceed d with probability $1 - \beta$. Then the required number of patients on each treatment

$$n = \frac{2p \times (100 - p)}{d^2} \times f(\alpha, \beta)$$

where the function f is as defined before (see table 9.1).

For example, suppose amitriptyline is expected to produce a favourable response (as measured by a specified reduction in Hamilton score) in about 70% of patients. In a randomized trial one could specify that a new antidepressant will only be considered acceptable if it can be demonstrated with 95% confidence that it is at worst 10% inferior to amitriptyline. Suppose one accepts a 20% risk that even if the drug is really equally effective one will fail to show it as acceptable in this sense. Then, $p = 70\%$, $d = 10\%$, $\alpha = 0.05$ and $\beta = 0.2$ so that $n = \dfrac{2 \times 70 \times 30}{10^2} \times 7.9 = 332$ patients needed on each treatment.

This example illustrates that *a very substantial number of patients are needed to establish with any confidence that two treatments have comparable efficacy.*

9.2 THE REALISTIC ASSESSMENT OF TRIAL SIZE

When statistical methods such as in section 9.1 are used as the scientific basis for determining trial size, it is a common experience for investigators to be shocked by the *unexpectedly large number of patients required.* One reaction can be to forget about such principles and just go ahead with the trial anyway and see how many patients turn up. Unfortunately, this 'head in the sands' approach is liable to result in a small trial of little scientific merit, and section 9.3 deals further with this problem of small trials. Instead, I feel that it is important that investigators should first make use of statistical methods for trial size since this will act as a preliminary, salutary exercise in providing some idea of the general order of magnitude that is needed. At this point, one will need to appraise the financial support and other resources available to cope with such a trial, though I consider the realistic evaluation of how many patients will be available as the issue of paramount importance.

Thus, the next step is to assess *the accrual rate* of patients into the trial which one anticipates will occur from the investigators currently envisaged as participants. Commonly, this is done by estimating how many eligible patients should present in a typical year. This obviously entails a certain amount of guesswork, but an examination of case records for the last year or two should be possible. The resultant estimate of the number of patients available per year usually ends up being larger than would actually occur. The reasons for this are:

(1) investigators may be overenthusiastic in their assessment
(2) some patients will not be eligible for the trial
(3) some eligible patients may not enter the trial or may not be evaluable.

It is hard to quantify the influence of these three issues, but my experience would suggest that the achievable accrual rate is often less than half what is estimated. In other words, investigators should 'bend over backwards' to ensure that the anticipated rate is a realistic figure.

Once the required trial size and the accrual rate have both been estimated, one divided by the other provides *the estimated time period* required for patient entry. This needs to be compared with what is conceived to be a maximum desirable period of patient accrual, bearing in mind that an additional period of patient follow-up for evaluation may be required. What is a reasonable accrual period depends very much on the nature of the disease. For instance, in a rare disease such as testicular cancer one inevitably expects slow accrual even in a multi-centre trial, so that investigators must accept that patient entry may take five years or more. However, for more common conditions such as hypertension it may be unrealistic for accrual to take more than a few months. For other diseases such as lung cancer or myocardial infarction it is common practice for patient accrual to last for one or two years. One must also bear in mind the trial's practical circumstances: the investigators' commitment to 'seeing the trial through' is important and if the accrual period is too long then enthusiasm will wane and both the quality of trial organization and the rate of patient accrual will decline. Thus, *as a general guideline I would suggest that the accrual period should not exceed two or three years* except for the unusual circumstance of a rare disease and/or experienced trial organizers whose track record is consistent with such a long-term commitment.

More often than not the estimated accrual period needed to meet the prespecified scientific objectives will turn out to be inordinately long, sometimes 10 years or more, in which case one will need to reassess the situation. Basically, there are three solutions here:

(1) increase the accrual rate
(2) relax the scientific requirements
(3) abandon the trial.

The first approach can best be achieved by *getting more investigators to participate*. For instance, one may first plan a trial in one hospital only to realize that it cannot achieve enough patients. If investigators in other hospitals can then be encouraged to collaborate and enter their patients in the same trial the 'numbers problem' can be overcome. The organization of such multi-centre trials is discussed in section 9.4. Another approach to increasing accrual is to review the eligibility requirements. Occasionally, one can become too 'pure' in one's objectives by restricting a trial to a particularly narrow class of patients. Relaxation of certain criteria (e.g. age limits, new cases only, severity or diagnostic classification of disease) may successfully increase patient numbers. For instance, the primary breast cancer trial in section 1.4 only became feasible when patients with fewer than four positive axillary nodes were also allowed in. Of course, one must avoid making the trial so general as to be meaningless. The essential feature is to make patients in the trial representative of all future patients who are liable to benefit from the trial's therapeutic findings.

The choice of scientific requirements for the statistical calculations of section 9.1 is clearly somewhat arbitrary, so that if the derived number of patients is incompatible with the feasible accrual rate, then one can review these specifications. For instance, in the method for comparing percentage successes on two treatments one can decrease the required number of patients either by:

(1) increasing the treatment difference in percentage successes $p_1 - p_2$ to be detected
(2) increasing the type II error, β, which is the chance of a false-negative result
(3) increasing the type I error α, which is the chance of a false-positive result.

For example, suppose the first specification for the anturan trial had been to be 95% certain of detecting a 20% drop in mortality on anturan (i.e. from 10% down to 8%) as being significant at the 1% level. Then, $p_1 = 10\%$, $p_2 = 8\%$, $\alpha = 0.01$, $\beta = 0.05$ so that the formula gives $n = 7280$ patients on each treatment. On paper the specification looks quite plausible since a 20% reduction in mortality after an infarct would be important enough to affect future clinical practice, but such a large trial size would be considered too expensive and unrealistic. Hence, by increasing $p_1 - p_2$ from 2% to 5%, β from 0.05 to 0.1 and α from 0.01 to 0.05 one was able to reduce n to 578 patients per treatment. In practice this estimate of just under 1200 patients in all was increased to 1500 to allow for the entry of some non-evaluable cases and to decrease the type II error. As it turned out, the placebo death rate was somewhat less than 10%, which in retrospect was another reason for increasing the sample size. In fact, the most striking treatment difference found in this trial has been in early sudden deaths which have still smaller numbers, 24 (3%) on placebo versus 6 (1%) on anturan in under six months, so that the large number of patients aimed for has been amply justified.

This re-examination of statistical specifications in order to reduce n can become ridiculous if carried to extreme. In the anturan trial, one could have specified a 50% chance of detecting an 80% drop in mortality as being significant at the 10% level (i.e. $p_1 = 10\%$, $p_2 = 2\%$, $\alpha = 0.1$ and $\beta = 0.5$) leading to $n = 46$ patients required on each treatment. However, such a small trial would be ludicrous since experience of secondary prevention trials in myocardial infarction indicates that such a dramatic reduction in mortality would be virtually inconceivable.

Thus, one must always choose a realistic value for the treatment difference $p_1 - p_2$. Clearly, there is no 'right answer' in any particular trial though in my experience clinical investigators, perhaps in discussion with a statistician, are usually able to agree on a sensible, clinically relevant goal in this context.

The type I error α is conventionally set at 0.05 and generally one should avoid larger values such as $\alpha = 0.1$. On occasions one may set $\alpha = 0.01$ in order to provide extra assurance that a detected treatment difference is indeed genuine, especially if the planned trial is a unique study of a major clinical issue.

An appropriate choice of β, the type II error, is generally in the range 0.05 to 0.2. Larger values of β, say 0.5, are not really acceptable since the chances of missing a major treatment difference become too high.

Evidently, there is no single clear-cut answer to the question 'How many patients are needed?' However, thoughtful use of statistical methods provides an objective scientific guideline with sufficient flexibility to fit in with a realistic accrual rate and period for patient entry.

I have so far said little about costing in relation to trial size. Obviously, large trials are expensive and any choice of patient numbers must be backed up by adequate funding for good organization and sufficient support staff. This issue is fundamental, but *lack of funds is no excuse for doing a trial of inadequate size.*

Earlier in this section I mentioned a third solution to the problem of inadequate patient accrual to meet the desired trial size: namely, to *abandon the trial before it starts.* This is not a facetious comment but a serious recommendation that if a trial will be too small to detect realistic and clinically relevant differences then one should avoid inconveniencing patients, and wasting funds and effort on an experiment which is scientifically inadequate. To be specific, if for a sensible choice of $p_1 - p_2$, $\alpha = 0.05$ and $\beta = 0.5$ the resultant number of patients per treatment n is still too large then there is little doubt that the trial should not go ahead.

Lastly, the discussion here is based on the idea of a fixed size of trial, whereas in many trials one expects to undertake interim analyses of results while patient accrual is still in progress. If such results show a major treatment difference one may have to stop the trial early. This issue is discussed in chapter 10. Thus, the size of trial decided at the planning stage might be considered as a maximum number of patients, since clearly there is an ethical need to stop earlier if a smaller number of patients ends up demonstrating a highly significant difference. Further discussion on the practicalities of sample size is given by Brown (1980).

9.3 THE INADEQUACY OF SMALL TRIALS

As already pointed out, a trial with only a small number of patients carries a considerable risk of failing to demonstrate a treatment difference when one is really present: i.e. *small trials have a large type II error.* Freiman et al. (1978) have illustrated this point by reviewing 71 'negative' trials in major medical journals each of which found no evidence of a treatment difference. They showed that 50 of these trials carried a 10% risk of having missed a 50% therapeutic improvement, thus demonstrating that the great majority of these trials were too small to reach a reliable conclusion. Furthermore, the situation may be worse than indicated by this review since many small trials reaching a negative conclusion will not be published at all.

In the field of cancer research Pocock et al. (1978) carried out a survey into the size of 50 randomized cancer trials, a random sample of trials registered with the Union Internationale Contre le Cancer. They found that the median rate of accrual was 33 patients per annum, which is unduly low given that most trial organizers had anticipated the need for over 100 patients on trial. Hence, although the planning of these cancer trials appeared generally of high quality, and many had used statistical calculations to estimate the trial size, the fact remains that in many cases patient accrual was generally too slow to complete the trial's objectives successfully. Similarly, Zelen (personal communication) has reviewed cancer trials published in the journal *Cancer* for 1977–1979 to find that the median size was 50 patients: this sort of trial size in cancer makes it extremely difficult to sift out the relatively small number of genuine therapeutic advances from the larger pool of treatments without improvement. This problem is discussed at greater length in section 15.2.

In a review of all British cancer trials Tate *et al.* (1979) provide some insight into why cancer research has difficulty in enrolling sufficient patients. They showed that for all sites of cancer (except leukaemia and Hodgkins lymphoma) less than 10% of British patients were being entered on clinical trials and in lung cancer only 1% were included in trials. Hence, for British trials in cancer as currently organized the major problem is the failure to enrol a higher proportion of available patients. As a consequence they found that trials often had a long period of patient intake of around five years or more.

As regards trials in other diseases I suspect *the tendency for too many small trials* is even more pronounced. If one is trying to establish that one therapy has greater effect than another, small trials are a hindrance to progress and may deter the development of new, more valuable regimens. However, in some diseases clinical trials are conducted in order to show that a new (conservative) treatment is of comparable effectiveness to a (more aggressive) standard treatment. The example of such a 'negative' trial at the end of section 9.1 indicated that one would need a substantial number of patients to demonstrate equivalence. Hence, there is the danger that potentially inferior drugs are being approved for marketing because adequate evidence of therapeutic equivalence cannot be obtained through the current tendency to unduly small trials. For instance, Bland *et al.* (1983) undertook a survey of 80 published trials of analgesic drugs recently approved for marketing and showed that less than 10% of trials exceeded 100 patients and over 70% have fewer than 50 patients.

Thus, while the pharmaceutical industry has generally accepted the need for randomized phase III trials, the major problem of getting enough patients remains largely unanswered. Until a greater effort is made to achieve larger numbers in all types of clinical trial, *much published clinical research remains essentially futile since it lacks the resources to answer the clinical questions being posed.*

9.4 MULTI-CENTRE TRIALS

Often any single source of patients (whether it be a hospital, general practice or some other clinical research base) may be insufficient to make a clinical trial of viable size. Sometimes this problem is clear-cut from the beginning but on other occasions a trial in a single centre lingers on with far too few patients and peters out as enthusiasm inevitably wanes. Thus, when planning a clinical trial it is important to recognize early on whether a single-centre study is feasible. If one does see the need for a multi-centre trial the pros and cons should be considered:

Advantages

(1) Evidently, the principal advantage of mounting a multi-centre trial is that

patient accrual is much quicker so that the trial can be made larger and/or the intended size can be achieved more quickly. The end-result should be that a multi-centre trial reaches more reliable conclusions at a faster rate so that overall progress in the treatment of a given disease is enhanced.

(2) The fact that a trial involves patients and clinicians from several centres means that any conclusions have a broader, more representative base than can be reached in a single centre. Hence, one may feel able to extrapolate one's findings to the whole population of such patients with greater confidence.

(3) Hopefully the collaboration of clinical scientists in a multi-centre trial should lead to raised standards in the design, conduct and interpretation of the trial.

Problems

(1) Clearly, the planning and administration of any multi-centre trial is considerably more complex than in a single centre and hence it is vital to have efficient centralized coordination of all trial activities.

(2) Multi-centre trials are very expensive to run, both as regards staff and resources, so that one must first obtain adequate funding for the study.

(3) It is important to ensure that all centres will follow the study protocol. Adequate communication across centres at the planning stage is needed to obtain prior agreement regarding the nature of the study. In particular, any potential investigators who cannot agree to the eventual design should be encouraged to exclude themselves from further participation in the study before problems of non-compliance arise.

(4) The need for quality control as regards any measurements, clinical observations and data recording requires prior recognition. Sufficient training and explanation should be given to ensure consistency across centres.

(5) The collection and processing of data poses especial problems in multi-centre trials which are often not anticipated. One needs a well-organized data centre which receives all data and provides prompt and reliable feedback to each participating centre of data requirements and problems.

(6) One particular difficulty is to motivate all participants in a large multi-centre trial to play an enthusiastic and responsible role. In a single-centre study the clinical investigators are continuously involved and publish the results themselves so that responsibilities and effort are clearly recognized. In a multi-centre study the individual clinician clearly has much less input into the trial's overall outcome so that it is important for trial organizers to maintain sufficient interest in the study by each investigator. In this respect, meetings of trial participants and feedback of general information on the trial's progress may help.

(7) A related issue concerns the desirability of each participant entering all eligible patients into the trial. It is advisable to avoid 'passive' investigators

who only enter the occasional patient, since the subsequent sample of patients in the trial may be highly unrepresentative.

(8) In general, the larger the number of centres in a trial the greater the above-mentioned problems are likely to be. Thus, in planning a multi-centre trial one may have to reach a compromise between quality and quantity of information: a few centres fully committed to the trial may be better than a larger number of centres giving half-hearted support, provided that the former can still provide enough patients in a reasonable time period.

(9) Lastly, multi-centre trials can sometimes degenerate into poor quality 'research by committee' by which I mean the trial may have no clear leadership and scientific goals and becomes a muddled compromise across a collection of separate proposals. Thus, I consider any multi-centre trial benefits enormously by having an experienced *principal investigator* or chairman who, while remaining responsive to the comments and desires of others, ensures that the overview of the trial's objectives is realistic and its execution is reliable.

Organization

To illustrate the complex structure that is required for a large multi-centre trial I will focus on one example: the British trial of treatment for mild hypertension as described by the Medical Research Council Working Party (1977). The trial is concerned with comparing two standard antihypertensive drugs with placebo in patients with a diastolic blood pressure in the range 90–109 mm Hg to see if there is a subsequent reduction in mortality and morbid events such as non-fatal stroke. The trial, involving 18 000 subjects, is one of the largest multi-centre trials ever undertaken in Britain so that its organizational structure, as explained below, is of particular importance:

(1) The Medical Research Council are funding the study and hence have reviewed the study design and are kept informed of study progress.

(2) The Trial Working Party and particularly its chairman and clinical secretary are responsible for organizing the trial in all its aspects.

(3) The Trial Monitoring Committee provides a group of experienced clinical researchers and statisticians who are called upon to oversee the trial's general progress (e.g. proposed changes in the protocol) but are not concerned with the day-to-day running of the study.

(4) The Ethical Committee is concerned with all ethical aspects of the study. Since the trial entails long-term treatment or placebo for subjects with mild hypertension who are otherwise healthy, these ethical issues are highly relevant.

(5) The Coordinating Centre consists of two clinical epidemiologists, a statistician and 12–15 technical and clerical support staff. Day-to-day activities are organized from this centre under the general supervision of the working party. In particular data collection, follow-up of subjects and evaluation of results are carried out from the centre.

(6) Trial Clinics, around 200 of them all over the country, are set up to screen middle-aged men and women to see if they are eligible and willing to participate in the trial. Such subjects, recruited from general practices and industrial work forces, are examined by a specially trained team of nurses.
(7) Central Laboratory Services are used for biochemical tests.

This trial is perhaps atypical as regards its large size but in terms of the organizational structure it provides a working model for multi-centre trials in general. Possibly in a smaller trial the working party and monitoring committee might be amalgamated. Further discussion of multi-centre trials is given by Freedman (1980).

Cooperative Groups

In some disease areas, notably in cancer, cooperative multi-centre trial groups have been set up as a somewhat more permanent body to undertake a continuing series of clinical trials. In chapter 2 the development of cancer cooperative groups in the United States was described. The administration of such groups is essentially the same as for any multi-centre trial, except that in addition to the structure for each separate trial there is an extra hierarchy of organization (e.g. group chairman, coordinating statistician, etc.) to ensure that all studies conform to the same overall system of patient registration, follow-up, data processing, reporting of results, etc.

Cooperative groups clearly provide an excellent opportunity to formulate a whole strategy for continuing clinical research and hence should be an improvement on the piecemeal approach of each trial as a separate entity, both in terms of efficient organization and scientific advances. However, I think there are real dangers that may counter these apparent advantages. Many cooperative groups are very large and require considerable funds so that there are problems in organization which can severely affect the quality and cost-effectiveness of research. Also, the sheer momentum of such groups may mean that trials continue to be undertaken in each specific disease regardless of whether there are any really good new ideas for improving therapy. As for multi-centre trials in general I feel one should not be overwhelmed by the scale of operation and an independent perspective is needed to assess the quality of research, both in organization and scientific merit.

The Pharmaceutical Industry

The way in which a pharmaceutical company organizes its large-scale clinical trial research programme for a new drug is often quite different from the type of multi-centre trial described above. One basic requirement in getting a drug approved for marketing for a common disease (e.g. rheumatoid arthritis, depression) is that it should be evaluated in phase III trials on a large number of patients. This cannot normally be achieved in any single trial, no matter how many centres participate and hence *the usual practice is to arrange for many different trials of a similar nature to be undertaken in different centres.* Each clinical investigator responsible for one such trial is able to evaluate and publish his results, with or without company assistance. As mentioned in section 9.3, each individual trial will often be very small such that when studied by itself it is hard to reach reliable conclusions.

However, the purpose of the pharmaceutical company is to combine all the results from these trials into one package of evidence to be presented to the regulatory bodies, such as the US Food and Drug Administration or the UK Committee on Safety of Medicines, in order to obtain approval to market the drug.

One advantage in this approach is that each investigator has the motivation to do a well-controlled trial which is publishable and recognized as his work. The disadvantage is that too many small trials scattered across the literature clearly make it difficult for other clinicians to evaluate the drug. However, another problem I see is the potential danger that a company could in theory select a rather unrepresentative collection of trials as its evidence.

For instance, it may turn out that some trials which fail to show adequate benefit for the new drug are not considered sufficiently interesting to merit publication by the investigating clinician, so that the published evidence is biassed in favour of the drug. One hopes that the pharmaceutical companies would still include such unpublished studies in their total evidence, but there is no guarantee that this is the case.

However, the system of multiple single-centre trials for a new drug may often be the only sensible way for pharmaceutical companies to proceed with a meaningful clinical research programme. Thus, to remain realistic I do not have any radical suggestions for changing the system. One possible improvement might be for pharmaceutical companies to maintain a register of *all* the trials undertaken for a given drug so that evidence to regulatory bodies is always based on the totality of research and not a selected sample of trials.

9.5 THE NUMBER OF TREATMENTS AND FACTORIAL DESIGNS

When a clinical trial is being proposed it is not uncommon to find that there are a substantial number of potential treatments that it is reasonable to consider. For instance, as regards adjuvant chemotherapy for primary breast cancer the promising improvements shown in the trials by Fisher *et al.* (1977) and Bonadonna *et al.* (1977) on two specific drug regimens have meant that anyone planning a subsequent trial has a glut of possible drug treatments to choose from, each of which might be just as effective.

However, one major problem is to avoid having too many treatments, since the power to detect treatment differences essentially depends on *the number of patients per treatment*, not the total number of patients in the trial. Since most trials experience difficulty in getting enough patients, one commonsense rule is to *avoid having more than two treatments* unless one is confident that sufficient patients per treatment can be obtained with three or more treatments.

Of course, there are exceptions to this rule. For instance, in advanced lung cancer there is no really effective chemotherapy but there are many new drugs which are worth trying. In randomized phase II trials one does not need a particularly large number of patients to evaluate each drug and with cancer cooperative groups there is no shortage of patients for such a common cancer. Hence, it is feasible to run a trial with say four new treatments which could accrue enough patients in a year. However, if the same sort of trial were planned in a single cancer centre one would have to argue against having so many treatments since the accrual rate could not justify it.

It can be frustrating to investigators with several therapeutic ideas to find themselves forced to condense them down to a two-treatment comparison, but the alternative of a multi-treatment trial, although scientifically and clinically sensible, can be an expensive mistake without enough patients.

In this situation, one needs to realize that any single trial should not be considered in isolation. The accumulation of knowledge about treatment of a given disease is usually obtained from a large number of trials taking place all over the world. Thus, anyone planning a trial must consider it in the broader context and see how that trial can best advance overall knowledge. Whereas initially one may think of the next trial as *the* means of answering all outstanding therapeutic problems, one will inevitably have to accept that in reality most trials need to answer just one question: Is new treatment A an improvement on standard treatment B?

Factorial Designs

Having presented this somewhat pessimistic outlook on number of treatments, I would now like to discuss one approach, the factorial design, which can sometimes be used to make two or more different therapeutic comparisons in the same trial without increasing the required number of patients.

For instance, Truelove (1960) describes a factorial therapeutic trial in chronic duodenal ulcer, which had three different types of treatments to evaluate:

S: stilboestrol 0.5 mg b.d.
P: phenobarbitone 65 mg b.d.
D: the Sippy diet (milk products at frequent intervals)

The conventional approach would have been to randomize patients to receive one or other of these treatments, perhaps with a randomized untreated control group as well. Instead, it was realized one could allow some patients to receive combinations of two or all these treatments. Hence, the trial was designed so that patients were randomized to receive one of the following eight treatment combinations:

S + P + D	S
S + P	P
S + D	D
P + D	or no treatment.

A total of 80 patients were entered in random permuted blocks of 8, so that each of the eight treatments was allocated once in each block of eight patients (see section 5.2).

The main advantage of such a factorial design is that each type of treatment (e.g. stilboestrol) is given to half the patients whereas in the conventional trial only a quarter of patients would be on any one treatment. Hence, the value of stilboestrol could be assessed by comparing the 40 patients on S, S + P, S + D or S + P + D with the 40 patients on no treatment, P, D or P + D.

In fact there were 1/40 clinical relapses within six months for such stilboestrol patients compared with 12/40 not on stilboestrol, a highly significant difference. Similar relapse comparisons for phenobarbitone versus no phenobarbitone and Sippy diet versus no Sippy diet showed no evidence of any difference.

Another advantage in a factorial design is that one can study whether any combinations of treatments are particularly effective or notably ineffective. For instance, did stilboestrol and phenobarbitone produce a better response than could be expected from the separate effects of stilboestrol alone or phenobarbitone alone. Of course, answers to such more detailed issues (commonly called treatment interactions) require large numbers of patients, which might explain why they were not studied in this trial. Cochran and Cox (1957, chapter 5) provide more extensive explanations of the design and analysis of factorial experiments.

The Canadian Cooperative Study Group (1978) describe another factorial trial to study the effects of aspirin (A) and sulfinpyrazone (S) in threatened stroke. 585 patients were randomized to one of four regimens: neither drug, A, S or A + S. To ensure that the trial was double-blind a placebo tablet was given for those not receiving S and a placebo capsule for those not receiving A. Those receiving neither drug were given both placebos.

The results of this trial illustrate one problem that can arise in interpreting a factorial design. The main outcome concerns the numbers (and percentages) of patients on each treatment experiencing stroke or death which were as follows:

Neither drug (N) 30/139 = 22 %   Sulfinpyrazone (S) 38/156 = 24 %
    Aspirin (A) 26/144 = 18 %   Both (A + S) 20/146 = 14 %

There appears substantial variation in the failure rates on different treatments. However, pairwise comparison of percentage failures on different regimens using χ^2 tests is not particularly helpful: the only significant difference between treatments was for A + S versus S alone ($P < 0.05$). But can one really recommend the combination of aspirin and sulfinpyrazone given that sulfinpyrazone alone had such a high failure rate? As mentioned in section 14.3, such multiple pairwise comparisons using significance tests can lead to awkward incompatibilities and hence are not generally to be advised. In this trial the authors decided to adopt an analysis based on the original factorial design. This is statistically somewhat complicated: to use statistical jargon, it is an analysis of survival data (i.e. time to stroke or death) using the logrank life-table method (as described in section 14.1) with significance tests for interaction between treatments (i.e. synergism or antagonism between the two drugs) and for the main effects of aspirin and sulfinpyrazone. The only interesting result here is that the main effect for aspirin was statistically significant and was estimated as a 31 % reduction in risk of stroke or death for aspirin as compared with no aspirin. The authors go on to show that this apparent benefit from aspirin showed up for men, but not women. However, their conclusion that aspirin is an efficacious drug for men with threatened stroke lacks some authority, given that the difference for men of 'aspirin alone' versus 'neither drug' was not statistically significant.

Overall, I would support the argument of Peto (1978) that *factorial designs have been much underutilized in clinical trials*. Of course, in many situations it would be practically infeasible to give some patients a combination of treatments either because of excessive toxicity, clinical impossibility or administrative complexity. An interesting example concerning such practical assessment is the MRC mild hypertension trial already mentioned in section 9.4. One suggestion was to have 1/3 of all patients randomly assigned to receive a daily dose of 300 mg aspirin in addition to the randomization to placebo or antihypertensive drug in the current protocol. Such a factorial design would mean that 1/3 of patients would receive no active treatment, 1/6 aspirin alone, 1/3 antihypertensive drug alone and 1/6 the combination. Such a proposal would have been scientifically efficient in enabling the effect on cardiovascular morbidity and mortality of both aspirin and antihypertensive agents to be explored without requiring any more patients than the current 'antihypertensive alone' design. However, this proposal really came too late and was not accepted since the trial had already been started and the administrative complications and risks of adding in an extra treatment were not to be underestimated. This illustrates that the scientific benefit of such designs must be balanced against the increase in organization required and the fact that any intervention in a smoothly running large multi-centre trial is not to be taken lightly.

CHAPTER 10

Monitoring Trial Progress

In most clinical trials patients are entered one at a time, so that their responses to treatment are also observed sequentially. In this chapter we consider the use of such accumulating information while a trial is still in progress and section 10.1 discusses the value of interim looks at data. Section 10.2 is concerned with the assessment of interim results to see if there is any evidence of treatment differences, with emphasis on practical issues. Section 10.3 deals with the problem of deciding when to stop a trial in the presence of a treatment difference and considers the use of repeated significance testing as a sensible stopping rule. Section 10.4 describes sequential methods for continuous monitoring of treatment differences, which have occasionally been used as a stopping rule.

10.1 REASONS FOR MONITORING

For trial organizers one of the most fascinating stages in a clinical trial is when evaluations of patient response begin to accumulate. After all the hard work involved in planning a study and getting it underway, investigators may be expected to display a certain degree of uncontrolled enthusiasm in poring over early results. However, any uncoordinated sifting through data is liable to present a somewhat confused picture of what is going on and hence it is advisable at a very early stage to plan how to handle trial results as they materialize. First, let us consider the reasons for monitoring trial progress:

(1) Protocol Compliance

One essential aspect is to check that investigators are following the trial protocol, and prompt inspection of each patient's results provides an immediate awareness of any deviations from intended procedure. This enables one to inform an investigator of such observed deviations thus reinforcing the need for protocol compliance. If early results indicate some general difficulties with compliance it may be necessary to make alterations to the protocol.

(2) Adverse Effects

One needs to monitor the reporting of side-effects, particularly severe toxic reactions to a new therapy, so that prompt action can be taken. Investigators need to be warned to look out for such events in future patients. Also, it may be necessary to define dose modifications. With a new therapy, it is advisable to report immediately any unusual toxic events rather than wait for case records to be completed.

(3) Data Processing

One common mistake is to let the patient records pile up for a while so that there is no organized check on trial progress in the early stages. It is better to organize the processing of data ready for statistical analysis from the very beginning: such prompt attention is needed to pick up any errors, inconsistencies or missing items on forms and have them corrected in time. Handling of data at the trial centre, whether on computer or otherwise, should be efficient enough to avoid undue delay when statistical analysis is required. Further details on data management are given in chapter 11.

(4) General Information

In order to maintain interest and to satisfy the natural curiosity amongst investigators one may wish to provide some general results on how the trial is progressing. Basic pretreatment information such as the numbers of patients and their distribution by prognostic factors should be made available. Also, overall data on patient response and follow-up for all treatments combined can provide a useful view of how the trial is proceeding.

(5) Treatment Comparisons

The main purpose in analysing interim results is to look for treatment differences which are sufficiently convincing and important to stop or change the trial. Although (1) to (4) above are important aspects of monitoring trial progress, they can generally be dealt with by common sense and efficient administration. However, the handling of treatment comparisons while a trial is still in progress poses some tricky problems, in medical ethics, practical organization and statistical analysis. Hence the remainder of this chapter focusses on those interim analyses of clinical trial data which are performed in order to look for possible treatment differences.

10.2 INTERIM ANALYSES

The primary reason for monitoring trial data for treatment differences is the ethical concern to avoid any patient in the trial receiving a treatment known to be inferior. In addition, one wishes to be efficient in the sense of avoiding undue prolongation of a trial once the main treatment comparisons are reasonably clear-cut. Hence *the assessment of interim treatment differences is of crucial importance if clinical trials are to be ethically acceptable.*

When undertaking analyses of interim data while a trial is still in progress there are two problem areas to consider: *how to organize* the handling of such interim results in the best interests of the trial as a whole and *how to interpret* and act upon any treatment differences allowing for the fact that one is taking repeated looks at the accumulating data. In this section, I will discuss nine principal issues which address both the organizational and interpretive aspects:

(1) Measures of Patient Response

One should decide in advance which patient outcomes are to be of value in interim comparisons. Once the trial is finished one may have a large number of outcome variables, but in interim analyses one should use only a limited number of major variables, since otherwise one has a problem in interpreting multiple comparisons. Indeed, it is advisable to concentrate on just one main treatment comparison for which a formal 'stopping rule' may be defined. Other treatment comparisons may then be used as a more informal check on the consistency of any apparent treatment difference.

Long-term measures of treatment effect such as patient survival, although ultimately very important, may be of no use in interim analyses. For instance, in cancer chemotherapy trials tumour shrinkage and drug toxicity give a quicker indication of potential treatment differences.

(2) Data Preparation

It is important that any interim analyses be based on data which are correct, complete and up-to-date. One should ensure that any delays and errors in the processing of patient evaluation forms are never so great as to distort the validity of any analysis. For instance, one needs to guard against the problem of 'bad news coming first'; investigators can return forms quickly for patients who fare badly and are taken off study early, whereas forms for patients who respond well and stay on treatment may not be returned for some time. Hence, intensive preparation may be needed prior to each analysis, especially for multi-centre trials. This could involve special requests to all investigators to complete interim evaluation forms on all patients who have been in the trial for a specified minimal period.

(3) Feasibility of Interim Analyses

There are three situations which can make interim analyses of little value. Firstly, interim analyses are liable to be of purely academic interest if a trial is of inadequate size, i.e. patient accrual is so slow that one will have difficulty in detecting clinically relevant treatment differences even when the trial is completed. Secondly, if the trial is badly organized interim analyses may be impractical or based on such biassed incomplete data as to be misleading. Thirdly, if the time lag between patient entry and observance of patient outcome is long relative to the total period of patient accrual then there will be insufficient data for any interim analyses to be worthwhile, especially if treatment is of short duration. For example, in a trial of simple versus radical mastectomy patient accrual may be completed before adequate data on disease-free interval or survival are available.

(4) The Decision-Making Process

The decision to stop or alter a trial should not be considered a purely statistical exercise. The magnitude and statistical significance of treatment differences must be considered in the light of other current knowledge, practical aspects of therapy (e.g. ease of administration, acceptability and cost), the degree of enthusiasm for the trial and future research ideas. Thus, the ultimate decision will be subjective though the statistical evidence, including the guideline of a formal stopping rule, should be a primary factor.

One does need clear definition of who is responsible for such decisions, e.g. a trial monitoring committee in multi-centre trials, so that interim analyses can lead to prompt action if necessary.

(5) Confidentiality of Interim Results

The circulation of interim results to a wide audience may have an undesirable effect on the future progress of a clinical trial. For instance, early interim results shown to an investigator could change his outlook and future participation. If there is little difference between treatments he may lose interest. However, a more serious situation arises if there are interesting but non-significant treatment differences. An investigator might then wish to drop out of the trial in the premature belief that there is a genuine treatment difference or he may continue half-heartedly with perhaps an increased risk of him adapting the supposedly inferior treatment, making premature withdrawals or worse still not accepting randomization. Undoubtedly, such interim knowledge does pose an ethical dilemma. Even if an investigator wisely avoids any over-reaction to early suggestions in the data of a possible treatment difference, it can still become difficult for him to obtain informed patient consent and to randomize the next patient.

Hence, some secrecy over interim results is advisable. For instance, in a multi-centre trial a monitoring committee may be supplied with full interim results to be interpreted confidentially while each investigator entering patients is not provided with data on treatment comparisons. Instead one could give to investigators background information on accrual, prognostic factors and overall outcome for all treatments combined with an assurance that no significant differences have arisen as yet.

An additional problem to avoid is the premature publication of interim results, either at scientific meetings or in a journal, while a trial is still in progress. This practice is liable to leave the whole medical community prejudiced towards one's interim conclusions and it is hard to correct for this with later publication. For instance, I know of one trial where an early significant treatment difference was published quickly, but when subsequent follow-up did not substantiate this finding considerable delay arose in publishing such a negative rebuttal of the preliminary finding.

(6) The Extent of Each Analysis

One should avoid making any interim analyses too elaborate, since they serve the limited objective of deciding whether a trial should continue in its present form and hence are of only passing interest. Often the data analyst is responsible for many studies and it would be inappropriate to devote a lot of time to such transient data. Indeed, interim analyses need only contain crude treatment comparisons on major end-points unless the results approach statistical significance, in which case some allowance for key prognostic factors may be worthwhile.

(7) Frequency of Analysis

Many of the statistical methods of sequential analysis for clinical trials (see section 10.4) are based on the premise that the accumulating data can be monitored continuously and any decision to stop the trial applied immediately. In practice such intensive surveillance and instant action are rarely feasible and instead it is usually more efficient and reliable to make a special effort to analyse interim results at periodic intervals, say every few months. The results of each analysis can be arranged to coincide with a meeting of trial organizers so that any necessary action can follow promptly. The time intervals between analyses depend on the rate of patient accrual, the time lag between entry and response evaluation and the practical arrangements for trial meetings. Also, as is shown in section 10.3, the statistical properties associated with repeated examination of accumulating data indicate that there is little advantage to be gained from carrying out a large number of interim analyses.

(8) Statistical Stopping Rules

One needs to decide in advance what is sufficiently strong evidence of a treatment difference to merit stopping the trial. Not only the magnitude of treatment difference must be considered but also the statistical significance. For instance, suppose a trial had 30% of patients responding on one treatment and 50% responding on the other. In most diseases this would be a highly relevant clinical finding if the 20% treatment difference was genuine. However, if there were only 10 patients on each treatment (i.e. 3/10 versus 5/10 responders) it would be very unwise to stop the trial: the difference would not be convincing since even if the treatments were truly equally effective such a difference is quite likely to occur by chance. At the other extreme, if there were 1000 patients on each treatment no-one would seriously dispute the genuineness of the 20% difference (provided the trial was properly designed) and it would be very unethical to continue the trial. Therefore, there comes some intermediate position where the size of trial becomes large enough for there to be sufficient evidence of a treatment difference. *Significance tests are a useful stopping criterion* whereby one can agree in advance that the trial should be stopped if the treatment difference for some major measure of patient outcome becomes statistically significant at some prearranged level, say $P < 0.01$.

The main problem with significance testing in interim analysis is that, even if the treatments are really equally effective, the more often one analyses accumulating data the greater the chance of eventually detecting a treatment difference significant at say the 5% level. That is, the type I error (as referred to in section 9.1) may be considerably increased and this fact will tend to contribute to the excess of false-positive findings in the clinical trial literature. Hence, for a sequence of interim analyses one must set a more stringent significance level than $P < 0.05$. This point is discussed further in section 10.3 but the following simple rule may suffice in many trials: *if one anticipates no more than 10 interim analyses and there is one main response variable, one can adopt $P < 0.01$ as the criterion for stopping the trial*, since the overall type I error (i.e. probability of a false-positive result) will not exceed 0.05.

(9) The Size of a Trial

The determination of trial size as described in section 9.1 was based on a fixed number of patients and this might appear rather inappropriate if one intends to apply a stopping rule to interim analyses. However, this contradiction between fixed design and flexible stopping in analysis is not of great practical import. The former is only intended to give a desired order of magnitude, not a precise target. In the presence of interim analyses one can look upon this fixed estimate as a maximum size of trial to be achieved if the trial does not stop early. In order to preserve the statistical properties (i.e. overall type I and type II errors) one then needs to increase this estimate slightly.

10.3 REPEATED SIGNIFICANCE TESTING: GROUP SEQUENTIAL DESIGNS

This section is concerned with precisely how to define a stopping rule for a clinical trial with interim analyses. The formulation is based on *repeated significance tests* and is sometimes called a *group sequential design*. All results are in terms of two-sided significance, though the possibility of one-sided tests is discussed in the last part of this section.

Risk of False-positive

First I return to the problem that repeated use of significance tests on accumulating data tends to increase the overall significance level, that is the probability of at least one significant difference when the treatments are really the same. Armitage *et al.* (1969) first tackled this problem and table 10.1 shows their numerical results. For instance, if one carries out 10 interim analyses the chances of at least one analysis showing a treatment difference significant at the 5% level increases to 0.19 even if the treatments are truly equally effective: that is, the overall type I error, or risk of a false-positive finding, would be increased to nearly 1 in 5 if one were to use $P < 0.05$ as a stopping criterion. Indeed, in a large trial if one analyses the data often enough one can expect to get $P < 0.05$ eventually regardless of whether there is a genuine treatment difference.

Table 10.1. Repeated significance tests on accumulating data*

No. of repeated tests at the 5% level	Overall significance level
1	0.05
2	0.08
3	0.11
4	0.13
5	0.14
10	0.19
20	0.25
50	0.32
100	0.37
1000	0.53
∞	1.0

* For two treatments, a normal response with known variance and equally spaced analyses, though broadly similar results for other types of data.

Nominal Significance Levels

The way round this problem is to choose a more stringent *nominal significance level* for each repeated test, so that the overall significance level is kept at some reasonable value, say 0.05 or 0.01. McPherson (1974) and Pocock (1978) discuss this problem and table 10.2 shows the required nominal significance levels for various numbers of repeated tests and for overall type I error = 0.05 or 0.01. The idea is that one decides in advance what is the anticipated maximum number of interim analyses and accordingly one makes the nominal significance level smaller. For instance, with at most 10 analyses and overall type I error = 0.05, one adopts $P < 0.0106$ as the stopping rule at each analysis for a treatment difference. In practice, this can be conveniently rounded to $P < 0.01$.

Table 10.2. Nominal significance level* required for repeated two-sided significance testing with overall significance level $\alpha = 0.05$ or 0.01 and various values of N, the maximum number of tests

N	$\alpha = 0.05$	$\alpha = 0.01$
2	0.029	0.0056
3	0.022	0.0041
4	0.018	0.0033
5	0.016	0.0028
10	0.0106	0.0018
15	0.0086	0.0015
20	0.0075	0.0013

* These nominal levels are exactly true for a normally distributed response with known variance, but are also a good approximation for many other types of data (see Pocock, 1977a).

With fewer interim analyses, say a maximum of three, the stopping rule is less stringent with $P < 0.022$ (perhaps rounded to $P < 0.02$) an indication of sufficient evidence of a treatment difference.

One should also consider whether an overall type I error $\alpha = 0.05$ is sufficiently small when considering a stopping rule. There are two situations where $\alpha = 0.01$ may be more appropriate:

(1) If a trial is unique in that its findings are unlikely to be replicated in future research, e.g. the clofibrate trial mentioned in section 9.1.
(2) If there is more than one patient outcome used in interim analyses and a stopping rule is applied to each outcome. However, one possibility would be to have one principal outcome with a stopping rule having $\alpha = 0.05$ and have other lesser outcomes with $\alpha = 0.01$.

It has been suggested that a very stringent stopping criterion say $P < 0.001$ be used, on the basis that no matter how often one performs interim analyses the overall type I error will remain reasonably small. It also means that the final analysis, if the trial is not stopped early, can be interpreted using standard significance tests without any serious need to allow for earlier repeated testing. However, such a stopping rule raises the ethical problem that a trial with a genuine treatment difference will continue for longer relative to the other rules mentioned above (see Pocock, 1982).

An Example

A trial in non-Hodgkins lymphoma compared two drug combinations CP (cytoxan-prednisone) and CVP (cytoxan-vincristine-prednisone) and the main criterion of response was tumour shrinkage. Patient accrual lasted over two years and around 120–130 patients were entered. It seems reasonable to plan for five interim analyses, i.e. one after about every 25 patients were entered. The consequent results are shown in table 10.3.

Table 10.3. Interim analyses for a trial in non-Hodgkins lymphoma

| | Response rates | | χ^2 (without continuity | |
	CP	CVP	correction)	
Analysis 1	3/14	5/11	1.63	
Analysis 2	11/27	13/24	0.92	
Analysis 3	18/40	17/36	0.04	
Analysis 4	18/54	24/48	3.25	$0.05 < P < 0.1$
Analysis 5	23/67	31/59	4.25	$0.016 < P < 0.05$

In the early stages of any trial the response rates can fluctuate wildly and one needs to avoid any over-reaction to such early results on small numbers of patients. For instance, here the first three responses occurred on CVP but by the time of first analysis the situation had settled down and the chi-squared test showed no significant treatment difference. By the fourth analysis the results began to look interesting but still there was insufficient evidence to stop the trial. On the final analysis, when the trial was finished anyway, the chi-squared test gave $P = 0.04$ which strictly speaking is not statistically significant being greater than the nominal level of 0.016 for $N = 5$ analyses. Of course, a totally negative interpretation would not be appropriate. From these data alone one could infer that the superiority of CVP is interesting but inconclusive. However, further data on response duration and survival eventually clarified that CVP did appear to be a better therapy.

Delayed Response

In principle, this example illustrates the ease with which group sequential methods may be applied. However, in practice one needs to allow for some time lapse between patient entry and the observation of response. In the above cancer trial it could take several weeks to observe a response. One solution is to fix a time, say three months in this case, to observe whether response occurs in each patient. Then interim analysis after each group of patients can take place three months after the last patient entry in the group. This unavoidable delay means that further patients will have entered the trial, and this raises complications if the nominal significance level is reached. If stopping the trial means that all patients still receiving the 'inferior' treatment are taken off it instantly then there will be no further direct data on treatment comparison and the conclusion remains unaltered. However, if it is thought appropriate for patients entered but not evaluated to continue their current treatment, there will be further response data which could alter the final treatment comparison. This can lead to contradictions if the results become less significant (as is likely to occur), but should not be a serious problem unless the delay to observe response is unduly long.

In this respect, there may be administrative delay in getting the observed response reported for inclusion in analysis. In multi-centre trials there is a danger that such delays could be a matter of months, in which case any stopping rule becomes greatly delayed and virtually irrelevant. For instance, the above example showed how one would have liked to conduct the ongoing analysis, whereas in practice the delays were such that final response data were not analysed until over a year after the last patient was entered. Thus, improvements in the feedback and processing of response data are a first priority before undertaking interim analysis.

Follow-up Studies and Survival Data

In many trials for chronic disease, the main measure of patient outcome is some time-related event: either time to death or recurrence of disease. Such treatment comparisons require methods of survival data analysis, as discussed in section 14.2. Here, I will consider a stopping rule for survival data based on the logrank test.

The group sequential methods described so far in this section require interim analyses at equally spaced numbers of patients, whereas for the logrank test it is more appropriate, and statistically equivalent, to *analyse at equally spaced numbers of deaths*. With some knowledge of the anticipated survival pattern and accrual rate, one can choose the number of such survival analyses (a maximum of, say, five will often suffice) and the number of deaths between analyses, whence the nominal significance levels in table 10.2 are applicable.

This approach should allow a reasonable time lapse between the start of the trial and the first analysis, but the time between analyses becomes shorter as more patients are entered and deaths occur more frequently. Hence, one avoids any unduly premature survival analyses based on very few deaths.

A significant treatment difference in interim survival analysis may just lead to cessation of patient entry but if treatment is continuous (e.g. long-term chemotherapy) the use of the inferior treatment may also cease, so that the whole trial is ended. In this latter case, no further data will be added to one's survival analysis, except as a result of administrative delay, but in the former case (e.g. in surgical trials) statistical interpretation will be more difficult as further survival follow-up continues. This problem of a stopping rule being followed by further data has not been satisfactorily resolved. One *ad hoc* approach is a conventional statistical analysis of the final data with informal acknowledgement that a stopping rule has been used. Canner (1977) and Gail *et al.* (1982) provide more theoretical descriptions of group sequential survival analysis.

Group Sequential Designs

Having defined the basic rules for repeated significance testing, let us now consider how they can be formulated into the design of a clinical trial, particularly as regards its required size. The two features to be decided at the start of such a group sequential trial are:

(1) How many significance tests should there be, i.e. what is the maximum number of interim analyses (or groups)?
(2) How many patients should be evaluated between successive analyses, i.e. what should be the size of each group?

The following theoretical argument explains how these issues may be answered by using power calculations. The non-statistical reader may prefer to skip to the next subsection.

Consider a trial with two treatments, $2n$ patients per group (n per treatment) and a maximum of N groups. This makes the maximum size of trial $= 2nN$ patients.

The method of determining the operating characteristics of designs with a variety of values for n and N is described by Pocock (1977a). Here we consider the simplest theoretical case of two treatments A and B for each of which we have a normally distributed response with means μ_A, μ_B and known variance σ^2. The conventional power calculation (as previously defined in section 9.1) here requires specification of an overall significance level α and power $1 - \beta$ for a specific alternative hypothesis $\mu_A - \mu_B = \delta$. Tables derived by numerical integration enable the required value of n for any given N to be determined, but for limitations of space let us here just consider results for $\alpha = 0.05$ and $1 - \beta = 0.9$ presented in table 10.4. Remember that the required nominal significance levels for any choice of N are to be found in table 10.2. Clearly, as the number of groups N increases, the number per group $2n$ decreases and the maximum number of patients $2nN$ increases.

Table 10.4. Group sequential designs for a normal response with known variance σ^2, overall significance level $\alpha = 0.05$ and power $1 - \beta = 0.9$ under H_A: $\mu_A - \mu_B = \delta$

Maximum no. of groups (N)	Required no. of patients per group ($2n$)	Maximum no. of patients ($2nN$)	Average no. of patients to termination of trial under H_A
1	42.04	42.04	42.04
2	23.12	46.24	32.60
3	16.11	48.33	30.29
4	12.43 $\times \dfrac{\sigma^2}{\delta^2}$	49.72 $\times \dfrac{\sigma^2}{\delta^2}$	29.33 $\times \dfrac{\sigma^2}{\delta^2}$
5	10.14	50.70	28.80
10	5.35	53.50	28.03
20	2.79	55.80	27.98

This means that the larger is N for a given α and β, the longer the trial will take to complete if the null hypothesis of no treatment difference appears to be true. Table 10.4 shows that in this situation 20% more patients will be needed for a design with $N = 5$ compared to a 'one-look' trial ($N = 1$).

However, this is compensated by the most important feature in a group sequential design, which is the extent to which it enables early termination of trial when the alternative hypothesis is true. This is indicated in the last column of table 10.4 by the average sample size. Evidently the greatest reduction is achieved by using a two-group design instead of a one-group (i.e. fixed sample size) design and there is virtually no extra reduction with more than five groups. This applies to any trial design based on $\alpha = 0.05$ and $1 - \beta = 0.9$, and similar examples could be evaluated for other values of α and β.

How Many Interim Analyses?

The above theoretical results indicate that there is little statistical advantage in having a large number of repeated significance tests. As a general rule, *it would seem sensible to plan on a maximum of five interim analyses.* The only advantage in having more analyses would be if it was feasible that an extremely large treatment difference could occur very early on in a trial, but in most trials one's prior knowledge and experience would indicate this to be very unlikely, especially in chronic diseases. McPherson (1982) provides further discussion and statistical modelling for this problem.

Many trials are currently undertaken without interim analyses. Such investigators should be encouraged to consider having just two analyses, one halfway through the trial and the other at the end. There can still be a major reduction in the number of patients exposed to an inferior treatment, since for such a trial with sufficient overall power there is a reasonable chance of being able to stop halfway through.

Varying Nominal Significance Levels

The methods described so far have been based on repeated significance testing at a constant nominal level. Such designs are primarily chosen for practical convenience and ease of comprehension, so that they have no obvious claims to optimality. Thus, it is relevant to consider whether there is any statistical advantage in varying the nominal significance levels for stopping a trial. For instance, should one have more stringent significance levels (say $P < 0.001$) early on in the trial and have levels nearer to 0.05 at later analyses?

There is no single answer to this question, but Pocock (1982) has produced the following results for a trial with five interim analyses. Consider again the theoretical model of a two-treatment trial with a normal response having known variance. Let $N = 5$ repeated significance tests and consider overall type I error $\alpha = 0.05$, as usual. Then, for a fixed overall power $1 - \beta$ for a certain alternative hypothesis H_A one can determine numerically the 'optimal' choice of nominal significance levels. That is, given N, α, β and H_A one can choose varying nominal significance levels to minimize the average number of patients when H_A is true, as shown in table 10.5.

For power $1 - \beta = 0.5$ this 'optimal design' has a marked increase in nominal levels from the first to the last analysis, similar to a proposed design of O'Brien and Fleming (1979). This indicates that for a trial with low power to detect a clinically relevant treatment difference, one should have a very stringent stopping rule for early interim analyses, e.g. $P < 0.0002$ at the first of five analyses. Power $1 - \beta = 0.5$ should generally be considered too low so that such designs are not to be recommended, but if one is forced into a trial of inadequate size, constant nominal significance levels may not be appropriate. A suitable compromise might be to choose a moderate variation in nominal levels, e.g. $P < 0.003$ for the first analysis increasing to $P < 0.03$ in the final analysis (the optimal design for $1 - \beta = 0.75$).

Table 10.5. 'Optimal' choice of nominal significance levels for group sequential designs with $N = 5$ interim analyses, $\alpha = 0.05$ and $1 - \beta = 0.5, 0.75, 0.9$ or 0.95

| Power $1 - \beta$ | Nominal significance levels | | | | |
	1st analysis	2nd analysis	3rd analysis	4th analysis	5th analysis
0.5	0.0002	0.004	0.010	0.018	0.042
0.75	0.003	0.011	0.016	0.019	0.031
0.9	0.010	0.017	0.017	0.017	0.021
0.95	0.015	0.016	0.016	0.016	0.017

For power $1 - \beta = 0.9$ or 0.95 the optimal set of nominal levels is nearly constant. Hence, for all practical purposes, if a trial is sufficiently large to have good power to detect clinically relevant treatment differences a stopping rule based on repeated significance testing at constant levels seems quite sensible.

Failure to Plan a Stopping Rule

Unfortunately, many investigators do not prepare in advance any formal stopping criterion. If they then undertake *ad hoc* interim analyses it is much more difficult to know what decisions to make when a treatment difference begins to show. For instance, Epstein *et al.* (1981) describe a trial of D-penicillamine versus placebo for primary biliary cirrhosis where patient survival was the main concern. During the summer of 1980 the organizers became aware of an increasing number of deaths in the control group so that they decided to see if the treatment difference was significant. There were 8/23 deaths on placebo compared with 2/37 on D-penicillamine. The trial was deliberately designed to have a lower proportion randomized to placebo (see section 5.4). A quick calculation ignoring follow-up times gave $\chi^2 = 8.81$, $P < 0.01$ and this level of significance was soon confirmed by a logrank test.

The problem was in deciding how to allow for the fact that the investigators had chosen to analyse the data because the results were getting interesting. Clearly, selective timing of analyses greatly increases the chance of a significant difference, whether true or false. If the results had only just been significant the decision over whether to stop the trial or not would have been very difficult, especially as this was a unique trial in a rare disease which was unlikely to be replicated elsewhere. However, since the difference was highly significant it seemed sensible to recommend that the trial be stopped. By the time of publication, the numbers of deaths were 10/23 on placebo, 5/37 on D-penicillamine. This slight reduction in the magnitude and significance of the difference is to be expected if more data are obtained after an initial positive finding.

Hence, *it is advisable to plan in advance when interim analyses should occur* and in particular the timing of analysis should not be influenced by the response data themselves. One can then ensure that statistical stopping rules provide a truly objective basis for the organizers' decisions.

One-sided Testing and Other Extensions

This section has dealt with two-sided significance testing as a stopping rule. In general I consider this more appropriate than one-sided testing, since treatment differences in either direction are usually relevant. However, on occasions when one is only interested in whether a new treatment does better than a standard treatment (i.e. it is inconceivable that it could do worse) then one-sided testing may be appropriate. Demets and Ware (1980) have reformulated group sequential methods for the one-sided case.

Another possibility is for a 'skew' design in which a less-stringent stopping rule is used if the new treatment appears worse than the standard, but this has not been evaluated theoretically for group sequential designs. However, simple rules could be devised: e.g. $P < 0.01$ for new treatment better than standard but $P < 0.05$ for new worse than standard. The high overall type I error for the latter would not be so important, since a new treatment of equal effectiveness to the standard may be of little interest anyway.

A further development would be to have early stopping rules for a negative result. There is no real ethical concern here, but more a sense of efficiency in reducing the size of a trial with a negative conclusion. One simple conservative rule is to stop if a significant difference could not be reached whatever happens to the remaining patients, but further research in this area would be useful.

10.4 CONTINUOUS SEQUENTIAL DESIGNS

Historically, the statistical theory for stopping rules in clinical trials has been largely concerned with sequential designs for the continuous monitoring of treatment differences. The basic principle behind such designs is that after every additional patient on each treatment has been evaluated, some formal statistical rule is applied to the whole data so far to determine whether the trial should stop. Armitage (1975) provides a clear exposition of many such designs, so that I will not attempt to describe them in any detail.

Instead, I will focus on *sequential designs for 'paired preferences'* as an illustration of the general approach. The idea here is that one has two treatments (say A and B) and patients enter the trial in pairs, one on each treatment. After response is evaluated one determines according to prearranged criteria which patient in each pair responded better. As the trial proceeds one may accumulate a certain number of excess preferences for treatment A or B. One then needs to devise an appropriate stopping rule based on such data, as in the following example.

Suppose one wishes to be 95 % sure of detecting a treatment difference if one treatment were truly better in 75 % of pairs. Also, if the two treatments were equally effective, i.e. truly 50 % preferences to each, one wishes only a 5 % chance of falsely finding a treatment difference. These specifications amount to a type I error $\alpha = 0.05$ and type II error $\beta = 0.05$ for the alternative hypothesis that the proportion of A (or B) preferences $\theta = 0.75$. Armitage (1975) describes three main sequential plans for this problem and they are shown in figure 10.1.

Each plan is to be used as a diagram of the excess preferences for A or B plotted against the overall number of preferences, which is to be filled out sequentially as successive pairs of patients are evaluated. Each plan has upper, lower and middle boundaries. The trial stops as soon as the plot of trial results reaches one of these boundaries. If the upper boundary is reached first one has evidence that A is better, and similarly the lower boundary indicates B is better. If the middle boundary is reached one declares there is no evidence of a treatment difference.

Open sequential plans, such as in figure 10.1(a), were the first to be developed. They have the desirable property that they minimize the average number of patients before stopping when the alternative hypothesis ($\theta = 0.75$ in this case) is true. Unfortunately, as indicated by the parallel line boundaries, they have no finite maximum number of patients and the distribution of sample size is skew. This potentially very variable length of trial is not really acceptable when planning a clinical trial so that *closed sequential plans*, as in figure 10.1(b) and (c) are generally preferred. The restricted plan (b) has upper and lower boundaries almost identical to (a) but the middle wedge boundary is altered to ensure a finite maximum size of trial (62 pairs of patients in this case). Plan (c) is an extension of repeated significance testing (RST) to continuous data analysis and has slightly curved outer boundaries.

Acute Leukemia Group B (1963) describe the results of a trial in acute leukemia comparing 6-mercaptopurine (6-MP) and placebo, in which the restricted plan was used. Patients in disease remission were randomly assigned to 6-MP or placebo and their subsequent duration of remission noted. For the sequential plan, patients were formed into matched pairs, one on each treatment, from the same institution and with the same initial remission state (partial or complete). A paired preference was then shown by whichever patient

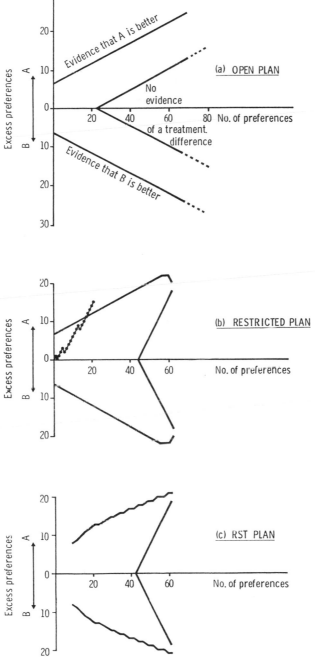

Fig. 10.1. Examples of sequential plans for paired preferences

had the longer remission duration. The results are plotted on figure 10.1(b) with A = 6-MP and B = placebo. The upper boundary was reached after 18 paired preferences (15 favouring 6-MP and 3 favouring placebo), evidence that duration of remission was longer on 6-MP.

This example, while successful in achieving a sensible decision to stop the trial early, also illustrates some of the problems in using continuous sequential designs. Since continuous analysis could not be linked to immediate decision making (the trial committee met every three months), three more pairs of patients were entered before the trial was stopped. Also, some randomized patients were not included in the sequential plan, presumably because they could not be formed into matched pairs.

In practice, continuous sequential designs have been applied to very few trials and hence it is relevant to consider some of their *theoretical limitations and logistic problems*:

(1) Pairing

Most sequential designs are for trials with two treatments and require that observations be made in pairs, one on each treatment. For within-patient comparisons (e.g. crossover trials, see chapter 8) there is a natural pairing of observations on the same patient, but for between-patient comparisons a more artificial pairing is required. Successive patients entering the trial may form a pair, the order of treatment allocation being at random. However, in many trials there are known prognostic factors affecting response so that one requires *matched pairs* of similar patients. Such pairing seems an unnatural restriction since it is not required by any other aspects of trial design and analysis. Also, if the trial is not double-blind the second in any pair has his treatment known in advance, and if matching is not complete there will be a certain waste of patient resources. Some recent theory in sequential methods (see Whitehead, 1982) does not require pairing and should increase the flexibility of continuous sequential designs.

(2) Types of Response

For trials in which each patient's response is simply some criterion 'success' or 'failure', the use of sequential methods is on a secure theoretical basis. However, the situation is more difficult for trials in which response is some measurable quantity. There exist sequential t tests, but these will prove unreliable if the data are not normally distributed. Such non-normality is less of a problem in the group sequential methods of section 10.3 since normal theory is more robust when applied to larger treatment groups. The sequential analysis of survival data is a recent development, with Jones and Whitehead (1979) deriving a sequential form of the logrank test.

(3) **Instant Evaluation**

Sequential designs generally make no allowance for the fact that patient evaluation is not achieved instantaneously. Not only does the observation of response take time (e.g. several weeks to observe tumour response in cancer chemotherapy trials) but there is often further delay by investigator and data centre before such results are added to the analysis. This means that sequential analysis is never quite 'on top of the data' since even if one reaches a stopping boundary there are usually further results 'in the pipeline'. For less-frequent interim analyses, the problem is partially overcome by making a special effort (e.g. reminders to investigators) in advance.

(4) **Constant Surveillance**

The essence of continuous sequential designs is that a constant vigil is maintained over the accumulating data. From a practical viewpoint this can pose an unnecessary burden on the trial participants and statistician. Actual decisions on stopping must be made by a meeting of the organizers and it is not easy to achieve prompt action based on sequential stopping rules.

(5) **Statistical Properties**

The purpose of any stopping rule is to try and reduce the number of patients exposed to any inferior treatment. Group sequential designs, as described in section 10.3, are an improvement on a fixed-size trial in that they do reduce the average number of patients to termination of a trial if a treatment difference exists. Now, to what extent can continuous sequential designs improve on this situation by allowing even earlier stopping? Pocock (1982) has compared group sequential and continuous sequential designs for one theoretical example of a normal response with known variance. In that instance, group sequential designs (say for five interim analyses) achieved on average almost as early a stopping rule as the continuous designs. Conversely, the latter required a larger maximum size of trial so that more patients were needed if there was no treatment difference.

It appears that continuous sequential designs may primarily be of value in the very early detection of extremely large treatment differences. However, in many trials it is more realistic to anticipate moderate improvements which may be more reliably established using a limited number of well-planned interim analyses.

CHAPTER 11

Forms and Data Management

One aspect of clinical trials which often receives inadequate attention is the recording and processing of patient data. The first fundamental is to design forms for recording information on each patient's evaluation and section 11.1 is devoted to this topic. The next requirement is to ensure efficient collection, checking and processing of all patient forms so that accurate data can be made available for statistical analysis. Section 11.2 deals with such issues of data management. The use of computers for processing of trial data and subsequent analysis is discussed in section 11.3.

11.1 FORM DESIGN

Decisions on what patient information to record in a clinical trial need to be stated in a study protocol (see sections 3.1 and 3.5). However, the accuracy and completeness of all such data are heavily dependent on the preparation of appropriate forms.

The design of good forms in clinical trials is often seen as a laborious and unattractive pursuit: trial organizers are anxious to get a trial underway and hence many trials are carried out with a woefully inadequate means of recording each patient's evaluation. Common problems are:

(1) too many data are collected on each patient
(2) the quality of recorded data often suffers as a consequence
(3) it is unclear precisely what information is required
(4) data are not recorded in a style suitable either for transfer to computer files or for statistical analysis.

My intention here is to elaborate on some of the principal issues to consider when designing forms. First, I will discuss the types of form required and then I will describe how to design such forms both as regards specific items and the general layout.

Types of Form

At the start of section 3.5 I classified patient evaluation into four categories and corresponding forms could be designed as follows:

Baseline assessment → on-study form

Principal ⎫
subsidiary ⎭ criteria of response → summary evaluation form

Other aspects of patient monitoring → flow sheets

Virtually every clinical trial requires an *on-study form*. In my experience, investigators have considerable difficulty in deciding what to include in such a form and are liable to produce a 'monster' form containing a large number of irrelevant questions. I recall one extreme case where I assisted in the design of a breast cancer on-study form. The first mistake was that there were too many collaborators involved in the form's design and secondly no-one seemed prepared to delete the unimportant questions. Some thought that the form provided an opportunity to collect epidemiological data for evaluating the natural history of breast cancer and so everyone's favourite questions seemed to get included. The end-result was four pages of close typing amounting to around 200 items of information for every patient. This all embracing approach to form design is ill-advised and nowadays I am more determined to ensure that only patient identification plus important baseline data on factors relevant to patient response get included on an on-study form.

As regards the specific content of an on-study form, information on personal characteristics and identification are relatively easy to obtain. Data on the patient's initial clinical condition and clinical history may present greater difficulty; a potentially complex clinical picture must be constrained into a series of specific requests for factual information so that consistent data recording takes place in a manner suitable for statistical analysis.

The recording of patient evaluation data once treatment is underway can be carried out in several different ways depending on the trial's structure. The above-mentioned approach, a *summary evaluation form* and *flow sheets*, is often realistic. For instance, in clinical trials of cytotoxic drugs for advanced cancer, flow sheets are used to record the patient's ongoing performance, the treatment received (including modifications), the results of biochemical tests, the incidence of side-effects and objective evaluation of the disease (tumour measurements, X-rays, bone scans, etc). Thus, flow sheets provide a means of recording routine patient evaluations as they are carried out at intervals specified in the study protocol. Such comprehensive data on each patient are valuable for patient monitoring but may not be directly suitable for the overall analysis and interpretation of results. Hence, it is sometimes useful to have a summary evaluation form which condenses these ongoing data into a series of relevant criteria of response. For instance, in a cancer trial one might wish to know about survival time, achievement of tumour response, duration of tumour response and the occurrence of certain side-effects. Flow sheets are available if

162

further details are needed, but it is helpful to summarize the actual criteria of response on a separate form.

Of course, the immense variety of clinical trials means that it is difficult to generalize about the type of form needed. If the duration of therapy or patient follow-up is long, then a single summary evaluation form may be infeasible: instead, interim summary evaluations may be completed so that interim analyses (see chapter 10) can be carried out.

In other trials where patient evaluation follows a regular pattern for a fixed time period, e.g. assessment every four weeks over a 20-week period, one can have a specific evaluation form for each assessment. However, one needs to be wary of generating too much data so that each repeat-assessment form should be as concise as possible. In those trials with fixed patterns of evaluation for all patients it is possible to supply investigators with identical *packages of forms* for every patient.

For instance, in a trial of antihypertensive therapy each patient was assessed for a total of 36 weeks, at two-weekly intervals in the first eight weeks and at four-weekly intervals thereafter. Each patient's package of case record forms was issued as a booklet prior to patient entry. It was clearly specified when each form was to be completed and despatched for data processing. Also pages of instructions were slotted in at important stages. For instance, for visit 3 the following instruction sheet was inserted:

STOP! Before continuing
(1) Is the patient eligible to continue?
(2) Have you given the patient a trial number and entered this on the register and *all* the forms?
(3) Have you given the patient therapy in bottle B?
(4) Have you sent off all the green copies of the forms using the pre-paid envelopes?
(5) Is the patient continuing with the trial? If not, specify reasons for withdrawal.

In this way, one can use the forms package to aid investigators in following the trial protocol.

In long-term follow-up studies patient evaluation after start of treatment may sometimes be kept on *forms for recording events*. For instance, in the UK-TIA study group aspirin trial (see Warlow, 1979), patients randomized to aspirin or placebo after a transient ischaemic attack are being followed at four-monthly intervals so that all myocardial infarcts, strokes and deaths are recorded. Here, the plan is for an evaluation form to be completed *every* four months, even though the great majority of patients will not have experienced any untoward events. Such regular submission of forms provides a check that patients are being evaluated regularly and hence is more reliable than allowing investigators to submit evaluations only when events occur.

This has been a brief and general comment on the types of form required. In some studies extra forms will be needed for recording information not available directly to the investigator. For instance, tumour pathology in cancer studies may be obtained at a separate pathology centre or X-ray evaluation may be determined by an independent panel of observers. Trial organizers need to ensure that forms for such data receive the same careful preparation as the main on-study and evaluation forms.

Layout and Question Design

It is essential to recognize that forms used in a clinical trial serve a different purpose from routine case notes. The latter often contain rather unstructured clinical comment on patient progress and are totally unsuitable for obtaining consistent data for objective comparison of groups of patients on different treatments. Thus, trial forms must confine attention to specific items of patient assessment as defined in the study protocol (see section 3.5).

I will begin discussion of each form's content by considering *patient identification* which must be given at the top of each form. At its simplest this consists of a trial number, assigned when the patient is registered in the trial, but this allows no check against errors so that, if confidentiality allows, I prefer to see the surname as well. Other identification (e.g. date of birth, hospital number, National Health Service or Social Security Number) is useful on the on-study form. In multi-centre trials, the investigator's name (or initials) and the hospital should also be recorded to aid identification.

In general the principal aim in collecting data on forms is for statistical analysis of treatment groups and not for perusal of individual experiences. Accordingly, virtually all questions should be constrained so that the answer can be given in *numerical form*. Furthermore, it is generally most reliable if answers are *recorded in boxes*.

For example, figure 11.1 lists a selection of questions which might be included in the on-study form of a hypertension trial. The list is not meant to be comprehensive but illustrates the form layout and type of question required. First, *actual measurements* such as blood pressure and pulse rate are easy to set out on a form. Three specific issues to consider are:

(a) make sure there are enough boxes for each item; e.g. most people have pulse rate under 100, but to allow for those few above 100 three boxes are needed
(b) the units of measurement (e.g. kg for weight) should be stated for each question
(c) items requiring decimal places (e.g. height) need to be absolutely clear where the decimal point is to be.

Many items seek *qualitative alternatives* (e.g. sex, grading of eye fundus) rather than quantitative measurements and here the standard approach is to associate each alternative with a number (e.g. male = 1, female = 2). Some questions require a straight yes/no answer and I prefer the convention no = 1, yes = 2. Since in general 'no' is the more common reply it is helpful if 'yes' requires the more distinguishable number '2'. For instance, in the last sequence

164

Patient's surname   _Davidson_

Patient's trial number | 0 | 3 | 2 |

Date of birth | | 5 | | 1 | 2 | 4 | 4 |
                                         D   M   Y

Date of randomization | | 8 | | 4 | | 8 | 3 |
                                         D   M   Y

Sex   (1=male 2=female) | 2 |

Body weight (kg) | | 6 | 1 |.| 4 |

Height (m) | 1 |.| 6 | 5 |

Supine blood pressure after 5 mins rest (mm Hg)

                        Systolic | 1 | 8 | 5 |

                        Diastolic | | 9 | 9 |

Pulse   (beats/min) | | 7 | 5 |

Eye fundus   right eye | 2 |
1=grade I   4=grade IV
2=grade II   5=normal   left eye | 1 |
3=grade III   6=not visualized

Previous treatment for hypertension | 1 |
        (1=no, 2=yes)

If yes,
a) Date of first hypotensive treatment | | | | | | | |
                                        D   M   Y
b) Details of previous hypotensive treatment (if known)

        Drug(s)   Inclusive dates
        | | |
        | | |
        | | |
        | | |

History of cardiovascular disease (1=no, 2=yes)

        Myocardial infarction | 1 |

        Angina | 2 |

        Stroke | 1 |

        Transient ischaemic attack | 1 |

        Other cardiovascular disease | 1 |

                specify _____

Fig. 11.1. Possible questions for a hypertension trial on-study form

of questions in figure 11.1 on previous cardiovascular disease, the great majority of patients will have had none at all in which case a sequence of 1's can be quickly entered. Note also that this sequence could not be combined into a single question since a patient could have experienced more than one item (e.g. myocardial infarction and angina). Another method of setting up yes/no questions is to use ticks and crosses but I think this is less reliable and more cumbersome for subsequent computer coding.

Another type of question concerns *dates* and *time intervals*. In general, it is more reliable to record dates rather than expecting the investigator to work out the time interval. For instance, in figure 11.1 we wished to know the time since first hypotensive treatment. Instead we obtain the date of first hypotensive treatment and the date of randomization. The difference can be worked out later by the trial staff or by a simple computer calculation if the data are transferred to computer for analysis. Similarly, it is better to record date of birth rather than age. One confusion to watch out for is that the American convention is to write month-day-year which differs from the order day-month-year in most other countries.

One basic rule is that *every question should require insertion of a number in the appropriate box*. That is why the answer 'no' to a yes/no item requires a definite reply, the number '1'. Otherwise, one would not be able to distinguish whether an empty box meant 'no' or 'I forgot to answer the question'. On occasions the answer to certain items is unknown. The convention for such *missing items* is to insert '9' in every box. For instance, if pulse rate was not taken one would insert '999'. Also, if the day of first hypotensive treatment is unknown but the month and year are known, one should insert '99' in the box for day. Alternatively, one could decide that recording day of onset is unnecessary precision and only provide boxes for month and year. Another convention is to insert '8' in boxes for inapplicable questions (e.g. date of first hypotensive treatment for patients not previously treated), but this is perhaps an unnecessary subtlety.

It sometimes occurs that certain information cannot be constrained into numerical answers. For instance, details of previous hypotensive treatment in figure 11.1 could involve so many different drugs, separately or in combination, that a more *open-style reply* is required. One needs to think carefully about the value of such information: it is difficult to incorporate in any analysis and hence is often kept as background data which may never get used at all. Thus, in general one should avoid using open-style replies unless they are the only way of collecting necessary data. Another circumstance for using open-style replies is in recording the patient's own assessment of side-effects (see section 3.5). The consequent record of events can subsequently be classified according to some prespecified list of numerical codes. This incurs extra work prior to transferring data off the form, but may be more reliable than asking each investigator to do the coding of side-effects himself.

The *appropriate wording* of questions requires considerable skill. This topic has received more extensive coverage in questionnaires for survey records but many of the same techniques apply to form design in clinical trials. The objective is obvious: each question needs to be unambiguous and clearly understood by the form-filler. Language should be as straightforward as possible and explanatory definitions need to be provided for any terms that might be confusing.

Any *general instructions* for completing a form should be given at the top of the form. Such matters as when the form should be completed and the convention for missing values fit in here. However, specific instructions and clarification for particular questions should be alongside the question itself. On evaluation forms it is particularly useful to summarize the definitions for any criteria of response. Most important is that such guidelines be on the form itself rather than relying on separate documents such as the study protocol.

After sorting out what items to include on a form, the *form layout* needs careful attention. The size of print and boxes needs to be adequate for legibility but not so large as to increase unnecessarily the overall size and number of forms. Also, it is better to use lower-case letters for text rather than capitals. Questions should be arranged so that the form can be answered by proceeding down the page, i.e. boxes should be in a vertical column as in figure 11.1. If questions are brief it may be convenient to have two columns of items on a page, the entire left-hand side being completed first. One needs to beware of cramping the form, but on the other hand it is useful to avoid multiple pages when possible.

Any form for use in a clinical trial requires *pretesting* to see that it actually works in practice. Thus, forms should be tried out on a few patients before the trial starts, preferably being completed by future trial participants, so that any flaws can be sorted out. No matter how experienced one may be in form design, only actual use can verify whether a form is workable. Those not so experienced will be surprised by the number of unexpected problems that pretesting can pick up.

Any form must be acceptable to the clinician and others responsible for its completion while also ensuring that it is suitable for subsequent extraction and analysis of data. Hence, *form design requires collaboration* between clinical investigators and those concerned with data processing and analysis (e.g. data managers, programmers or statisticians).

Further discussion on the design of forms for clinical trials is given by Wright and Haybittle (1979) and Gore (1981b).

11.2 DATA MANAGEMENT

The main purpose of having well-designed forms is so that patient evaluations can be made suitable for statistical analysis (see chapter 13). However, before analysis can take place, *all data have to be collected, checked and organized*. Such data management activities often receive inadequate attention in clinical trials with the danger that subsequent analysis may be delayed and/or based on erroneous or incomplete data. Hence, the aim of this section is to stress the need for efficient data management. The role of computers is discussed in section 11.3.

The first step is to arrange for each investigator to have the appropriate forms for every patient he enters in the trial. *Distribution of forms* should be done before the trial starts and each investigator should be kept supplied with additional forms as necessary. Instructions about which forms should be completed and at what time should be in the protocol, but could also be reinforced when each patient enters the trial. It should also be made clear who is responsible for completing each form. It is sometimes more appropriate and reliable for nursing or clerical staff to be specifically assigned the task rather than leaving it entirely to 'busy' clinicians, many of whom are not very adept at form-filling.

I will now concentrate on *multi-centre trials* since they present greater problems of data management, though many of the principles also apply to smaller trials in one institution. Preferably each institution in a multi-centre trial should have an on-site *data handler* who is responsible for sending completed forms at the appropriate times. All forms should be collected at the trial *coordinating centre* (see sections 3.2) and there should be close liaison between the on-site data handler and the data management personnel in the coordinating centre.

Multiple copies of each form are usually needed. Certainly the local institution and the coordinating centre should have copies and sometimes further copies are needed. For instance, in the Eastern Co-operative Oncology Group a copy of each patient's forms is also sent to the study chairman so that he can check the validity of tumour responses, etc. Although Xerox copies can be made if necessary it is advantageous to have printed carbonless multi-copy forms. This also allows use of different colours and separate labelling for each copy so that it is clear which copy goes where.

The handling of clinical trial data at the coordinating centre requires administrative and clerical skills which should not be the priority of clinicians or statisticians. Hence, in the last decade it has been recognized that one needs specially trained *data managers* whose job it is to get all trial data in good shape ready for statistical analysis. As each form arrives at the coordinating centre, the data manager should carry out a series of checks:

(a) *General checks* Has the form been sent at the right time, have all previously required forms for that patient been received and is the patient's trial number stated correctly?

(b) *Missing data* Are there any specific items or whole sections of the form which have not been answered?

(c) *Range checks* Are there any items which do not fall within the appropriate range of replies? e.g. errors such as sex recorded as 0 when the codes for male and female are 1 and 2; diastolic BP recorded as some ridiculously high value, say 195 mm Hg.

(d) *Logical checks* Are there any inconsistencies in replies to different questions? For instance, slip-ups such as date of tumour response being before date of randomization or diastolic BP > systolic BP need to be picked up.

Any problems identified by these checks should be conveyed back to the local institution so that corrections can be made. Many of these checks can also be carried out as the data are transferred to computer files (see section 11.3), but it is certainly useful if errors can be picked up by the data manager as soon as the form is received.

It is useful if data managers are actively involved in seeking forms from the institutions. If a clinical investigator is left in peace it is quite likely that he will forget to submit forms as required. Hence, the coordinating centre should send *requests for patient forms* when they are overdue so that the data available at the coordinating centre do not lag too far behind the actual patient evaluation. As regards the timing of such requests, one should bear in mind when the data are next to be analysed. Thus, it may be useful to send out requests for all missing forms some appropriate interval (say two months) before the intended analysis date. Similarly, in follow-up studies one should seek an update on each patient's survival status (dead, alive or lost to follow-up; date of death or date last known alive) at regular intervals.

Data managers will also be concerned with the subsequent data processing which often requires use of a computer (see section 11.3 for details). It is important that all forms received be kept in a readily accessible order. Usually one has a folder for each patient's records, these folders being ordered either by trial number or patient's name. Since identical surnames are quite common, ordering by trial numbers is more reliable. Patient registration and randomization (see section 5.1) is another aspect of the trial to be carried out by a data manager. The difficulty and importance of a data manager's duties is often underestimated. Indeed, some trials proceed without anyone specifically delegated to this role and this fact alone is a major cause of the chaotic circumstances surrounding the analysis of many studies.

11.3 THE USE OF COMPUTERS

Many people not directly concerned with computers are inclined to overrate what they can do. In clinical trials it is a common fallacy to believe that once the data are collected all one needs to do is get it onto a computer and, as if by magic, the required results will be produced. In reality, *the use of computers for data processing and analysis requires careful planning and execution by experienced personnel.* For any large trial, or a collection of trials coordinated at one centre, one generally needs the skills of data manager, computer programmer and statistician in collaboration if satisfactory results are to be obtained. For smaller trials the process may be so simplified that a single person, perhaps a statistician or even a clinician prepared to acquire such skills, can adequately process and analyse the data. Indeed, for any small trial one should think twice about whether a computer is needed at all, but more on this later.

Now, my aim here is to describe the *three main aspects of computing* for a clinical trial:

(1) Data transfer
(2) Data file handling
(3) Statistical analysis

I shall mainly concentrate on the full-scale use of a computing system, though later I will also refer to the more limited use of microcomputers for specific tasks of analysis. I shall not explain the details of computer hardware and programming, nor cover the more general topic of computer applications in medicine; see Kember (1982) for details of the latter.

(1) **Data Transfer**

The first step in using the computer is to transfer the data. The traditional way is to use 80-column *punch cards*. The numerical information on each patient's form is transferred in the same fixed sequence as on the form itself. That is, each box on the form has a corresponding column on the punched card. In order to indicate the exact card columns intended, a form can have the column numbers printed in small type after each row of boxes. For instance, figure 11.2 shows how part of figure 11.1 should be if these numbers are added. Sometimes rather than giving the range for each row of boxes (e.g. 11–16 for date of randomization) only the first number (11) or the last number (16) is recorded. It can be somewhat annoying to have a form cluttered up with such numbers. To avoid this, one could instead provide the card punch operator with a transparent overlay with the number codes for each form.

Note that each card needs to indicate which form it relates to and this requires a card number following the patient's trial number. In figure 11.2, the on-study form is coded '1' in column 4. If there were more than 80 columns of

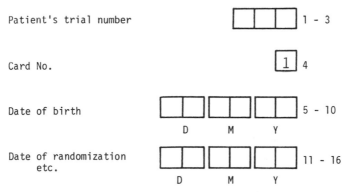

Fig. 11.2. The start of an on-study form with column codes for computer transfer of data

data on this form then a second card, with '2' in column 4, would be required. Subsequent forms for that patient would start with different numbers in the fourth column. Every form should begin with the patient's identification number, e.g. columns 1–3 in figure 11.2. If the trial is one of a sequence to be processed together, then an additional number identifying the trial would be required on each card.

Although most information transferred onto cards is numerical and in fixed format it is sometimes useful to include other items such as the patient's name. This can be done by setting aside a fixed number of columns, e.g. columns 17–26 for punching the first 10 letters of the surname. However, confidentiality of patient records may prohibit use of names on computer files.

With many computing installations it is now possible to transfer data by *key-to-disk* instead of punch cards. This means that the data are stored directly onto a magnetic disk rather than on cards, which allows greater speed and flexibility in computer processing. The same basic principles apply, except that the restriction to 80 columns is removed. Whichever method of transfer is used, errors are liable to happen. Hence, *it is advisable to have the data verified*: that is, a second dummy run of punching is carried out, any differences from the first run picking up potential errors. If possible, data transfer should be done by trained punch operators since they are considerably more reliable than amateurs trying their luck.

Once data are on cards or disk, a series of *checks for accuracy and completeness* should be carried out. Although data should have been checked by the data manager prior to punching (see section 11.2), checks programmed on the computer can provide a more rigorous detection of errors or missing data. Again the checks should be for inappropriate or missing forms, missing items, range checks and logical checks. It is helpful to have a program package available for data checking, otherwise the programming required for each trial gets too extensive. All the acceptable ranges and logical consistencies required in the data must be specified in advance. Although range checks are relatively simple to set up, it is often more difficult to define all the logical checks that could be made. Hence, certain errors in the data may only be revealed with statistical analysis. However, it would be unwise to delay data checking until analysis begins since it is then more difficult and time consuming to contact investigators and get corrections made.

(2) **Data File Handling**

The simplest situation as regards data handling for a clinical trial is where:

(a) all patients have exactly the same type and number of records and
(b) the information on all patients is to be processed and analysed once only when the trial is completed.

This is most likely to arise in small trials for short-term evaluation of therapy for a common ailment. One has to decide whether data are to be stored on cards, tape or disk and arrange for appropriate back-up copies (e.g. a spare data tape) in case the main file gets lost by accident. Otherwise, there are no real problems beyond routine programming for analysis of equal length records.

However, for many clinical trials the data handling on computer becomes more complicated, the main problems being that:

(a) patients have *unequal length records*
(b) the file of patient records accumulates gradually and this entails repeated *sorting and merging* of records.

As an illustration, consider data file handling for a typical trial in advanced cancer. For each patient the sequence of events for receipt of data might be as shown in figure 11.3. Immediately after randomization (by telephone) a *preliminary record* of patient's name, trial number, date of randomization and assigned treatment is entered on the data file. The *on-study form* should be completed and added to the file soon afterwards. The *first patient evaluation form* may be expected to arrive some three to six months after randomization. *Subsequent evaluation forms* may also follow at intervals of several months until information on treatment and response is completed. Updates on the patient's *survival status* will be obtained at intervals for as long as the trial follow-up is maintained.

At any particular moment in the trial the amount of data received for patients will vary. For instance, some patients will have just started treatment (steps 1 and 2), others will have had their first evaluation report (step 3) while others who have completed therapy will be followed for survival only (step 5). Thus, unequal length records will inevitably occur as the trial goes along. One must also decide how to handle repeat evaluation forms as in step 4 of figure 11.3. One approach is to make sure that the latest evaluation incorporates all previous evaluations so that each patient's data include only one fixed length evaluation record. *Updating by replacement* is relatively easy to handle computationally and makes for easier interpretation of data. In cancer studies it is quite practicable because one usually wishes to update qualitative assessments such as side-effects, tumour response and time intervals such as duration of response and survival time.

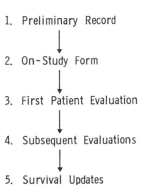

1. Preliminary Record

2. On-Study Form

3. First Patient Evaluation

4. Subsequent Evaluations

5. Survival Updates

Fig. 11.3. The sequence of data for each patient in a typical trial for advanced cancer

Another approach is to accumulate on the data file *separate records for each evaluation*. For instance, in a trial of secondary prevention for myocardial infarction one might wish to evaluate certain risk factors (e.g. blood pressure, smoking, serum cholesterol) at regular intervals. This will further complicate data file handling since patients may drop out of the trial after differing numbers of follow-ups. Indeed, one might consider keeping such complicated background data on a separate subsidiary file so that the main file can contain the more essential data on survival and recurrent infarcts.

As new data arrive they need to be merged into the main data file and this is best done using a sort-merge program which most computers have available. It is usual to have the file set up so that each patient's records are together and in correct sequence: indeed it is useful if the computer file is in exactly the same order as the data forms which the data manager should preserve as a manual reference (see section 11.2). Until recently there has been a lack of data base management computing packages suitable for scientific studies, so that data handling for clinical trials has often been somewhat primitive compared with (say) commercial data processing. However, SIR (Scientific Information Retrieval) is one widely available package which does offer the data management facilities appropriate to clinical trials; see Robinson *et al.* (1980) for details.

Statistical Computing

The methods of statistical analysis for clinical trials are described in chapters 13 and 14. The aim here is to discuss the use of computers to perform the appropriate numerical calculations. It is fundamental to recognize that the required analyses must be precisely specified in advance by the statistician (or others responsible for analysis). One cannot simply instruct the computer to 'analyse the data', though I fear that many people use computers in a rather carefree and uninformed manner so that the saying 'garbage in—garbage out' applies to the computer-assisted analysis of all too many trials.

Statistical packages such as SPSS, BMDP and SAS can greatly ease the burden of analysis. Indeed, nowadays it should be rather unusual for anyone to need to write their own computer programs specifically for a particular trial. Thus packages exist for performing virtually all the methods in chapters 13 and 14: a short sequence of instructions to identify the appropriate variables and required analysis is sufficient to produce the results whether it be a simple tabulation of mean response by treatment or a complex life-table analysis of survival adjusting for prognostic factors. Thus, for any centre concerned with analysing clinical trials it is essential to have available suitable statistical package programs for the types of analysis envisaged. There is a wide range of statistical packages available, so that I do not intend to make any specific recommendations. Another aspect to consider is that many packages take up sizeable computer core which is presently beyond the scope of many mini-computers. Many trial centres acquire their own mini-computer: this is ideal as regards having instant access, but may restrict the range of analyses one can perform. The alternative is to make use of a larger time-sharing computer.

I would like to refer briefly to the frequent *misuse of statistical packages*. Since they make each analysis task so easy to perform, there is a real danger that the user requests a whole range of analyses without any clear conception of what he is looking for. The user and his colleagues may be mistakenly impressed by the sheer quantity of results generated, though they may have little idea what to do with it all. Thus, my main message here is that *use of computers is no substitute for clear thought*. Each analysis performed should have a predefined purpose, usually to clarify a specific hypothesis concerning comparison of treatments.

In my experience it pays to be economical in computer analysis. Only perform analyses you are really interested in and allow adequate time after each analysis to interpret the findings properly. The user who continually rushes from one program to the next cannot clearly understand the consequences of his frenetic activity. Similarly, I find interactive statistical computing of limited value. While data transfer, checking and file handling may well be enhanced by interactive programs, I feel that statistical analysis for clinical trials generally proceeds more satisfactorily with batch processing.

Some statistical packages generate more results for each specific analysis than are required by the user. For instance, let us consider the most widely used package SPSS. The routine CROSSTABS may be used to produce a table of response (yes or no) by treatment. However, SPSS can produce this table of numbers along with three sets of percentages and nine different statistical tests (including chi-squared, Cramer's V, Kendall's Tau, Somers' D) most of which are not needed and probably not understood by the user (nor by me, incidentally). Hence, the user of a statistical package should aim to suppress superfluous information from the computer output and certainly ignore it when it cannot be omitted. The art of statistical computing is to concentrate on what *you* really need to know and not to get side-tracked into more obscure aspects of analysis.

One danger in using a computer for analysis is that the whole process can become so automated that one never really gets a feel for the data. The computer user can get accustomed to certain routine analyses which he applies to each data set regardless of what is appropriate. The computer should be a valuable tool not a rigid straitjacket, so that it can take away the burden of calculation while still allowing imagination and flexibility in one's approach to analysis. One should not be afraid to do some analysis by hand. For instance, graphical display of results is often best achieved by hand, since in my experience few computers have really good facilities for producing exactly the graphs you want. Also, I find that computer line-printer output is usually not a very effective means of communicating results to interested colleagues. It is usually difficult to follow, containing superfluous information and giving inadequate description, so that one should aim to transfer relevant information into a more intelligible display of results.

Data files with unequal length records (i.e. differing quantities of data per patient) are usually not directly accessible by statistical packages, although one or two packages (e.g. SAS, PSTAT) can cope with this situation. Hence, one may need a program prior to analysis which converts the data (or a subset of them) into records of fixed length per patient. Alternatively, one could arrange to store the data in fixed length records by adding blank records for each patient with less than the maximum amount of data, though this may lead to an unreasonably large data file.

Analysis without Major Computer Facilities

For any large-scale trial it would be futile to attempt analysis of results without using a computer. However, many trials are quite small, both as regards the number of patients and the amount of data per patient, and in this situation it is worth considering whether analysis really needs a computer. Of course, if the equipment and skilled personnel are readily available then it might still be silly to avoid computer analysis. However, many centres (e.g. local hospital research groups, small pharmaceutical companies) do not have ready access to computing facilities.

For instance, consider a crossover trial comparing two steroid inhalers for treatment of asthma (see sections 8.2 and 8.3 for the design and analysis of this trial). The trial recruited 27 patients each of whom had peak flow rate (PEFR) measured daily for a four-week period on each inhaler. The pharmaceutical company running this trial did not have computing facilities available, so what could be done? Well, the first step was to summarize the data on each patient by calculating his mean PEFR for each two-week period. Then, the summarized data were transferred onto a *large sheet of paper*, each row representing a patient and each column representing a variable (e.g. mean PEFR in the first two weeks, second two weeks, etc.). The necessary analyses (e.g. frequency distributions, means and standard deviations, *t* tests and confidence limits) could all be performed easily with the aid of a calculator. The analysis of other lung function tests (e.g. forced expiratory volume) measured every two weeks was also done this way.

Such 'hand analysis' can be assisted by having a pocket calculator which includes statistical functions (e.g. mean and standard deviation). Better still, a *desk-top microcomputer* can be used for basic statistical methods such as *t* tests. The idea is that one calls upon an already programmed statistical routine and types the data in for each specific analysis task. I have found a microcomputer very useful as a sort of 'glorified calculator' for analysing small data sets. This is evidently a much more limited use of a computer compared with full-scale data processing and analysis described earlier.

Now, some statisticians might claim that the above hand analysis is reminiscent of the 'dark ages' but I would disagree with such a scornful outlook. *Hand analysis for small trials has one big advantage: it allows one to get to know the data* in a way which is hard to achieve with computers.

The use of computers by pharmaceutical companies varies. The large companies tend to have their own installations while many smaller companies obtain help from *commercial computing agencies*. My limited knowledge of this field leaves me with the impression that such agencies are not the panacea for analysing trial data that they might wish to appear. I think it is important that computer processing and analysis of data be done by people who have a close appreciation of other aspects of a clinical trial. An agency's computing service may be provided in the abstract with the consequent risk that the quality and relevance of the results may not be as one would wish.

I cannot give a single, dogmatic answer regarding the role of computers in clinical trials. One must react to individual circumstances in recognizing that sophisticated computing systems can be of immense value especially for large trials, while noting that considerable expenditure and frustration can be incurred by the inexperienced using computers inappropriately.

This chapter has covered the basic principles of form design, data management and computing. The Cancer Research Campaign Working Party (1980) discusses these topics further in the context of multi-centre trials.

CHAPTER 12

Protocol Deviations

Any carefully planned clinical trial is intended to provide a proper assessment of treatment efficacy while ensuring that each patient's individual needs are catered for. No matter how meticulously one plans the trial protocol, it is almost inevitable that some patients' requirements will deviate from the protocol specifications. Also, protocol violations can arise if the patient or investigator fails to follow correct trial procedure.

There are innumerable ways in which things can go wrong in a clinical trial. Global catastrophes do occasionally happen: I recall one trial in which the active drug was prepared in an unstable form so that in reality placebo was compared with placebo, and another instance where an investigator made up fictitious results. More commonly, protocol deviation occurs for an individual patient because some aspects of the patient, his treatment and/or evaluation fail to conform to the prespecified trial design. The aim of this chapter is to deal with three aspects of such individual deviations from protocol: how to minimize their occurrence, how to detect them when they do occur and how to incorporate them in the analysis or interpretation of results. *The underlying objective is to try and avoid protocol deviations biassing any therapeutic comparisons.*

Section 12.1 is concerned with the problem of ineligible patients being included in a trial. The need for all eligible patients to be included is also discussed. Section 12.2 tackles the problems of patient non-compliance with therapy and incomplete patient evaluation. Section 12.3 provides guidelines on how drop-outs, i.e. patients who did not complete therapy and/or evaluation, should be considered in the analysis of trial results.

12.1 INELIGIBLE PATIENTS

Any trial requires a precise definition of which patients are eligible for inclusion; see section 3.3 for details. Ideally, the specification of eligibility criteria in a study protocol should be sufficient to ensure that investigators do exclude ineligible patients from the trial, but in practice one will usually find that a small proportion of ineligible patients are included by mistake.

If the proportion of ineligible patients becomes unduly large, say 10% or more, this may reflect a generally poor standard of trial organization which needs tightening up. On the other hand it can indicate that the trial's eligibility criteria are too restrictive, so that investigators are finding that many patients they consider suitable are not actually eligible. In such circumstances one may need to broaden eligibility criteria to include a more representative cross-section of patients.

The main priority should be to reduce the number of ineligible patients. First, the definition of patient eligibility can be clarified by using a check-list in the protocol; see section 3.3. Each investigator should then be encouraged to run through this check-list every time he is about to enter a patient. However, it is better still if patient registration and randomization incorporate a formal check on eligibility (see section 5.1). For instance, Pocock and Lagakos (1982) in an enquiry into randomization methods for cancer trials found that some multi-centre cooperative groups instituted formal *eligibility checks* as the first step in their telephone randomization procedure. This meant that for each patient the person at the coordinating centre read off the check-list of eligibility criteria so that the investigator could confirm or deny that patient's acceptability for the protocol. Such intensive checks can help to make ineligibility a rare event. One other cancer centre without such checks at randomization reported that 7% of patients were known to be ineligible while another 3% were considered ineligible because no on-study form was received. I have known this figure become higher still in some cancer trials.

One of the first steps in processing patient records should be to try and detect any ineligible patients. It is helpful if the patient's on-study form (see chapter 11) contains the relevant information. For instance, if the trial is for squamous cell lung cancer patients under age 70 without previous chemotherapy, then the on-study form should include questions about cell type, age and previous therapy. In practice, the list of eligibility criteria may be considerably longer.

If possible, each patient's eligibility should be checked before that patient's response data become available. Otherwise, any decision on eligibility may be influenced by how poorly or well the patient responded with the obvious danger of biasing treatment comparisons. In particular, a patient should never be declared ineligible because he responded differently from what was expected. For instance, the cancer patient who dies the day after treatment started, with or without evidence of toxicity, should not be declared ineligible. Such cases are considered further in sections 12.2–12.3.

The detection of an ineligible patient should immediately be reported back to the responsible investigator. It is quite likely that he was unaware of the error or had thought it unimportant, so that such prompt feedback will reduce the chances of further ineligible patients being entered.

Another problem is when ineligibility is discovered retrospectively as additional information comes to light. For instance, in many cancer studies the histological classification of a malignancy may determine whether a patient is eligible. In some multi-centre trials histology is finally determined by a central pathologist some weeks after patient entry and only then may ineligible patients be identified. I think such late ineligibles should generally be counted as eligible since otherwise the trial becomes too far removed from clinical reality.

The next issue is whether ineligible patients should be included in the analysis of trial results. Firstly non-randomized patients mistakenly included in a randomized trial should be declared ineligible and totally excluded from analysis. Failure to randomize is a clear protocol violation which could seriously bias results; see chapter 4. As regards other ineligible patients there is some diversity of opinion. Pocock and Lagakos (1982) found that most cancer trial centres excluded ineligible patients but one or two centres kept them in the analysis. The argument for excluding them is that the trial was designed to answer a therapeutic issue specific to eligible patients and analysis should be restricted accordingly. The contrary arguments are that (a) a trial's findings are to be extrapolated to future clinical practice in which eligibility for a given treatment is less-strictly defined and (b) inclusion of all randomized patients guards against any bias incurred by subjective choice of ineligible patients.

I prefer to exclude ineligible patients from analysis, provided that the eligibility criteria are absolutely clear and objective. Any suggestion of individual judgement being required would change this opinion for any given trial. In particular, if a trial is double-blind one can safely exclude ineligible patients since decisions on eligibility should be made without knowing each patient's treatment. It is useful to decide on an exclusion policy when the trial is being planned. One should avoid duplicate analyses, with and without ineligible patients, since this would only confuse interpretation and give scope for emphasizing whichever analysis gave the greater treatment difference. In addition, any trial report should mention the numbers of ineligible patients on each treatment and the reasons for ineligibility.

I now wish to discuss the 'reverse problem' of *how to ensure that a high proportion of all eligible patients are included in a study.* For instance, Mather *et al.* (1976) in a trial comparing home and hospital care for myocardial infarction patients reported that only 31 % of eligible patients were randomly assigned to home or hospital care. This pioneering study into a difficult issue of patient management was a great achievement in that it took place at all. However, interpretation of the results (essentially no evidence of a survival difference between home and hospital care) is made difficult since such a selective group of randomized patients cannot really be considered representative of all myocardial infarction patients.

At least Mather *et al.* kept a record of all patients who elected for home or hospital care without randomization so that the problem was explicitly defined. Unfortunately, in most studies such information is not available. For instance, the Anturane Reinfarction Trial Research Group (1980) reported a trial in which 1558 patients with myocardial infarction were randomly assigned to sulfinpyrazone or placebo. Hampton (1981) comments that 'the total number of patients from which these were recruited is unknown, but from the text it is clear that each centre was admitting only a few patients to the trial each month. What distinguished these patients from the others is unknown.'

Sylvester *et al.* (1981) have also studied this problem in multi-centre cancer trials. They showed that those institutions which contributed only a small number of patients to a study tended to provide a much poorer quality of participation. That is, there were more ineligible cases, more deviations from protocol treatment and more missing data forms. Such minor participants presumably failed to include a large proportion of their eligible patients and this reflected an inadequate commitment to the trial. Sylvester *et al.* comment that 'the minor participants were actually detrimental to the study from both scientific and administrative viewpoints'. These results suggest that institutions should not participate in multi-centre studies unless they can enter some predetermined minimal number of patients per year.

These examples lead me to make *two general recommendations*:

(1) A record should be kept of all patients eligible for a study but who for one reason or another are not included. The numbers and characteristics of such patients enable one to assess the representativeness of the sample of patients who are included.
(2) Investigators should be actively encouraged to include as many eligible patients as possible since it will then be easier to generalize trial findings to the population of future patients.

12.2 NON-COMPLIANCE AND INCOMPLETE EVALUATION

In this section I intend to discuss the various types of protocol deviation that can occur after a patient has entered the trial. The consequences for analysis and interpretation of trial results are discussed in section 12.3.

Basically, any departure from the intended treatment and/or evaluation constitutes a protocol deviation. The problem can range in severity from early patient withdrawal (i.e. neither treatment nor evaluation was carried out) to minor lapses from the treatment or evaluation schedule. The aim should be to *identify* each protocol deviation, to try and explain why it occurred and more generally to *prevent* unnecessary deviations occurring in the future. Wolf and Makuch (1980) drew up a useful classification of deviations:

(1) *Protocol violations* which were caused by or could have been prevented by the investigator and which materially affect the study results
(2) *Major deviations* which could not be prevented
(3) *Minor deviations* which are not likely to affect the evaluation of treatment efficacy.

The repeated occurrence of protocol violations may indicate that the trial is poorly administered with low cooperation from investigators and/or patients. If major deviations are frequent one should consider whether the protocol as specified is impractical and fails to fit in with acceptable clinical practice. In either case one should take steps to improve study design and execution rather than proceed with the mistaken hope that statistical analysis can 'sort out the mess'.

Let us now consider one or two specific types of protocol deviation:

Non-compliance

The fact that some patients fail to adhere to their prescribed treatment is a common experience in general clinical practice so that it would be naive to anticipate perfect patient compliance in clinical trials. Nevertheless, one should aim at a high degree of patient compliance as being one important aspect of a well-administered trial.

The issue of non-compliance is most evident for trials of out-patients involving repeated dosage of *oral drug therapy* administered by the patient himself. Trials of antihypertensives or antidepressants are two common areas particularly prone to non-compliance problems.

The first step in reducing non-compliance is when patients are being entered into the trial. Careful explanation to the patient of his treatment schedule and the trial's objectives would seem essential in achieving full patient cooperation. In addition to verbal explanation by the attending physician (which is often not well remembered) and *legible labelling* of dose schedules on the medicines provided, it may also be helpful to prepare an *explanatory pamphlet* for each patient to keep. Nursing or pharmacy staff can also help to encourage cooperation. Essentially a caring and well-organized treatment team is a valuable start to patient compliance.

Regular check-ups and reinforcement of compliance should be undertaken at *follow-up examinations*. The simplest check is to ask the patient to bring his tablets to each examination and then count the number of remaining tablets to see if this agrees with the intended dose schedule. This will aid both detection and prevention of non-compliance. Too few or too many remaining tablets are a clear indication of non-compliance which should be pursued by further questioning. If the tablet count is correct there is no guarantee that compliance is occurring: the astute non-complier can easily dispose of tablets to achieve the right number. Hence, it may still be worth asking every patient about adherence to the correct schedule. This can conveniently follow any routine enquiry into side-effects.

One needs to draw a distinction between *non-compliance* attributed to lack of patient cooperation or genuine misunderstanding and *cessation or modification of therapy* because of adverse reactions or disease progression. The latter is a necessary component of treatment policy and an important aspect of clinical evaluation (see section 3.4) while the former reflects problems of patient management. Unfortunately, this distinction may be unclear in many cases, e.g. individual reaction to minor side-effects will vary depending on the patient's desire to comply.

In some instances, patient compliance can also be checked by blood or urine tests. For instance, Hjalmarson *et al.* (1981) were able to check compliance with metoprolol therapy after myocardial infarction by using assays of metoprolol in urine. One might also get an indication of overall compliance in a group of patients by the occurrence of predictable side-effects, e.g. use of oral beta-blockers should tend to lower pulse rate. However, lack of side-effects is not reliable evidence of individual non-compliance.

For long-term drug therapy one needs to decide on *appropriate intervals between repeat drug supplies* and follow-up examinations. Too long an interval between visits may lead to a steady fall in patient compliance due to lack of encouragement while too short an interval may prove a nuisance and reduce cooperation. Thus, in a trial of antihypertension therapy lasting several months, repeat prescriptions and visits every two weeks may be a suitable choice. The actual interval may also be determined by the need to monitor response (e.g. by measuring blood pressure and heart rate) and the availability of resources.

The issue of patient compliance also needs consideration when defining a treatment schedule. For instance, it may be pharmacologically superior to have drug therapy four times daily but this will reduce compliance compared with a larger once-daily dose. Also, if making a trial double-blind requires extra placebo capsules this may affect compliance. Accordingly, *an appraisal of potential non-compliance when planning a study may deter unrealistic protocol specifications.* Indeed, for any major trial it may be useful to have a pilot study to assess compliance.

Patient Withdrawals and Incomplete Evaluations

The ultimate in non-compliance is for a patient to withdraw totally from the trial. This arises either because of *patient refusal* to participate further or *clinical judgement* that the patient should be transferred to alternative therapy. Though each patient must be ethically entitled to withdraw from a trial one should naturally keep refusals to a minimum. A substantial number of refusals may indicate something seriously wrong with the protocol. Of course, some refusals may be unavoidable (e.g. if the patient moves away).

As regards clinical judgement for withdrawal, this should normally be based on reasonable evidence that it is in the patient's best interests to change treatment, e.g. excessive toxicity or disease progression in advanced cancer indicates cessation of cytotoxic treatment is required. If such evidence is lacking, one may conclude that the investigator violated the protocol by prematurely withdrawing the patient.

Withdrawals on the basis of sound clinical reasoning are an important indication of treatment efficacy. Other (non-medical) withdrawals are less easily interpreted, though they are often associated with a poor response to treatment.

For trials involving seriously ill patients (e.g. secondary prevention trials of acute myocardial infarction) one should generally expect very few non-medical withdrawals. However, in less serious conditions the anticipated withdrawal rate may be much higher, especially if therapy is prolonged. For instance, in the clofibrate trial (see Committee of Principal Investigators, 1978), subjects with high cholesterol were randomized to clofibrate or placebo. Over 20 % failed to continue treatment for the intended five years, not a surprising proportion given that subjects were essentially disease-free.

Withdrawal from treatment, whatever the reason, should not preclude a patient from subsequent evaluation. Indeed, it may be vital for the study that evaluation continues; see section 12.3. For instance, Epstein et al. (1981) in a trial of primary biliary cirrhosis had several patients withdraw from D-penicillamine therapy because of side-effects. Such patients were still followed for reporting of morbidity and mortality. Of course, if patients refuse to continue, further evaluation becomes impossible except that subsequent mortality can still be obtained from national or state registers of deaths.

A lesser problem concerns patients who have not withdrawn but have incomplete data for evaluation. For instance, some patients may fail to attend all follow-up examinations or certain measurements may not be recorded. Such missing data may be due to poor patient cooperation or be simply an oversight. Either way it is a considerable nuisance when analysing the results. Generally, one would like to assume that any missing values occur at random so that analysis of the available data remains unbiassed. However, if patients miss appointments or are not subjected to certain tests because of ill-health there is an obvious bias which should be noted.

12.3 INCLUSION OF WITHDRAWALS IN ANALYSIS

Firstly, all protocol violations and major deviations should be recorded as they occur and investigators should aim to provide an honest account of such events in any report of trial findings. Not to mention the existence of patients who withdrew from therapy or otherwise deviated from protocol is a serious failing which can lead to exaggerated claims about treatment efficacy.

However, should such patients with protocol deviations be included in the main treatment comparisons *or* should they simply be noted as being deviates and be excluded from subsequent results? In most circumstances I think the first approach is required; that is, *all eligible patients, regardless of compliance with protocol should be included in the analysis of results whenever possible.* This 'pragmatic approach' is sometimes called 'analysis by intention to treat' and is normally preferred since it provides a more valid assessment of treatment efficacy as it relates to actual clinical practice. The alternative 'explanatory approach' would confine analysis to patients who received therapy according to protocol, i.e. 'analysis of compliers only', but this can distort treatment comparisons.

For instance, a randomized double-blind trial compared low and high doses of a new antidepressant with amitriptyline. Fifty patients were entered but 15 had to withdraw due to possible drug side-effects. For the remaining 35 patients the clinician's global assessment of treatment effect is shown in table 12.1.

The initial interpretation was that high dose produced the highest proportion

Table 12.1. Clinical assessment of treatment effect in an antidepressant trial

	Low dose	High dose	Amitriptyline
Very effective	2	8	6
Effective	4	2	8
Ineffective	3	2	0
Total assessed	9	12	14
Withdrawn patients	6	8	1
Total randomized	15	20	15

of 'very effective' assessments, i.e. 8/12 on high dose versus 6/14 on amitriptyline. However, patient withdrawals were 6, 8 and 1 on low dose, high dose and amitriptyline respectively, so that when these additional 'treatment failures' are included the proportion of 'very effective' is equal on high dose and amitriptyline. However, 14/15 on amitriptyline were rated as 'effective or very effective' which is a significantly higher proportion than high dose (10/20) or low dose (6/15), $P < 0.01$ in each case. Thus, the trial's conclusions were completely reversed once withdrawals were taken into account.

Sackett (1981) illustrates the same principle with a trial by Fields *et al.* (1970) comparing surgical versus medical therapy in bilateral carotid stenosis. Each patient was assessed for a recurrent transient ischaemic attack, stroke or death. Here, the explanatory approach restricts attention to compliers, i.e. patients who left hospital free of stroke, as shown in table 12.2(a).

This analysis appears to produce a significant risk reduction on surgical treatment, but it excludes 16 patients who died or had a stroke before leaving hospital, all but one of whom were randomized to surgical treatment. Including such patients in an analysis by intention to treat produces the results in table 12.2(b).

Table 12.2. Comparison of surgical and medical therapy for bilateral carotid stenosis

Treatment	Recurrent TIA*, stroke or death
(a) Excluding deaths or strokes while in hospital	
Surgical	$43/79 = 54\%$
Medical	$53/72 = 74\%$ $\left.\right\}\chi^2 = 5.98, P = 0.02$
(b) Including all patients	
Surgical	$58/94 = 62\%$
Medical	$54/73 = 74\%$ $\left.\right\}\chi^2 = 2.80, P = 0.09$

* TIA = transient ischaemic attack.

The risk reduction on surgical treatment is no longer statistically significant. This example emphasizes that no matter how early a patient withdrew he can still be included in analysis. Some patients randomized to surgical treatment had a stroke before surgery could begin. Even these patients should be included since, if they had been assigned to medical treatment, their therapy would have begun sooner and might have affected the outcome. Furthermore, the preponderance of withdrawals on one treatment is itself an indication that their exclusion from analysis would bias treatment comparison.

The exclusion of withdrawals from statistical analysis does not often make such a dramatic difference. Rather it creates a feeling of uncertainty whereby the reader does not quite know how much to trust the trial's conclusions. For instance, the Anturane Reinfarction Trial Research Group (1980) comparing anturan against placebo for survival after myocardial infarction adopted rather a curious presentation of results. Deaths were classified as 'analysable' or 'non-analysable' according to whether patients continued on treatment or withdrew. Hampton (1981) provides an interesting review of how results should be presented for such trials. Of relevance here are the results shown in table 12.3.

Table 12.3. Mortality in the anturan trial for patients who continued on therapy and for patients who withdrew

| | Anturan | | Placebo | |
	Continued	Withdrawn	Continued	Withdrawn
No. of patients	563	220	580	195
No. of deaths	44	20	62	23
Percentage mortality	5.4%	9.0%	7.6%	11.7%
		7.8%		10.4%

Although the inclusion of withdrawals did not really alter the treatment difference, the exclusion of 30% of patients from the main analysis would justifiably cast doubt on the findings especially since there were more exclusions on anturan than on placebo. However, once one accepts the idea of including all patients in the main analysis of results, an additional analysis providing separate comparison for those continuing and withdrawn can provide valuable extra insight. Note that patients who withdrew from treatment had a higher mortality than compliers, even in the placebo group.

One might consider analysing patient response according to duration of time the patient stayed on treatment. However, this is a particularly confusing approach which is open to misinterpretation. For instance, Costello (1974) studied tumour response for patients with malignant melanoma randomized to two cytotoxic drugs (DTIC or TIC mustard). Response rates by treatment duration are shown in table 12.4.

Table 12.4. Response rates in a trial for malignant melanoma according to duration of treatment

| | Duration of treatment | | | |
	Less than 5 days	5–34 days	35–64 days	65 or more days
DTIC	0/15 patients	2/20	3/13	10/15
TIC mustard	1/19	1/28	0/2	1/2

Evidently patients who stayed on DTIC longer had a better response rate. This does not mean that patients should stay on treatment longer in order to improve response. Instead, it simply shows that patients who are able to respond can consequently cope with treatment for longer. This is an obvious finding applicable to just about any treatment, so that such an analysis is of no real value.

In some trials it is not easy to include withdrawals in the main analysis since a quantitative measurement forms the basis of patient evaluation. For instance, Cook et al. (1982) describe a randomized trial of morphine and buprenorphine for analgesia after abdominal surgery. Their main findings concern the respiration rate of patients after operation and are shown in table 12.5.

These results seem to show that respiration rates on both drugs are raised immediately after operation followed by a subsequent decline. However, for buprenorphine the rate eventually fell to a level which was undesirably lower than initially. Table 12.5 necessarily excludes seven withdrawals of whom five, all on burprenorphine, had to be taken off the trial because of respiratory depression. Thus, the pattern of withdrawals is consistent with the results for patients who stayed in the trial. One could argue for including the last recorded respiration rate for withdrawals as a substitute for their missing rates at later times, but I am rather against this because the quoted mean respiration would then lack reality. Another possibility is to do an analysis based on the lowest recorded respiration rate of each patient. Instead, I think where withdrawals

Table 12.5. Respiration rates after abdominal surgery for patients given morphine and buprenorphine

| | | Morphine | | Buprenorphine | |
	Hours	No of patients	Respiration rate (mean ± SD)	No. of patients	Respiration rate (mean ± SD)
Before operation		24	17.7 ± 1.8	23	18.7 ± 1.9
After operation	0	24	22.2 ± 6.4	23	21.5 ± 5.8
	6	23	21.9 ± 4.5	21	18.3 ± 6.0
	12	23	20.0 ± 3.1	17	18.8 ± 3.7
	18	23	19.5 ± 2.8	17	17.2 ± 3.7
	24	23	18.1 ± 3.5	17	16.8 ± 4.1

cannot be included directly in analysis they need to receive appropriate emphasis and explanation in any report.

Sometimes withdrawn patients can be included in some parts of the analysis but not in others. For instance in the clofibrate trial (see Committee of Principal Investigators, 1978, 1980), patients who withdrew from treatment (clofibrate or placebo) for any reason were no longer followed for occurrence of cardiovascular morbidity but subsequent mortality data were available. Hence, the first publication focussed on morbid and/or fatal events while patients were still complying with treatment. That is, every patient's experience while on treatment was included in the results, using appropriate methods of analysis (e.g. the life-table approach described in section 14.2) to allow for differing periods on treatment. The second publication is a mortality analysis according to 'intention to treat'. That is, all deaths up to the end of 1978 were included regardless of whether patients were still on treatment.

Hence, lack of response data once a patient is withdrawn leaves one no alternative but to exclude such a patient from any corresponding analyses. However, are there any other circumstances where a non-compliant patient's follow-up evaluation data should not be included? I see two main situations which are exceptions to the general rule of 'include withdrawals when possible':

(1) *Patients who withdraw before treatment is even started* may sometimes be excluded from analysis. However, one should check that the time lapse between randomization and start of treatment is comparable for all treatments and that the numbers and reasons for such withdrawals show no marked treatment differences. Note this was not the case in the trial by Fields *et al.* (1970) mentioned earlier and hence no patients were excluded.

(2) *Phase I and early phase II trials* are concerned with exploring the properties of treatment in idealized conditions. Such early clinical evaluation of a new drug is more akin to closely controlled preclinical laboratory experiments. At that stage one is not immediately concerned with the overall evaluation of a treatment policy in clinical practice. Instead one wishes to study the effects of treatment when taken as specified. In such circumstances, one might exclude non-compliant subjects from analysis. However, such early trials require a high compliance rate to be successful. There should not be many non-compliers otherwise serious bias may occur.

Armitage (1980) and Sackett and Gent (1979) provide further insight on how to deal with protocol deviations when analysing results. The philosophical distinction between explanatory and pragmatic approaches to clinical trials was developed by Schwartz and Lellouch (1967) and is explored further by Schwartz *et al.* (1980).

CHAPTER 13

Basic Principles of Statistical Analysis

The aim of this chapter is to explain the main statistical principles required in the analysis and interpretation of data from clinical trials. The exposition is deliberately non-technical since I feel it is more important to concentrate on the underlying purpose of statistical methods than it is to provide a 'cook book' of statistical recipes. Nevertheless, a few fundamental statistical techniques are described.

Section 13.1 deals with *descriptive statistics*, i.e. how to get a feel for the data and express the basic results comparing treatments in a comprehensible manner. There is a need to infer whether any observed difference in treatments is genuine or could reasonably have arisen by chance. *Significance tests* have become the most commonly used method of statistical inference in clinical trials and section 13.2 describes their purpose with examples of certain basic significance tests and also discusses their possible abuse. One should also estimate the magnitude of treatment difference, rather than merely assess its statistical significance. *Confidence limits* are a useful method of statistical estimation and section 13.3 illustrates their value. The clear presentation of results is obviously desirable and section 13.3 also discusses the problem of communicating statistical findings.

Certain more complex issues in statistical analysis are described in chapter 14. Even so, I cannot hope to provide a fully comprehensive introduction to the subject of statistics in the available space and hence the reader may wish to refer to other texts devoted to statistical methods in medicine. Many clinicians have found Swinscow (1977) a useful elementary book, though it is more geared to technical description rather than underlying principles. Colton (1974) provides a more rounded understanding of basic statistical methods, while Armitage (1971) is a more advanced and comprehensive text. In addition, Gore and Altman (1982) discuss many of the principles and problems associated with statistical methods.

187

13.1 DESCRIBING THE DATA

Planning

One fundamental principle is that the statistical analysis of results, no matter how cleverly done, can never rescue a poorly designed study. Of course, inadequate statistical presentation can impair interpretation but the quality of a clinical trial is also heavily dependent on good planning and proper execution. Hence, it is very useful to think about statistical analysis when designing a trial. Indeed, it helps to be quite specific early on as to which statistical tables and graphs one intends to produce since this will focus trial plans on achieving such essentials. While wishing to maintain sufficient flexibility in analysis one should realize the benefits of advance preparation. Particular attention should be given to obtaining adequate personnel and equipment for handling data and to ensuring data are as correct and complete as possible (see chapter 11). One common failing is not to allow enough time for analysing the results. No matter how efficiently the trial is organized, good-quality statistical analysis cannot be achieved overnight so that an adequate provision of time for the analysis and interpretation of trial data should be recognized when planning a trial.

Types of Data

For each patient in a clinical trial one collects three types of data:

(1) *Treatment* The patient's assigned treatment and the actual treatment received
(2) *Response* Measures of the patient's response to treatment including side-effects
(3) *Prognostic factors* Details of the patient's initial condition and previous history upon entry into the trial.

Use of prognostic factors in analysis is discussed in section 14.1 so that here we concentrate on response data for comparing treatments in which all patients on each treatment are combined to form a *treatment group* for statistical analysis.

Problems of patients being ineligible, not receiving their assigned treatment or withdrawing from treatment have already been discussed in chapter 12. In particular, one needs clear-cut rules about which patients to include, and in general as few patients as possible should be excluded from the analysis of each treatment group's results.

There are basically *three types of response data* in clinical trials:

(1) qualitative response
(2) quantitative response
(3) time to relapse

I will now discuss each of them in turn.

(1) Qualitative Response

Each patient is classified into one of several response categories according to some predefined evaluation criteria. At its simplest one can have two response categories, which might be labelled 'success' or 'failure', response or no response. Consider the following examples:

Hodgkins lymphoma   'success' = disappearance of all tumours for at least four weeks

Myocardial infarction   'success' = survival for one year

Hypertension   'success' = blood pressure below 160/90 after four weeks' therapy

Tuberculosis   'success' = considerable X-ray improvement.

Also, most side-effects are recorded in this way, e.g. alopecia while on cytotoxic therapy for lung cancer is noted as present or absent.

Sometimes one can achieve a slightly more detailed classification by having more than two categories of response. For instance, Ezdinli *et al.* (1976) in a trial of chemotherapy for lymphocytic lymphoma had four categories of antitumor response:

Complete remission = complete disappearance of all lesions

Partial remission   = 50 % reduction in sum of lesion surface areas and no new lesions

Progression   = increase of 25 % in sum of lesion surface areas and/or appearance of a new lesion

No change   = the remainder

This can be termed an *ordered* qualitative response since there is a natural ordering of 'success', complete remission, partial remission, no change, progression.

The same authors also reported side-effects as ordered qualitative variables. For instance, each patient's lowest white blood cell count (WBC) and platelet count while on treatment were converted to the following five-point scale of haematologic toxicity:

Grade	WBC		Platelets
0 absent	≥ 4000	and	$\geq 90\,000$
1 mild	3000–4000	or	70 000–90 000
2 moderate	2000–3000	or	50 000–70 000
3 severe	1000–2000	or	30 000–50 000
4 life-threatening	< 1000	or	$< 30\,000$

Qualitative measures of response are often used in trials when it is difficult to measure precisely how well each patient is responding. For instance, in the above lymphoma trial, the complex and varied ways in which the disease may progress force the investigators to adopt a relatively simple response classification. Similarly, in trials for relief of essentially unmeasurable symptoms, e.g.

pain in rheumatoid arthristis, one has to adopt rather crude qualitative assessment scales (e.g. very effective, effective, not effective) for patient and/or clinician.

(2) Quantitative Response

Use of a qualitative response classification implies some loss of detail in evaluating each patient. For instance, simply to classify hypertensive patients after four weeks' therapy into responders or non-responders according to diastolic BP < or $\geqslant$ 90 mm Hg does not fully utilize the available data. No distinction is made between patients with diastolic BP of 90 and 120 mm Hg: both could be classified as non-responders. Hence, when a reliable quantitative measure of response does exist it is usually best to use its actual numerical value for each patient in the results.

Sometimes the same quantitative measurements can also be taken before treatment commences, and these *baseline data can be used in assessing the magnitude of each patient's response*. Suppose in a hypertension trial one has diastolic BP measured before and after four weeks' treatment. Then, there are three basic options for measuring response:

$$BP_{after}$$

$$BP_{before} - BP_{after} = \text{difference}$$
$$\text{or}$$
$$\frac{BP_{after}}{BP_{before}} = \text{ratio}$$

The ratio may also be converted to a

$$\text{percentage change} = \left(\frac{BP_{after}}{BP_{before}} - 1 \right) \times 100.$$

To ignore the baseline values may be wasteful of information: a final diastolic BP of 85 represents a much better response if the initial diastolic was 125 rather than 105. Hence, one's analysis should also focus on some measure of change. This becomes particularly important if there are baseline differences between treatment groups (e.g. by chance one treatment group may have higher initial mean diastolic BP than the other).

One needs to choose whether the difference or ratio should be used in analysis. On statistical grounds, if the fall in blood pressure is likely to be greater for patients with high initial blood pressure then the ratio may be more appropriate. A scatter diagram of each patient's difference plotted against his initial reading will help to determine if they are associated. If the differences are not related to initial readings then the difference is preferred. However, there may also be clinical reasons for preferring the simple difference as providing a more straightforward description of patient improvement. For a reasonably large trial, the choice between difference or ratio is unlikely to affect the conclusions.

With quantitative response measures such as blood pressure, heart rate or lung function tests, it is often possible to obtain repeated observations during the course of treatment. For instance, in a trial of steroid inhalers for asthma it is possible for patients to measure their peak flow rate twice daily. This can generate a wealth of data which require careful analysis, as is discussed in section 14.3.

(3) Time-to-relapse

In some trials the main evaluation of therapy is in terms of the time to some major event, e.g. death or disease recurrence. For instance, in trials for patients with myocardial infarction one may be interested in

(a) time to death from whatever cause or
(b) time to fatal or non-fatal recurrent myocardial infarction.

Of course many patients have not died or have not had an infarct by the time the results are analysed, so that one cannot use time to death as a conventional quantitative variable. An alternative is simply to define death within some specified time period since start of treatment (e.g. one year) as a qualitative variable (yes or no). However, this has two drawbacks: it fails to utilize information on when each patient died and also some patients may not have been followed for the whole period. Hence, the analysis of time-to-relapse data, usually called *survival data* for simplicity, poses special problems which are considered in section 14.2.

Describing Qualitative Data

Here one first needs to calculate for each treatment the numbers of patients in each response category. These numbers (frequencies) can then be converted into percentages of the total for each treatment in order to aid the comparison of treatments. For instance, Ezdinli *et al.* (1976) compared cytoxan + prednisone (CP) and BCNU + prednisone (BP) in lymphocytic lymphoma. Table 13.1 shows the tumour response data for each treatment.

Table 13.1. Tumour response in a trial of lymphocytic lymphoma

| | Treatment* | | Total |
	BP	CP	
Complete response	26 (19%)	31 (23%)	57 (21%)
Partial response	51 (37%)	59 (44%)	110 (40%)
No change	21 (15%)	11 (8%)	32 (12%)
Progression	40 (29%)	34 (25%)	74 (27%)
Total no. of patients	138 (100%)	135 (100%)	273 (100%)

* BP = BCNU + prednisone, CP = cytoxan + prednisone.

When using percentages to present qualitative results it is essential to record the *total number of patients* on each treatment since otherwise one cannot reliably interpret the results. It makes a great difference to know if a 50% response rate is based on 10 or 1000 patients. Otherwise, it is a matter of style whether one quotes the numbers or percentages or both for each response category. Table 13.1 shows the maximum information one could display, including the results for both treatments combined. If preferred one could condense the table by eliminating the 'total' column and all percentages. Possibly the percentage complete or partial response, 56% on BP versus 67% on CP, could then be added as the most useful overall comparison of response rates.

The next step is to assess to what extent any treatment difference in the observed response pattern (as shown in Table 13.1) provides evidence of a genuine difference in treatment efficacy. This requires chi-squared significance tests as described in section 13.2.

Describing Quantitative Data

With any quantitative response I find it a useful preliminary to study the spread of observed values on all patients as one group, regardless of treatment. Thus, I obtain a listing of individual patient values and a detailed frequency distribution, i.e. an ordered list of observed values from lowest to highest giving the frequency with which each occurred. In particular, one can check that the lowest and highest values are clinically feasible and valid thus reducing the possibility of erroneous extreme results. If the trial is small or computing facilities are limited (or non-existent) one may prefer simply to scan one's eye over the list of patient values rather than form a frequency distribution. Either way, I think it is important to get an initial look at the sort of individual data one is dealing with before ploughing into statistical analysis.

For comparison of treatments the simplest summary is to compute the *mean response* for patients on each treatment. For instance, Cockburn *et al.* (1980) report a clinical trial for prevention of infant hypocalcaemia in which pregnant women receiving vitamin D supplement were compared with untreated women. The infant's plasma calcium concentration measured six days after birth was of principal interest. The means were 9.36 and 9.01 mg per 100 ml for vitamin D and control women, respectively, which suggests that the infant calcium tends to be higher in the vitamin D group. However, before jumping to the premature conclusion that vitamin D causes raised infant calcium levels one needs to answer three additional questions:

(1) How many patients were in each group? In this case, 233 on vitamin D and 394 controls.
(2) How much did infant serum calcium levels vary within each group?
(3) How strong is the evidence that the mean difference between treatments is genuine rather than due to chance or factors other than treatment?

This last question requires a significance test, the two-sample t test, as described in section 13.2.

As regards the second question one can usually summarize individual variation by the *standard deviation* defined as $\sqrt{\dfrac{\text{sum (value} - \text{mean})^2}{\text{no. of patients} - 1}}$. Here, the standard deviation of infant calcium was 1.15 and 1.33 mg per 100 ml for vitamin D and control patients, respectively. The standard deviation gives some idea of the extent to which individual values differ from the mean. Some patients will differ from the mean by at least one standard deviation. More precisely, if the variable being measured is normally distributed (see Swinscow, 1977, chapter 2), then about 5 % of values will be more than two standard deviations from the mean. The standard deviation is also needed for significance tests and confidence limits, (see sections 13.2–13.3).

It is helpful to present the means, standard deviations (SD) and numbers of patients in a simple table (see table 13.2). Evidently, the difference in means looks less impressive now that the standard deviations are given alongside.

Table 13.2. An example of summarizing quantitative data

Treatment	No. of patients	Infant 6th day plasma calcium (mg per 100 ml) Mean	SD
Vitamin D	233	9.36	1.15
Control	394	9.01	1.33

Although to summarize extensive data by such a concise table is often useful, one must recognize a need to provide further insight into a quantitative treatment comparison. In particular, means and standard deviations do not elucidate what actually happens to individual patients so that some *graphical display of individual data* may be called for.

For instance, Lebrec *et al.* (1980) investigated whether propranolol could reduce portal hypertension in cirrhotic patients. Sixteen cirrhotic patients were randomized to receive either propranolol (eight patients) or placebo (eight patients) and the difference between wedged and free hepatic venous pressures (WHVP − FHVP, a measure of portal hypertension) was measured before and during treatment in each patient. Mean of WHVP − FHVP was 2.5 kPa both before and during placebo treatment but fell from 2.4 kPa to 1.8 kPa during propranolol. An appropriate significance test (see section 13.2) indicates strong evidence for propranolol reducing portal venous pressure. However, the authors made their conclusions more convincing by displaying the individual data as shown in figure 13.1. It was then easy to observe that WHVP − FHVP fell substantially in all eight propranolol patients whereas only two placebo patients showed any drop at all.

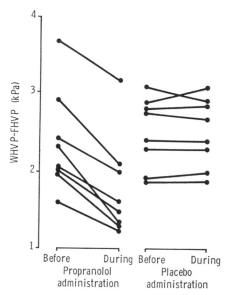

Fig. 13.1. Individual values for gradient between wedged and free hepatic venous pressures (WHVP-FHVP) before and during administration of propranolol or placebo

Only in relatively small trials, say <30 patients per treatment, is it feasible to display graphically the exact response of every patient. Instead, for large trials one can display the distribution of response by treatment using *histograms* or *cumulative frequency distributions*. Figures 13.2 and 13.3 show such graphical alternatives for infant serum calcium in the vitamin D trial mentioned earlier. One can then see that the difference in means is primarily due to a higher percentage of low plasma calcium in the control group. The choice between histograms and cumulative frequency distributions depends on personal preference. The former gives a clearer idea of the distribution's shape but I often favour the latter as being more concise and giving a more direct treatment comparison. It also enables one to read off the medians or the percentages below a certain point. For instance, vitamin D and control groups had 6% and 13%, respectively, below 7.5 mg per 100 ml.

Graphical data description serves two main purposes:

(1) *Data exploration* enabling investigators to understand their own data, particularly in the early stage of statistical analysis.
(2) *Presentation of findings* in the formal publication of results.

The former may entail a multitude of roughly drawn sketches conveying useful impressions of the data, whereas in publications one is often severely limited to at most one or two precisely drawn graphs. If the full distribution of individual data cannot be shown, it may be useful just to give percentages of patients on each treatment exceeding some clinically relevant cut-off value of a quantitative

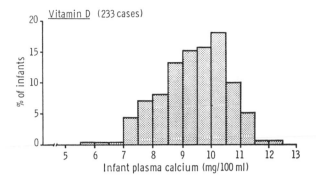

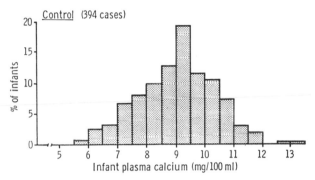

Fig. 13.2. An example of histograms for displaying individual data

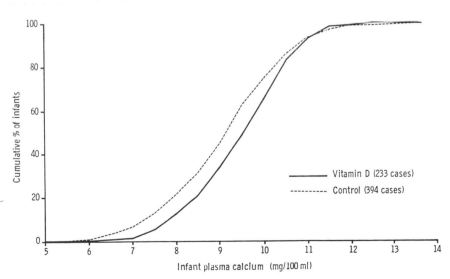

Fig. 13.3. An example of cumulative frequency distributions

measurement. For instance, plasma calcium below 7.5 mg per 100 ml is used to indicate neonatal hypocalcaemia and above 160 mm Hg is an oft-quoted reference level for systolic hypertension. This helps to clarify the relevance of a difference in treatment means to the experience of individual patients.

Using the mean as a summary of quantitative response may be inappropriate if the data have a skew distribution. For instance, Shaper *et al.* (1983) studied the distribution of gamma-glutamyl transpeptidase (GGTP), a measure of liver function affected by alcohol consumption, in 7613 middle-aged men, as shown in figure 13.4. The distribution is very skew: the great majority of men are in the range 5–20 IU/litre but a few exceed 100 IU/litre. The mean GGTP = 19.2 IU/litre which is not a very suitable 'average' measure since only a quarter of men exceed the mean. Furthermore, *t* tests based on the mean become unreliable with such skew data (see section 13.2). The problem can be alleviated by applying a *log-transformation* to the data. As seen in figure 13.4, the distribution becomes less skew and statistical methods more reliable using log (GGTP). In this context the geometric mean = antilog (mean of logs) = 15.6 IU/litre for GGTP is a useful substitute for the conventional (arithmetic) mean. Gore (1981c) discusses further the transforming of data.

The median is another useful summary of quantitative data particularly if the distribution is skew. It is defined as that value which splits the distribution in half. Ranking observations from lowest to highest,

$$\text{the median} = \begin{cases} \text{the middle value, for an odd number of cases} \\ \text{mean of middle two values for an even number} \end{cases}$$

An example is given by Gralla *et al.* (1981) in a randomized trial to evaluate the antiemetic efficacy of metoclopramide compared with placebo for cancer patients on cytotoxic drugs. The distributions of number of emetic episodes and volume of emesis were both highly skew so the authors used the summary of results shown in table 13.3. For both measures the median on placebo exceeds the highest value on metoclopramide, a fairly strong indication of a treatment difference.

Table 13.3. Summary of results for a trial comparing antiemetic effects of metoclopramide and placebo

	Metoclopramide (11 patients)	Placebo (10 patients)
No. of emetic episodes		
Median	1	10.5
Range	0–9	5–25
Volume of emesis		
Median	20	404
Range	0–225	250–1870

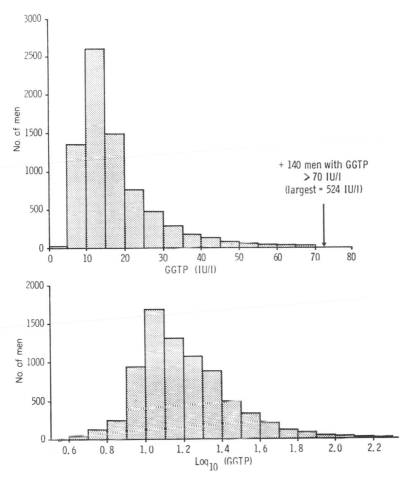

Fig. 13.4. Distributions of GGTP and $\log_{10}$ GGTP for 7613 middle-aged men

13.2 SIGNIFICANCE TESTS

As illustrated in section 13.1, simple data description should reveal whether
there is an interesting difference between treatments worthy of further statistical
investigation. The next issue is to decide whether the apparently better response
on one treatment compared with the other is genuine or could have arisen by
chance. Significance tests are of value here in applying probability theory to
work out the chances of getting a treatment difference as large as that observed
even if the two treatments are really equally effective.

My objective now is to explain the logical reasoning behind significance tests
and to describe the main basic tests (e.g. chi-squared test, two-sample t test and
Wilcoxon test) for comparing two treatments. I will also discuss some of the
problems associated with their use and interpretation.

Comparing Two Percentages: the χ^2 Test

I think the concept of significance testing is best introduced by an example of one specific test, rather than by general, theoretical explanation. The simplest test is a χ^2 test for comparing two percentage response rates (χ = greek letter 'chi' pronounced as in 'kite'). I will now explain how it can be applied to a randomized trial by Hjalmarson *et al.* (1981) studying the effect on mortality of metoprolol or placebo after an acute myocardial infarction.

Table 13.4 shows the death or survival of each patient 90 days after his/her entry into the trial. Mortality on metoprolol is only 5.7% compared with 8.9% on placebo, which is about one-third fewer deaths. If this reduction were actually caused by metoprolol it would represent a major improvement in the treatment of heart attacks. But how strong is this evidence of lower mortality on metoprolol?

Table 13.4. Mortality within 90 days of patient entry in a
trial for acute myocardial infarction

	Treatment Placebo	Metoprolol	Total
Died	62 (8.9%)	40 (5.7%)	102 (7.3%)
Survived	635	658	1293
Total	697	698	1395

The χ^2 significance test proceeds by first considering the *null hypothesis* that metoprolol and placebo are equally effective. If the null hypothesis were true, then for the population of all patients with myocardial infarction eligible for the trial, metoprolol and placebo would have identical percentage mortality. That is, each patient has the same chance of surviving on either treatment.

Question: If the null hypothesis is true, what are the chances of getting as big a difference in percentage mortality as that observed? That is, what is the probability of getting a treatment difference as large as (or larger than) 8.9% versus 5.7%?

This probability, commonly denoted by P, is determined as follows:

$$\text{Observed difference in percentages} = 8.9\% - 5.7\% = 3.2\%$$

Combining both treatments, the overall percentage

$$\bar{p} = 102/1293 = 7.3\%.$$

The standard error of the difference in percentages

$$= \sqrt{\bar{p} \times (100 - \bar{p}) \times \left(\frac{1}{n_1} + \frac{1}{n_2}\right)}$$

$$= \sqrt{7.3 \times 92.7 \times \left(\frac{1}{697} + \frac{1}{698}\right)} = 1.4\%$$

This standard error expresses how accurately the percentage difference has been estimated and is explained more fully in section 13.3.

Now, $$\chi^2 = \left[\frac{\text{observed difference in percentages}}{\text{standard error of difference}}\right]^2 = \frac{3.2^2}{1.4^2} = 5.2$$

The interpretation of χ^2 is as follows. *The larger the value of χ^2, the smaller the probability P and hence the stronger the evidence that the null hypothesis is untrue.* This general statement can be made more precise by referring to a table which converts specific values of χ^2 into corresponding values for P, as shown in table 13.5. For instance, $\chi^2 = 3.84$ means that $P = 0.05$. Hence if χ^2 exceeds 3.84 it follows that P is less than 0.05.

Table 13.5. The χ^2 test: conversion of χ^2 to a P-value

χ^2	P
0.46	0.5
1.64	0.2
2.71	0.1
3.84	0.05
6.64	0.01
10.83	0.001

In this case $\chi^2 = 5.2$ so that the probability P lies somewhere between 0.05 and 0.01. This is usually written $0.01 < P < 0.05$. That is, if metoprolol and placebo were really equally effective, the chances of getting such a big percentage difference in mortality are less than 1 in 20 but more than 1 in 100.

Since P is less than 0.05 one can say that the difference in percentages is statistically significant at the 5 % level, which is generally considered as evidence of a genuine treatment difference. There exist tables for computing a more precise value for P (here $P = 0.023$ in fact). Some would argue that such exact P-values should be quoted, but since most significance tests require approximations or certain assumptions I think such precision is somewhat illusory.

Some people have an intuitive feel for *the meaning of P < 0.05* so that detailed explanation may be unnecessary. Nevertheless, the following brief definition may help. Suppose the null hypothesis (no treatment difference) is true and consider the hypothetical situation where one repeats the whole clinical trial over and over again with different patients each time. Then on average 5 % of such repeat trials would produce a treatment difference large enough to make $\chi^2 > 3.84$ and hence $P < 0.05$. Note that one common pitfall is to misinterpret P as being the probability that the null hypothesis is true.

In practice, the *calculation of χ^2* can be done more simply and reliably by first constructing a table of responses by treatment as follows:

| | Treatment | | |
	A	B	Total
Response	a	b	$a + b$
No response	c	d	$c + d$
Total no. of patients	$a + c$	$b + d$	N

Then,
$$\chi^2 = \frac{(a \times d - b \times c)^2 \times N}{(a + b)(c + d)(a + c)(b + d)}$$

Hence, from our example in table 13.4

$$\chi^2 = \frac{(62 \times 658 - 40 \times 635)^2 \times 1395}{102 \times 1293 \times 697 \times 698} = 5.15$$

The two formulae are mathematically equivalent. This method gives a less intuitive feel of what χ^2 means but is quicker and less subject to rounding errors in calculation.

Let us consider another example, the lymphoma trial whose results were given in table 13.1. The percentages of patients with complete or partial response were 56 % on BP and 67 % on CP. Here χ^2 is calculated to be 2.15 so that $0.1 < P < 0.2$. Since P exceeds 0.1 this is generally regarded as insufficient evidence for a genuine treatment difference and one may declare that the difference in response rates on BP and CP is *not statistically significant*.

Now, it is often the case that a simple χ^2 test can be improved upon by more complex significance tests. For instance, in the lymphoma trial there were four ordered grades of response and there exists another method, the χ^2 test for trend in proportions (see Armitage, 1971, section 12.2), which takes account of this more detailed response classification. Hjalmarson *et al.* (1981) in the metoprolol trial actually used Fisher's exact test (see Armitage, 1971, section 4.8). This test computes P more precisely, especially in small trials, but the extra calculation was not really needed in this case. They then undertook tests for comparing two survival curves (see section 14.2 for details) which took account of when each death occurred. Also, other patient factors (e.g. age) could be allowed for in more complex χ^2 tests (see section 14.1). Some people prefer to modify χ^2 by using Yates's correction but I think this is not appropriate (see Grizzle, 1967).

Of course, statistical refinements are of value when done properly and explained clearly, but in general a straightforward χ^2 test is the most useful significance test which usually provides a valid and meaningful assessment of the evidence for a difference in two percentage response rates.

Comparison of Two Means: The Two-Sample *t* Test

Let us return to the example in table 13.2 comparing women on vitamin D with untreated controls for the prevention of neonatal hypocalcaemia. A two-sample t test to assess the evidence for mean plasma calcium being genuinely higher after vitamin D proceeds as follows.

First, consider the *null hypothesis* that vitamin D does not affect infant plasma calcium. Then, if the null hypothesis is true, what is the probability P of getting a difference in treatment mean plasma calcium as large as (or larger than) that observed?

Observed difference in means $= 9.36 - 9.01 = 0.35$ mg per 100 ml.

Standard error of the difference in means

$$= \sqrt{\frac{s_1^2}{n_1} + \frac{s_2^2}{n_2}}$$

where s_1, s_2 and n_1, n_2 denote the standard deviations and numbers of patients on each treatment.

$$= \sqrt{\frac{1.15^2}{233} + \frac{1.33^2}{394}} = 0.10 \text{ mg per } 100 \text{ ml}$$

Again, this standard error expresses how accurately the mean difference is estimated (see section 13.3 for clarification).

Now, $\quad t = \dfrac{\text{observed difference in means}}{\text{standard error of difference}} = \dfrac{0.35}{0.10} = 3.5$

The larger the value of t (whether $+$ or $-$) the smaller the value of P and hence the stronger the evidence that the null hypothesis is untrue. To be more precise, table 13.6 lists certain values for t and their corresponding values for the probability P. The style of interpretation is much the same as the χ^2 test mentioned earlier. For instance, if the null hypothesis is true the magnitude of t exceeds 1.96 with probability $P = 0.05$. Hence, *if t is greater than 1.96 then P is less than 0.05 and the treatment difference is significant at the 5% level.*

In this case, $t = 3.5$ so that $P < 0.001$. That is, under the null hypothesis the chances of getting such a big mean difference are less than 1 in 1000. This is very

Table 13.6. The two-sample t test: conversion of t to a P-value

Magnitude of t	P
0.67	0.5
1.28	0.2
1.64	0.1
1.96	0.05
2.33	0.02
2.58	0.01
3.29	0.001

strong evidence of a genuine difference between vitamin D and control groups and one declares that the mean difference in plasma calcium is significant at the 0.1 % level.

For the two-sample t test, if the standard deviations of the two groups are similar one can use a different formula for the standard error of the difference in means as follows:

Standard error of difference in means

$$= \sqrt{\left[\frac{(n_1 - 1) \times s_1^2 + (n_2 - 1) \times s_2^2}{n_1 + n_2 - 2}\right]} \times \sqrt{\left[\frac{1}{n_1} + \frac{1}{n_2}\right]}$$

The first part of this product is called the 'pooled' standard deviation. The real two-sample t test uses this more complicated formula, though in practice the simpler formula (sometimes called the z test) is usually accurate enough, and often more reliable if the two standard deviations do differ.

Whichever test formula is used, if there is only a small amount of data one requires somewhat larger values of t to achieve a given P-value. This depends on the degrees of freedom $v = n_1 + n_2 - 2$. For instance,

if $v = 20$ one requires $t > 2.09$ for $P < 0.05$
if $v = 10$ one requires $t > 2.23$ for $P < 0.05$

See Armitage (1971, section 4.6 and table A3) for details.

The two-sample t test is used to compare means obtained on two different groups of individuals. If one needs to compare means of two measurements obtained on the same individual as in a crossover trial then the t test for paired differences is required (see section 8.3).

Now the t tests only give correct P-values if the data follow a normal distribution. However, they are a good approximation if the data are on a reasonable number of patients, say >20 in all, and the distribution is not too skew. Otherwise, with data which are very skew or based on few patients one should use a Wilcoxon test instead:

Comparisons of Two Distributions: the Two-sample Wilcoxon Test

Karpatkin et al. (1981) conducted a clinical trial to see if giving steroids to pregnant women with autoimmune thrombocytopenia could raise the infant platelet count. Table 13.7 shows the infant platelet counts for 12 mothers given steroids and seven mothers not given steroids. One could calculate means and standard deviations and perform a two-sample t test, but the resultant P-value would be unreliable because of the small size of trial and the presence of one unduly high platelet count (399 000). Instead one can perform a two-sample Wilcoxon test as follows:

Rank all 19 observations on both treatments from lowest to highest, as in table 13.7.

Obtain the sum of the ranks T on one of the treatments

$$T = 1 + 3 + 11 + 4 + 6 + 5 + 2 = 32$$

Let n_1 = the number of patients on that treatment

n_2 = the number of patients on the other treatment.

Now, consider the null hypothesis that steroids do not affect infant platelet counts. That is, if one were to obtain the distributions of infant platelet counts for very large numbers of mothers with and without steroids, they should be the same.

If the null hypothesis is true T has an expected value

$$= n_1 \times (n_1 + n_2 + 1)/2$$
$$= 7 \times 20/2 = 70$$

Then, what is the probability P of getting a value of T so far removed from its expected value, if the null hypothesis is true?

One computes
$$z = \frac{T - \text{expected value}}{\sqrt{\dfrac{n_1 \times n_2 \times (n_1 + n_2 + 1)}{12}}}$$

$$= \frac{32 - 70}{\sqrt{\dfrac{7 \times 12 \times 20}{12}}} = -3.21$$

Table 13.7. Effect of maternal steroid therapy on platelet counts of newborn infants

	Infant platelet count after delivery (per mm^3)	Rank
Mothers given steroids		
	120 000	12
	124 000	13
	215 000	18
	90 000	9
	67 000	8
	126 000	14
	95 000	10
	190 000	17
	180 000	16
	135 000	15
	399 000	19
	65 000	7
Mothers not given steroids		
	12 000	1
	20 000	3
	112 000	11
	32 000	4
	60 000	6
	40 000	5
	18 000	2

The value of z is then interpreted in the same way as the value of t was earlier in order to obtain limits for the P-value. In this case, referring to table 13.6, we note that the magnitude of z lies between 2.58 and 3.29 so that $0.001 < P < 0.01$. Thus, the two-sample Wilcoxon test comparing the distributions of infant platelet counts with and without steroids is significant at the 1 % level.

Obtaining P-values from the above formula for z is an approximation which becomes less reliable the fewer patients one has. Instead, one can use statistical tables converting values of T to P-values (see Geigy, 1970, pp. 124–127). In this example, the tables agree with the above use of z.

Another problem occurs if two or more patients have exactly the same observations (e.g. identical platelet counts). Such ties require their ranks to be averaged: e.g. in table 13.7 if the infant with a count of 60 000 had 65 000 instead both infants with 65 000 would be recorded as having rank $6\frac{1}{2}$. Ties also require a slight reduction in the denominator of z; see Armitage (1971, section 13.3) for details.

This two-sample Wilcoxon test is sometimes called the Wilcoxon rank sum test and gives identical answers to the Mann-Whitney U test. Siegel (1956) provides further explanation of this and other non-parametric tests based on the ranking of observations.

Interpretation of Significance Tests

The purpose of significance testing is to assess how strong is the evidence for a genuine superiority of one treatment over another. This strength of evidence is quantified in terms of probabilities, P-values, such that the smaller the value of P the less likelihood there is of a treatment difference having arisen by chance. However, one must note that a small P-value is not absolute proof of a treatment's superiority.

For instance, the χ^2 test showing metoprolol had a significantly lower mortality than placebo ($P = 0.02$) *does not prove* that metoprolol causes a reduction in mortality. Instead, $P = 0.02$ indicates that such a difference is rather unlikely to occur by chance so that there is reasonable evidence of benefit on metoprolol. Nevertheless, one should remember that for every 100 clinical trials using a significance test to compare *identical treatments* one can expect five to have $P < 0.05$. That is, *if $P < 0.05$ is one's criterion for evidence of a treatment difference one in every 20 truly negative trials produces a false-positive finding*. If one performs multiple significance tests for each trial the chance of false-positives may be considerably increased (see section 14.3). On the other hand, if a treatment comparison does not produce a significant difference, i.e. P is greater than 0.05, this does not prove that the two treatments are equally effective. For instance, the χ^2 test comparing CP and BP for lymphoma showed no significant difference in response even though CP had 11 % more responses than BP. This negative finding merely indicates that there is insufficient evidence of a difference: one might exist in reality but it cannot be shown on the available data.

Another issue is that *statistical significance is not the same as clinical importance*. For instance, if the above lymphoma trial were done on 100 000 patients then even a 1% difference in response rate would be significant at the 5% level whereas with only 20 patients a 40% difference would not be. Hence, the larger the trial the greater the chance of showing a certain treatment difference as statistically significant. The clinical relevance must then be assessed in terms of the magnitude of difference and here confidence limits (section 13.3) are of use.

It is common practice to focus on certain specific significance levels: that is $P < 0.05$, $P < 0.01$ or $P < 0.001$ are used as conventional guidelines for conveying results of significance tests. The choice of such levels is entirely arbitrary and has no mathematical or clinical justification. They are merely convenient reference points for displaying findings. In particular, $P < 0.05$ has become unduly emphasized as the level needed to declare a positive finding: some use the phrases 'accept or reject the null hypothesis' according to whether P is greater or less than 0.05. I think such wording gives a false impression of significance tests since it mistakenly attempts to express the inevitable uncertainty of statistical evidence in terms of concrete decisions. In practice, one must recognize that there is precious little difference between $P = 0.06$ and $P = 0.04$.

Now there are three factors which may contribute to an observed treatment difference in response:

(1) *chance* variation
(2) *treatment* itself
(3) *bias* due to other factors.

Significance tests enable one to assess whether the first factor, chance variation, could reasonably explain the difference. Once a significant difference is found one then needs to consider whether the third aspect, bias, could be relevant. Much of this book is concerned with the avoidance of bias. Chapters 4, 6 and 12 on randomization, blindness and patient withdrawals illustrate some means of avoiding potential bias. Two of the trials analysed in this section were non-randomized: the trial of vitamin D for hypocalcaemia (table 13.2) and the trial of steroid therapy for autoimmune thrombocytopenia (table 13.7). Hence the highly significant results achieved in these two trials require a somewhat more cautious interpretation since one is unable to quantify the possible bias due to not randomizing (see chapter 4).

One final technical point on significance testing concerns the use of *one-sided* or *two-sided* tests. The latter have been used throughout this section and are based on the prior assumption that a treatment difference could occur in either direction. The former are based on the premise, preferably decided before the trial begins, that one treatment (A say) cannot be worse than the other (B) so that the significance test assesses the evidence for A better than B *or* A equivalent to B. This implies that if A ended up significantly worse than B one would attribute this to chance since A *cannot* be worse than B. As a consequence the *P*-value is half that for a two sided test, e.g. $0.05 < P < 0.1$ becomes $0.025 < P < 0.05$. To my mind, the use of one-sided tests is generally inappropriate since it prejudges the direction of treatment difference (usually new treatment better than standard) and there have been many trials where a new treatment has fared worse.

13.3 ESTIMATION AND CONFIDENCE LIMITS

The main purpose of a clinical trial should be to estimate the magnitude of improvement of one treatment over another. Although significance tests give the strength of evidence for one treatment being better they do not tell one *how much better*. Hence, significance tests are not the finale of analysis but should be followed by statistical estimation methods such as confidence limits, which are now described in terms of some of the trials already mentioned in section 13.2.

Confidence Limits for Percentages

Let us return to the metoprolol trial data in table 13.4. Percentages dying were 8.9% on placebo and 5.7% on metoprolol, a different of 3.2%. Such a *point estimate* of treatment difference is a useful starting point, especially since the difference is significant ($P < 0.05$). However, each percentage is subject to random variation: one cannot *exactly* determine what the true percentage mortality on metoprolol would be in the long run. Hence the true mortality reduction due from the experience of 700 patients to metoprolol may differ somewhat from the observed 3.2%. The statistical approach to this problem proceeds as follows:

For $n = 698$ patients on metoprolol, $p = 5.7\%$ died within 90 days.

We need to assume that these 698 patients were representative of all myocardial infarction patients who would be eligible for inclusion in the trial's protocol. In fact we assume they are a *random sample* of such patients. We are only interested in this *sample* of 698 patients in so far as they represent the *population* of all such patients.

The estimated standard error of the percentage dying

$$= \sqrt{\frac{p \times (100 - p)}{n}} = \sqrt{\frac{5.7 \times 94.3}{698}} = 0.88\%$$

Then, the *95% confidence limits* for the true percentage dying on metoprolol
$= $ sample % $\pm 2 \times$ standard error of %
$= 5.73 \pm 2 \times 0.88 = 4.0\%$ and 7.5%

That is, we are 95% sure that if the whole (infinite) population of all eligible myocardial infarction patients were given metoprolol the true percentage dying within 90 days lies somewhere between 4.0% and 7.5%.

Similarly, the 95% confidence limits for the percentage dying on placebo are 6.7% and 11.1%.

Before further interpretation of the standard error and confidence limits, let us consider the difference in percentages in a similar way.

The estimated *standard error of the difference in percentages* (as previously defined in section 13.2)

$$= \sqrt{\bar{p} \times (100 - \bar{p}) \times \left(\frac{1}{n_1} + \frac{1}{n_2}\right)} = 1.39\%$$

where $\bar{p}$ = the overall percentage dying on both treatments = 7.3%

95% confidence limits for the difference in percentage mortality

= observed % difference $\pm$ 2 $\times$ standard error of % difference

$= 3.2\% \pm 2 \times 1.39\% = 0.4\%$ and 6.0%.

This formula is an approximation which is reliable except for trials with a small number of patients. Hence, *we are 95% sure that the true percentage reduction in mortality on metoprolol compared with placebo is between 0.4% and 6.0%.*

Here I have introduced confidence limits for the difference in percentages $= p_1 - p_2$ whereas one can also obtain confidence limits for the percentage difference in two percentages $= \dfrac{(p_1 - p_2)}{p_1} \times 100$, as illustrated in figure 15.1.

Interpretation of Standard Error and Confidence Limits

Firstly, *the standard error of a percentage* indicates how precisely the population percentage has been estimated. Theoretically, if one were to repeat the whole myocardial infarction trial over and over again each time using the same number of patients on metoprolol, then the variability in the percentage dying in such repeat trials could be summarized by calculating the standard deviation of all these percentages. This hypothetical standard deviation has been renamed the standard error of the percentage dying and is estimated by the above formula. The standard error of the difference between two percentages can be defined in similar fashion.

One main use of standard errors is to obtain confidence limits as seen above. The whole purpose of *confidence limits for a percentage* is to give some idea of what the true percentage in the whole population of future patients might be. Conventionally, 95% confidence limits are used, these limits for the percentage dying on metoprolol being 4.0% and 7.5%. This means that provided the 698 patients on metoprolol were representative of future patients then with probability 0.95 the true percentage dying on metoprolol lies between those limits. However, every time one calculates such 95% confidence limits there is a 1 in 20 chance that the true percentage for future patients does not lie between those limits.

In clinical trials one is usually more interested in *confidence limits for the treatment difference in percentages*, for which the same style of interpretation applies. People not used to such methods are often surprised by how wide the confidence interval is between the limits. For instance, in the metoprolol trial based on over 1000 patients one has to accept that metoprolol might reduce mortality by anything from 0.4% to 6.0%. The difference is quite likely to be around 3% but could be almost nothing or nearly double that. This illustrates why clinical trials need such large numbers of patients (see chapter 9).

Another example is the lymphoma trial in table 13.1. Here the 95% confidence limits for the difference in percentage complete or partial response are −0.8% and +22.6%. That is, at one extreme BP may be 1% better than CP and at the other CP may be 23% better than BP. The observed difference was 11% in favour of CP, but this was not statistically significant. These two examples illustrate the link between confidence limits and significance tests: *if the test is significant at the 5% level then the two 95% confidence limits will be in the same direction*, otherwise the limits will be in opposite directions, indicating that the absence of a treatment difference is plausible.

One problem in using confidence limits is that the patients in a clinical trial may not be representative of future patients: sometimes they may be a selected group of predominantly good risk or poor risk patients whose response data may be atypical. Confidence limits will then be misleading (the true percentage difference will have more than a 1 in 20 chance of being outside the limits), but then so might be any analysis based on unrepresentative patients.

It is standard practice to use 95% confidence limits. If one wishes to use 90% or 99% confidence limits then one replaces the number 2 in each formula by 1.64 or 2.58, respectively. Confidence limits are a valuable tool for displaying the uncertainty still present after a trial is completed. I feel they could be used beneficially in many more clinical trials, since they convey much more information than significance tests which are all too often used as a convenient shorthand for not looking properly at the data.

Now we go on to the equivalent methods for quantitative data, standard errors and confidence limits for a mean.

Confidence Limits for Means

Consider the vitamin D trial data in table 13.2. For the 233 patients on vitamin D the mean and standard deviation of infant plasma calcium = 9.36 and 1.15 mg per 100 ml. We are really interested in what the mean infant plasma calcium might be if all pregnant women were given vitamin D. The estimated *standard error of the mean*

$$= \frac{\text{standard deviation}}{\sqrt{\text{no. of patients}}} = \frac{1.15}{\sqrt{233}} = 0.075 \text{ mg per 100 ml}$$

Theoretically, this means that if one took a large number of repeated random samples of 233 pregnant women and gave them vitamin D and worked out the mean calcium level for each such sample, then the hypothetical standard deviation of these repeated means is called the standard error of the mean. In practice, we can think of it as assessing how accurately we know the true mean for the population of all pregnant women assuming the sample of 233 women is truly representative.

The *95% confidence limits for the true (population) mean* on vitamin D = sample mean $\pm$ 2 $\times$ standard error of the mean = 9.36 $\pm$ 2 $\times$ 0.075 = 9.21 and 9.51 mg per 100 ml. Hence there is a 1 in 20 chance that the true mean is outside these limits.

The 95% confidence limits for the mean of untreated patients are 8.88 and 9.14 mg per 100 ml. The two 95% confidence intervals do not overlap and this indicates a significant difference ($P < 0.05$ at least). Note that non-overlapping intervals can also sometimes occur when P is less than 0.05.

However, a more direct comparison is to compute the *95% confidence limits for the difference in means*

= observed difference $\pm$ 2 $\times$ standard error of difference

$$= \text{mean}_1 - \text{mean}_2 \pm 2 \times \sqrt{\frac{s_1^2}{n_1} + \frac{s_2^2}{n_2}}$$

using notation previously defined in the two-sample t test (section 13.2). In this example the limits are 0.35 $\pm$ 2 $\times$ 0.10 = 0.15 and 0.55 mg per 100 ml.

Even though the difference in means is highly significant ($t = 3.5$, $P < 0.001$) the confidence limits are still fairly wide, indicating that the magnitude of benefit from vitamin D cannot be accurately determined by a trial of this size.

Sometimes it is useful to present a *graphical comparison* of the means of quantitatives responses, especially if there are more than two treatments. In addition to the mean one can show either the standard deviation, the standard error of the mean or the 95% confidence limits and these three options are shown in figure 13.5(a)–(c) for the vitamin D trial:

(a) *The standard deviation* is the largest of the three and summarizes individual variation about the mean. It does not provide a direct indication of whether there is a genuine difference between treatments. Unless there is an extremely marked treatment difference, use of standard deviations will show that there are high and low values on both treatments, which can be a useful reminder that any treatment has limited ability to affect individual response.

(b) *The standard error of the mean* is the smallest of the three and is therefore perhaps the most tempting for investigators wishing to show a marked treatment effect.

(c) *The 95% confidence limits* are, however, of more direct relevance in providing a valid graphical comparison of treatment means and they are my usual preference.

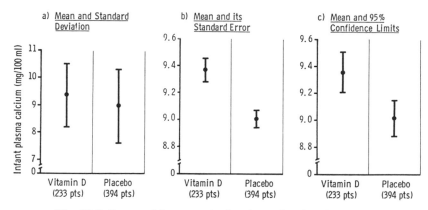

Fig. 13.5. Summarizing quantitative data: the vitamin D trial

If results are given in a table (as in table 13.2), one faces the same choice: perhaps the standard deviation is then the most useful since it summarizes the data prior to statistical inference and allows the reader more easily to check or calculate any significance tests, etc. It is most important that the reader knows *which* is being used since it is a common error to confuse the standard deviation and the standard error of the mean. Also, one should always include the number of patients on each treatment.

Communication of Statistical Findings

This chapter has presented the fundamentals of statistical analysis which I feel anyone concerned with clinical trials would benefit from understanding. Of course, there exist many more complex procedures which generally require the skills of a trained statistician, but the basic findings of most well-designed clinical trials can be successfully revealed with this limited repertoire of techniques plus a good grounding of common sense.

The essence of good data analysis is the effective communication of clinically relevant findings. Hence, one's presentation should always be such that the clinical reader with a rudimentary statistical knowledge should be able to understand the results. More advanced techniques such as analysis of co-variance or statistical models for survival data (see chapter 14) can be of use in clarifying the validity and nature of a treatment difference, but only if their conclusions are interpreted in a non-technical manner.

Further Aspects of Data Analysis

In the analysis of clinical trial data there are many practical and technical issues one could discuss. However, having established the basic principles in chapter 13 I now wish to focus on just three main aspects each of which is commonly encountered. Further developments in statistical methods, especially of a technical nature, are covered in many other texts specifically devoted to such topics.

For each patient one often has information on factors which may affect his or her prognosis and section 14.1 considers how such ancillary data can be incorporated in analysis.

In section 14.2 I deal with the analysis of survival data, where patient outcome is assessed by the time to some event, e.g. disease recurrence or death.

It is quite common to generate a large amount of trial data. One may have several treatments to compare, many different measures of patient outcome, repeated measurements over time or many prognostic factors to consider. Section 14.3 deals with various ways of handling such a multiplicity of data.

14.1 PROGNOSTIC FACTORS

When each patient enters a clinical trial it is often sensible to collect information on personal characteristics (e.g. age, sex), current disease status and previous history of disease/treatment.

The recording of such on-study (baseline) data is discussed in sections 3.5 and 11.1. Its chief value is that some of the patient factors may be related to the patient's subsequent response to treatment. For instance, the prognosis for a myocardial infarction patient tends to be poorer if he has also had a previous infarct. Also, tumour response to chemotherapy of advanced cancer tends to be better if the patient is ambulatory prior to treatment. Here I wish to describe how such prognostic factors can be used in the analysis of results, especially for comparing treatments. I shall use two main examples: *the metoprolol trial* by Hjalmarson *et al.* (1981) and *the vitamin D trial* by Cockburn *et al.* (1980). The basic results of both trials have already been given in chapter 13 and familiarity with those findings may help the reader before proceeding further.

Comparable Treatment Groups

The first step is to check that there are no major dissimilarities in treatment groups as regards prognostic factors. For instance, table 14.1 shows patient characteristics for both treatment groups in the metoprolol trial. For qualitative

Table 14.1. Characteristics of patients on placebo or metoprolol

Characteristics	Treatment group	
	Placebo ($n = 697$) (%)	Metoprolol ($n = 698$) (%)
Sex		
Male	76.2	75.5
Female	23.8	24.4
Age		
<65 years	65.0	66.5
65–74 years	35.0	33.5
Clinical history		
Previous infarction	22.7	21.2
Angina pectoris (5)*	34.7	35.7
Hypertension	29.7	29.1
Therapy before admission		
Digitalis (6)	12.9	12.5
Diuretics (5)	18.7	18.7
Beta-blockers	25.4	25.2
Clinical status at entry		
Pulmonary râles	9.0	11.6
ECG signs of infarction (1)	47.8	49.9
Heart rate >100 beats/min (1)	6.2	4.7
Systolic blood pressure <100 mm Hg (2)	4.4	3.3
Dyspnoea at onset of pain (29)	30.8	28.8
Treatment in hospital before blind injection		
Morphine (3)	53.9	53.6
Atropine (3)	3.5	2.9
Isoprenaline or analogues (2)	0.0	0.0
Diuretics (3)	9.8	10.8
Digitalis (3)	1.9	2.3
Lignocaine (3)	2.7	2.3
Beta-blocker or verapamil (5)	1.6	2.2
Mean age ± SEM	60.0 ± 0.3	60.0 ± 0.3
Mean time from onset of symptoms to blind injection ± SEM (16)	11.4 ± 0.4	11.1 ± 0.4

* Numbers in parentheses are numbers of patients for whom data were missing.

factors (e.g. previous infarction) percentages on each treatment are compared while means and their standard errors are given for quantitative features, e.g. time from onset of symptoms. Age is compared both using means and percentages over 65. A useful extra was to record the number of cases with missing data.

These data show close agreement as regards the types of patients on metoprolol and placebo which reassures that the simple mortality comparison in table 13.4 could not be attributed to any lack of comparability in prognostic factors. In randomized clinical trials one can generally expect treatment groups to be fairly well matched but occasionally one will be unlucky and discover some factor which differs substantially between treatments. This is more likely to occur if the trial is small. When a difference in a prognostic factor is found one might consider whether it is just due to chance or possibly something wrong in the randomization procedure. The risk of any imbalance in prognostic factors can be reduced by using a stratified randomization (see section 5.3).

In non-randomized trials it is particularly important to check for imbalance since one reason for considerable scepticism about non-randomized comparisons is that patient selection may differ enormously between treatments (see chapter 4, particularly comments on the vitamin D trial which was not randomized).

Subgroup Analyses

It is often natural to enquire whether the response difference between two treatments depends on the type of patient. This can be investigated by dividing patients into different subgroups and comparing treatments within each subgroup. However, this does pose problems of interpretation. For instance, in the vitamin D trial one can study the treatment difference in infant plasma calcium separately for breast-fed and artificially fed babies, as shown in table 14.2. Breast-fed babies have higher mean calcium levels than artificially fed babies both for vitamin D and control groups. Also, the treatment difference appeared greater for artificially fed babies which implies that vitamin D may be more advantageous if the baby is not going to be breast-fed. However, one can check this hypothesis by performing the following *significance test for an*

Table 14.2. Infant plasma calcium by treatment and infant feed

| | Artificially fed | | Breast-fed | |
	Vitamin D	Control	Vitamin D	Control
No. of infants	169	285	64	102
Mean plasma calcium (mg per 100 ml)	9.20	8.78	9.79	9.64
Standard deviation (mg per 100 ml)	1.10	1.28	1.17	1.26

interaction between treatment and type of feed. The statistical term interaction is used to describe the situation where the impact of one factor (treatment) on response depends on the value of another factor (type of feed).

Consider the null hypothesis that there is no interaction between treatment and type of feed. Then, we calculate the following:

Mean treatment difference for artificially fed − mean treatment difference for
$$\text{breast-fed} = (\text{mean}_{A1} - \text{mean}_{A2}) - (\text{mean}_{B1} - \text{mean}_{B2})$$

where suffices A and B refer to subgroups (A = artificially fed, B = breast-fed) and suffices 1 and 2 refer to treatments (1 = vitamin D, 2 = control)

$$= (9.20 - 8.78) - (9.79 - 9.64) = 0.27 \text{ mg per } 100 \text{ ml}$$

$$\text{Standard error of this difference} = \sqrt{\frac{s_{A1}^2}{n_{A1}} + \frac{s_{A2}^2}{n_{A2}} + \frac{s_{B1}^2}{n_{B1}} + \frac{s_{B2}^2}{n_{B2}}}$$

$$= \sqrt{\frac{1.10^2}{169} + \frac{1.28^2}{285} + \frac{1.17^2}{64} + \frac{1.26^2}{102}}$$

$$= 0.22 \text{ mg per } 100 \text{ ml}$$

$$t = \frac{\text{subgroup difference in mean treatment difference}}{\text{its standard error}}$$

$$= \frac{0.27}{0.22} = 1.23$$

This t value can be converted to a P-value using table 13.6. Hence $P > 0.2$, which indicates there is no evidence of an interaction. Thus, although it looks as if the treatment effect is greater for artificially fed babies such an interaction could easily have arisen by chance.

One common error in this situation is to perform separate significance tests comparing treatments for each subgroup. For instance, t tests comparing vitamin D and control groups lead to $t = 0.78$, $P > 0.2$ for breast-fed infants and $t = 3.70$, $P < 0.001$ for artificially fed infants. One may feel that these results show that the treatment difference is only present for the artificially fed, but this is too dogmatic an interpretation. *Separate significance tests for different subgroups do not provide direct evidence of whether a prognostic factor affects the treatment difference*: the above test for interaction is much more valid.

Remember that the statistical significance of a treatment comparison depends on the magnitude of difference and the numbers of patients. The fewer patients the less chance there is of a genuine treatment difference being statistically significant. Hence, consider the situation where subgroup A had many more patients than subgroup B but the observed difference in treatment means was greater in subgroup B. Then it would be possible for the smaller difference in subgroup A to be highly significant while the larger difference in subgroup B was not significant. Such conflicting findings will not help one's understanding of prognostic factors. Hence separate significance tests comparing treatments within subgroups should be avoided unless there is a highly significant interaction test.

As another example, let us consider the metoprolol trial mortality results in three age-groups as shown in table 14.3. Mortality rates increase with age in

Table 14.3. Mortality results in three age-groups in the metoprolol trial

| | No. of deaths/no. of patients (and %) | |
	Placebo	Metoprolol
Age 40–64	26/453 (5.7%)	21/464 (4.5%)
Age 65–69	25/174 (14.4%)	11/165 (6.7%)
Age 70–74	11/70 (15.7%)	8/69 (11.6%)

both treatment groups. Unfortunately, these data could be manipulated using χ^2 tests for comparing treatments in various combined age-groups. For instance, age 40–64 has $P > 0.2$ and age 65–74 has $P = 0.03$ which appears to suggest metoprolol is better in the elderly. But age 40–69 has $P = 0.04$ and age 70–74 has $P > 0.2$, which implies metoprolol is better in the younger patients! Again, we get into trouble using separate tests within subgroups. This particular confusion arises because the mortality difference was greatest in the middle age group 65–69. Such a curious age-dependence for the metoprolol effect appears highly implausible, and Hjalmarson et al. (1981) sensibly concluded that 'from the present material we cannot claim that metoprolol has a more beneficial effect on mortality in any particular age-group'.

In this situation a test for interaction could have been performed and would produce a non-significant finding. Unfortunately, with qualitative data interaction tests are complicated to perform (see Halperin et al., 1977), and hence one may prefer to use them only when there is a strong indication that a genuine interaction might exist. This was not so in the metoprolol trial.

In a trial with several prognostic factors one can produce a subgroup analysis for each one. For instance in the metoprolol trial subgroup analyses, such as for age in table 14.3, were also given for previous infarction (yes or no), previous beta-blocker (yes or no) and diagnosis (definite myocardial infarct or others). In this way, one can study treatment results on the same patients classified in several different ways. One needs to be careful not to over-interpret such multiple breakdowns of the trial data. Although it may be useful to display subgroup data it should be looked upon as subsidiary information which is of secondary interest to the overall comparison of treatments. Occasionally, a treatment's effect may be genuinely confined to some subgroup of patients, but this is the exception rather than the rule, so that one should proceed cautiously in interpreting subgroup analyses and refrain from emphasizing factors which do not produce a significant interaction.

Adjustment for Prognostic Factors

I return to the main issue of providing an overall treatment comparison, but now wish to consider how one can make allowance for prognostic factors. If one has comparable treatment groups, as discussed earlier in this section, then any adjustment for prognostic factors will scarcely affect the magnitude of treatment difference but may improve the precision of one's estimate, e.g. by narrowing the confidence interval. However, if treatment groups differ with respect to some prognostic factors then both the magnitude and significance of treatment differences may be altered (i.e. they are determined more correctly) by adjustment for prognostic factors. In particular, if randomization was not used it is important to allow for prognostic differences.

Multiple Regression

For a *quantitative response, multiple regression* is the most common method of statistical adjustment. In this context it is sometimes called analysis of covariance. As an example, let us consider the vitamin D trial. Prior to analysis it was thought that infant calcium levels might be influenced by treatment and also several prognostic factors, as listed on the left of table 14.4(a). First one needs to convert each factor i into a numerical variable, x_i. For some quantitative measurements such as birth weight this is obvious. For other quantities, skewness in the distribution may be diminished either by transformation or truncation. For instance, parity > 3 was set equal to 3. For qualitative factors (e.g. sex) one needs to create *dummy variables* (e.g. male = 0, female = 1). For an ordered qualitative factor such as social class one can either create an artificial numerical variable (e.g. classes I to V score as 1 to 5) or a series of dummy variables. Treatment also needs to be expressed as a dummy variable: control = 0, vitamin D = 1.

An additive model is then proposed for how the infant calcium, y, can be predicted by the numerical variables. That is, for each infant

$$\text{predicted } y = c_0 + c_1 x_1 + c_2 x_2 + \ldots + c_{11} x_{11}$$

where $c_0, c_1, \ldots, c_{11}$ are numerical constants called *regression coefficients* to be estimated from the data. For any choice of c_i values one could calculate the predicted y for each infant. Multiple regression determines that choice of c_i values which minimizes the standard deviation of (actual y − predicted y). In that sense, it provides the best fit between the response y and the variables x_i for prognostic factors and treatment. Computer programs for performing multiple regression are readily available.

Table 14.4(a) shows the results for the vitamin D trial. Each variable x_i has an estimated regression coefficient with its standard error. A significance test for whether a variable contributes to prediction is obtained by computing

Table 14.4. Factors affecting infant calcium level: a multiple regression analysis

Factor (i)	Numerical variable (x_i)	Regression coefficient (c_i)	Standard error	
(a) *Full model*				
1. Treatment group	Control = 0, vitamin D = 1	+0.354	0.103	$P < 0.001$
2. Type of feed	Artificial = 0, breast = 1	+0.717	0.115	$P < 0.001$
3. Sex of infant	Male = 0, female = 1	+0.256	0.100	$P = 0.01$
4. Maternal age	Age in years	−0.225	0.270	
5. Total parity*	Parity, except set equal to 3 if parity > 3	−0.014	0.058	
6. Social class	Classes I to V scored 1 to 5, unmarried women scored as 3	−0.067	0.054	
7. Marital status	Married = 0, unmarried = 1	−0.025	0.192	
8. Birth weight	Weight in kilos	+0.070	0.120	
9. Gestation period*	Gestation in weeks, except set equal to 37 if gestation < 37	+0.053	0.047	
10. Special care unit (SCU)	Not in SCU = 0, in SCU = 1	−0.254	0.170	
11. Pre-eclamptic toxaemia (PET)	No PET = 0, PET = 1	−0.425	0.470	
		Constant term, $c_0 = 7.488$		
(b) *Condensed model*				
1. Treatment	Control = 0, vitamin D = 1	+0.336	0.101	$P < 0.001$
2. Feed	Artificial = 0, breast = 1	+0.771	0.111	$P < 0.001$
3. Sex	Male = 0, female = 1	+0.254	0.098	$P = 0.01$
		Constant term, $c_0 = 8.686$		

* To prevent undue influence of extreme values (e.g. parity 8, gestation 32) these variables have been restricted to a certain range of values.

t = regression coefficient ÷ standard error and using the same P-values as for the t test in table 13.6.

The regression coefficient for treatment is of particular interest. Here it is +0.354 which indicates that the mean increase in plasma calcium using vitamin D, adjusting for prognostic factors, is estimated as +0.354 mg per 100 ml. t = 0.354/0.103 = 3.44 so that $P < 0.001$, indicating that the treatment difference after adjustment remains highly significant. 95% confidence limits for the adjusted mean difference are +0.354 ± 2 × 0.103 = 0.15 and 0.56 mg per 100 ml, which agree very closely with the unadjusted limits calculated in section 13.3. This shows that in a well-balanced trial adjustment for prognostic factors usually makes little difference. However, it does provide reassurance that the unadjusted treatment comparison was valid: that is, knowledge that prognostic adjustment has been looked into gives credibility to the simpler analyses such as in chapter 13.

As regards the prognostic factors in table 14.4(a) only two, sex and type of feed, had regression coefficients significantly different from zero. Hence, there is no evidence that the other factors affect infant calcium levels and one should consider whether it is relevant to keep them in the multiple regression. Accordingly, table 14.4(b) shows the multiple regression for just three factors (treatment, sex and feed). This condensed model is perhaps a more convenient summary of the data. It informs one that for each infant the

> predicted plasma calcium level = 8.686 + 0.336 if given vitamin D
> + 0.771 if breast-fed
> + 0.254 if female

The standard error of prediction (= 1.220 mg per 100 ml) is approximately the standard deviation of (actual − predicted value) and gives an idea of individual variability unexplained by these three factors. Armitage (1971, sections 10.1–10.2) gives further details on the use of multiple regression.

Multiple Logistic Model

For a *qualitative response*, where each patient is classified as achieving some response or not, one can use a *multiple logistic model* as being the equivalent to multiple regression for a quantitative response. Again one first needs to express the prognostic factors (and treatment) as numerical variables x_i using dummy variables when necessary. For example, in the clofibrate trial (Committee of Principal Investigators, 1978) men with high cholesterol were randomized to clofibrate or placebo. Table 14.5 lists treatment and five prognostic factors with their numerical variables x_1 to x_6. One qualitative response of particular interest was whether each subject subsequently suffered from ischaemic heart disease (IHD).

Each patient has a certain probability p of achieving a response. In the clofibrate trial let us consider p as the probability of getting ischaemic heart disease, an unfavorable response in this instance. Then, one can define the following multiple logistic model for how p depends on the prognostic variables x_i:

$$\log\left(\frac{p}{1-p}\right) = c_0 + c_1 x_1 + c_2 x_2 + \ldots + c_6 x_6$$

where as before $c_0 \ldots c_6$ are numerical constants called *logistic coefficients*. $\text{Log}\left(\dfrac{p}{1-p}\right)$ is called the *log odds* of getting IHD and is the most statistically manageable way of relating probabilities to explanatory variables. One can apply the statistical method called maximum likelihood to estimate the c_i values and again computer programs are widely available.

Table 14.5. Multiple logistic model for incidence of ischaemic heart disease in the clofibrate trial

Factor (i)	Numerical variable (x_i)	Logistic coefficient (c_i)	t-value
1. Treatment	0 = placebo, 1 = clofibrate	−0.32	−2.9
2. Age	$\log_e$ (age)	3.00	6.3
3. Smoking	0 = non-smoker, 1 = smoker	0.83	6.8
4. Father's history	0 = father alive, 1 = father dead	0.64	3.6
5. Systolic BP	Systolic BP in mm Hg	0.011	3.7
6. Cholesterol	Cholesterol in mg/dl	0.0095	5.6
	Constant term, $c_0 = -19.60$		

Table 14.5 shows the results for the clofibrate trial. Each variable x_i has a logistic coefficient and also its standard error can be used to obtain t-values as for multiple regression. In this case all six variables have t greater than 2.58 so that each makes a separate significant contribution to a patient's probability of IHD ($P < 0.01$ in each case).

The logistic coefficient for treatment is negative indicating that the log odds, and hence the probability, of IHD is smaller on clofibrate. The other five coefficients are all positive indicating that the chances of getting IHD increase with age, smoking, high blood pressure, high cholesterol and poorer heredity (as measured crudely by father being dead). One can use the logistic coefficients to quantify the impact of each factor. For instance, $e^{c_1} = 0.73$ is the estimated relative risk of getting IHD on clofibrate compared with placebo: that is, the odds of getting IHD were 27% lower on clofibrate, after allowing for prognostic factors. The standard error of $c_1 = 0.11$ so that 95% confidence limits for c_1 are $-0.32 \pm 2 \times 0.11 = 0.10$ and 0.54. Hence e^{c_1} has 95% confidence limits $e^{-0.1}$ and $e^{-0.54} = 0.90$ and 0.58 so that 95% confidence limits for the reduction in odds of getting IHD due to clofibrate are 10% and 42%.

Further details on the use of multiple logistic models are given in Armitage (1971, section 12.5) and Walker and Duncan (1967). It is a relatively complex statistical method which enables one to adjust for prognostic factors in assessing both the magnitude and significance of treatment effect on a qualitative response. However, a simpler method is possible if one has just one or two qualitative prognostic factors to adjust for and one wishes only to assess the significance, not the magnitude, of a treatment difference. This is called the *Mantel-Haenszel test* and proceeds as follows.

Mantel-Haenszel Test

First one classifies patients into several different prognostic categories. For instance, in table 14.3, patients in the metoprolol trial were divided into three age-groups. One could include more than one prognostic factor, e.g. previous infarct (yes or no) could have been added to produce six categories, with or without previous infarct separately for each age-group. However, let us keep to just three age-groups for this illustration.

The null hypothesis is that metoprolol makes no difference to the chances of dying after an infarct. *For each age-group* it is useful to introduce the following notation for the mortality results:

	Placebo	Metoprolol	Total	e.g. Ages 40–64 Placebo	Metoprolol	Total
Dead	a	b	$a + b$	26	21	47
Alive	c	d	$c + d$	427	443	870
Total	$a + c$	$b + d$	N	453	464	917

For ages 40–64, observed deaths on metoprolol $= b = 21$. If the null hypothesis is true, expected deaths on metoprolol

$$= \frac{(a + b) \times (b + d)}{N}$$

$$= \frac{47 \times 464}{917} = 23.78$$

$$\text{Variance} = \frac{(a + b)(c + d)(a + c)(b + d)}{N^2 \times (N - 1)}$$

$$= \frac{47 \times 870 \times 453 \times 464}{917^2 \times 916} = 11.16$$

This calculation is repeated for each age-group.

Then
$$\chi^2 = \frac{[\text{sum (observed} - \text{expected)}]^2}{\text{sum (variances)}}$$

$$= \frac{[(21 - 23.78) + (11 - 17.52) + (8 - 9.43)]^2}{11.16 + 8.06 + 4.13}$$

$$= 4.93$$

The value of χ^2 is then converted to a P-value in the same way as the standard χ^2 test in section 13.2, by referring to table 13.5. In this case P is less than 0.05 so that after adjusting for age the mortality difference between treatments remains statistically significant. Since the age distributions on metoprolol and placebo were very similar, this agreement between the Mantel-Haenszel test and the simple unadjusted χ^2 test is only to be expected. Cox (1970, section 5.3) and Mantel and Haenszel (1959) give further details of this useful test.

Further insight into the rationale and statistical methods for handling prognostic factors is given by Armitage and Gehan (1974). One issue I have not dealt with is the fact that analysis of patient outcome by prognostic factors can give valuable results on factors other than treatment influencing the course of disease. For instance, Stanley (1980) has combined results of several trials in inoperable lung cancer to study prognostic factors for survival. However, such information is not the prime purpose of a clinical trial and hence is not emphasized here.

14.2 THE ANALYSIS OF SURVIVAL DATA

For clinical trials into potentially fatal chronic diseases, e.g. cancer and ischaemic heart disease, the main evaluation of patient outcome is whether the patient dies or not and the time from entry into the trial until death. The analysis of such survival data requires specific techniques which are described in this section. The same methods are applicable if patient outcome is the time to some other measure of patient relapse, e.g. time to disease recurrence in leukemia or time to occurrence of a stroke for patients with transient ischaemic attack.

The first step in analysis is to record for each patient

(a) whether he is still alive or dead, *and*
(b) his *survival time* = time from trial entry to death or time from trial entry to when last known to be alive.

For instance, Kirk *et al.* (1980) randomized 44 patients with chronic active hepatitis to either prednisolone or an untreated control group. Their survival data are listed in table 14.6, in increasing order of survival time ready for analysis. Such individual data can also be displayed graphically, as done by Kirk *et al.* Note that one patient on prednisolone was lost to follow-up 56 months after randomization. He might have since died but since we have no further knowledge we record him as last known to be alive with a survival time of 56 months.

Initial data inspection can elucidate a few basic facts. For instance, 11 prednisolone patients and 16 controls had died. One could compare these using a χ^2 test ($\chi^2 = 2.4$, $P > 0.1$) but this takes no account of when the deaths occurred and how long each patient was followed for. After all, we all die eventually! Hence, it is preferable to make fuller use of the data by using (a) a *life table* to display graphically a treatment comparison and (b) a *logrank test* to see if there is evidence of a treatment difference.

Table 14.6. Survival data for 44
patients with chronic active hepatitis
(D = dead, A = still alive)

Control survival times (months)	Prednisolone survival times (months)
2 Dead	2 Dead
3 D	6 D
4 D	12 D
7 D	54 D
10 D	56 Alive
22 D	68 D
28 D	89 D
29 D	96 D
32 D	96 D
37 D	125 A
40 D	128 A
41 D	131 A
54 D	140 A
61 D	141 A
63 D	143 D
71 D	145 A
127 Alive	146 D
140 A	148 A
146 A	162 A
158 A	168 D
167 A	173 A
182 A	181 A

Life-table Survival Curves

The purpose of a life table is to estimate for each treatment group the percentage of patients surviving any given period of follow-up. In the control group this is easy to do since all patients still alive have longer survival times than the patients who have died. Thus, 100% survived up to 2 months, $21/22 = 95.5\%$ survived beyond 2 months, $20/22 = 90.9\%$ survived beyond three months and so on down to $6/22 = 27.3\%$ survived beyond 71 months. This can be drawn as a life-table survival curve, as shown in figure 14.1. Note that it is drawn as a step function, that is the percentage surviving falls at each month when a death occurs and remains unchanged during months when no deaths occur.

For the prednisolone group the calculation becomes more complicated since some patients who died had a longer survival time than some patients who were still alive. This is often the case and the method is as follows. Working through the death times in ascending order, then

$p(T)$ = estimated percentage surviving beyond death time T

$$= \frac{\text{no. of patients surviving beyond } T}{\text{no. surviving beyond } T + \text{no. dying at } T}$$
$$\times \text{ estimated percentage surviving up to time } T$$

Then, $\quad p \text{ (2 months)} = \dfrac{21}{21 + 1} \times 100 = 95.5\%$

$p \text{ (6 months)} = \dfrac{20}{20 + 1} \times 95.5 = 90.9\%$

$p \text{ (12 months)} = \dfrac{19}{19 + 1} \times 90.9 = 86.4\%$

$p \text{ (54 months)} = \dfrac{18}{18 + 1} \times 86.4 = 81.8\%$

$\leftarrow$ 1 patient still alive at 56 months

$p \text{ (68 months)} = \dfrac{16}{16 + 1} \times 81.8 = 77.0\%$

$p \text{ (89 months)} = \dfrac{15}{15 + 1} \times 77.0 = 72.2\%$

$p \text{ (96 months)} = \dfrac{13}{13 + 2} \times 72.2 = 62.6\% \leftarrow$ 2 deaths at 96 months

$\leftarrow$ 5 patients still alive, at 125, 128, 131, 140 and 141 months

$p \text{ (143 months)} = \dfrac{7}{7 + 1} \times 62.6 = 54.8\%$

and so on. The resultant survival curve is shown in figure 14.1. This is sometimes called the Kaplan-Meier method of life-table estimation. Note that it is identical to the simpler approach, used above for controls, until one reaches the death times which are beyond the smallest survival time for patients still alive.

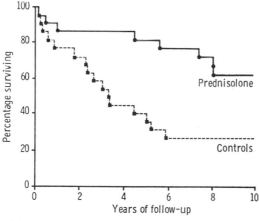

Fig. 14.1. Life-table survival curves for control and prednisolone-treated patients

Figure 14.1 indicates that patients on prednisolone tended to survive longer than controls. For instance, the estimated percentages surviving 10 years were 63% and 27% for prednisolone and controls, respectively. When displaying survival curves one needs to decide what is an appropriate maximum period of follow-up to show. Here 10 years was chosen since, although one or two deaths occurred after that, the life-table estimates become increasingly unreliable since many of the patients had not yet been followed much beyond 10 years. If one shows too great a period of follow-up there is a danger of overemphasizing later treatment differences based on very few patients. For instance, Lebrec *et al.* (1981) compared propranolol and placebo for recurrence of gastrointestinal bleeding in patients with cirrhosis. Life-table survival curves for the percentage free of rebleeding were shown for up to one year even though the majority of patients still free had been followed for less than six months.

In large clinical trials with many deaths, detailed survival curves showing every death time may be conveniently replaced by showing just percentages surviving at certain equally spaced follow-up times. An example was shown earlier in figure 1.2.

The Logrank Test for Comparing Two Survival Curves

The visual comparison of two survival curves is an informative but subjective pastime. One also needs a significance test to provide a more objective means of assessing the evidence for a genuine treatment difference in survival. Historically, people have simply compared the percentages surviving for some fixed time period, say five years. However, this is somewhat unsatisfactory since

(a) the choice of time period is usually arbitrary,
(b) one may be tempted to exaggerate the treatment difference by selecting *post hoc* that time point with the largest difference between survival curves,
(c) one is not making full use of the precise survival times for each patient.

Hence, it has become standard practice to use a logrank test which essentially compares the observed deaths on each treatment with the deaths to be expected if the two treatments were really equally effective (i.e. under the null hypothesis of truly identical survival curves). I now describe this test using the data in Table 14.6 for the trial in chronic active hepatitis.

The main task is to calculate the number of deaths expected on each treatment if the null hypothesis is true. One first needs to rank the survival times of all deaths (both treatments combined) in ascending order. Then for each death time, T, one needs to record the number of deaths at that time d_T (usually just one) and the number of patients alive up to that death time on each treatment, say n_{AT} and n_{BT} for the treatments A and B. Let control = A and prednisolone = B. e.g. for $T = 96$ months, we have $d_T = 2$, $n_{AT} = 6$ and $n_{BT} = 15$.

Then for each death time there are small contributions e_{AT} and e_{BT} to the expected deaths for A and B, respectively, defined as

$$e_{AT} = \frac{n_{AT}}{n_{AT} + n_{BT}} \times d_T \quad \text{and} \quad e_{BT} = \frac{n_{BT}}{n_{AT} + n_{BT}} \times d_T$$

For $T = 96$ months

$$e_{AT} = \frac{6}{6 + 15} \times 2 = 0.57 \qquad e_{BT} = \frac{15}{6 + 15} \times 2 = 1.43$$

Then the expected deaths on A, E_A = sum of e_{AT} for *all* death times T.
The following table, derived from table 14.6 may clarify the calculation:

Death time T in months	d_T	n_{AT}	n_{BT}	e_{AT}
2	2	22	22	1.0
3	1	21	21	0.50
4	1	20	21	0.49
6	1	19	21	0.48
7	1	19	20	0.49
$\vdots$				$\vdots$
96	2	6	15	0.57
$\vdots$				$\vdots$
168	1	1	3	0.25

Hence, $E_A = 1.0 + 0.50 + \ldots + 0.25 = 10.62$ deaths.
One does not have to repeat the whole calculation for treatment B since E_B – total observed deaths – E_A

$$= 16 + 11 - 10.62 = 16.38$$

Let O_A and O_B be the observed numbers of deaths on treatments A and B.

Then
$$\chi^2 = \frac{(O_A - E_A)^2}{E_A} + \frac{(O_B - E_B)^2}{E_B}$$

$$= \frac{(16 - 10.62)^2}{10.62} + \frac{(11 - 16.38)^2}{16.38}$$

$$= 4.49$$

This χ^2 value is converted to a *P*-value in the same way as a conventional χ^2 test (see section 13.2). Hence, using table 13.5 we have $P < 0.05$ so that the logrank test has shown a significant survival difference between prednisolone and control groups.

Peto *et al.* (1977) in a comprehensive practical guide to survival data provide further details of life tables and logrank tests. Suitable computer programs are usually required to ease the burden of calculation.

Survival Data and Prognostic Factors

The use of prognostic factors in clinical trials was discussed in section 14.1. The same general principles apply to survival data, so here I will concentrate on the actual statistical methods available.

First, if one divides patients into several different subgroups using prognostic factors then life tables and logrank tests could be used for separate treatment comparisons within each subgroup. This can generate a lot of results which are difficult to interpret, as mentioned in section 14.1, so that one should think more towards statistical methods of *adjusting for prognostic factors* when comparing treatments for survival.

The logrank test is readily adaptable for this purpose if patients are divided into subgroups. For instance, Kirk *et al.* (1980) in the trial of prednisolone for chronic active hepatitis looked at survival by sex and treatment. The results of logrank tests done separately for each sex are then combined to produce 'sex adjusted' expected numbers of deaths for each treatment as shown in table 14.7.

Table 14.7. Observed and expected numbers of deaths by treatment and sex in the trial for chronic active hepatitis

	Control		Prednisolone	
	Observed deaths	Expected deaths	Observed deaths	Expected deaths
Male	6	3.01	2	4.99
Female	10	7.53	9	11.47
Total	16	10.54	11	16.46

Then χ^2 is calculated as before except we use these sex-adjusted expected totals instead.

Hence
$$\chi^2 = \frac{(16 - 10.54)^2}{10.54} + \frac{(11 - 16.46)^2}{16.46} = 4.64$$

which is slightly larger than χ^2 for the unadjusted logrank test.

This is a useful adjustment method for survival data but does have its limitations:

(1) It cannot be used for quantitative prognostic factors (e.g. age) except by forming them into categories (e.g. broad age-groups).
(2) Patients can be subdivided by more than one factor, but one has to beware of having too many small subgroups.
(3) It is primarily a significance test and does not estimate the magnitude of treatment difference.

Hence one would really like a statistical method for survival data which was equivalent to multiple regression (analysis of covariance) for a quantitative response or the multiple logistic model for a qualitative response (as described in section 14.1). The most successful approach in this direction is by Cox (1972) using what is called 'the proportional hazard model' defined as follows:

Consider a patient who is still alive after being followed for time t. He has a certain (unknown) probability of dying before any subsequent time $t + \delta$, say. The hazard function $\lambda(t)$ for a patient alive up to time t is defined as:

$$\text{the limit of } \frac{\text{probability of dying before time } t + \delta}{\delta} \text{ as } \delta \text{ tends to 0.}$$

One can think of it as the instantaneous death rate at time t and it is sometimes called the 'force of mortality'. Then if treatment and prognostic factors are converted to numerical variables $x_1, \ldots, x_k$ the proportional hazard model is $\log \lambda(t) = c_0(t) + c_1 x_1 + \ldots + c_k x_k$.

$c_0(t)$ represents the fact that the hazard function varies over time, whereas the constants c_i indicate the extent to which the risk of dying is affected by treatment and prognostic factors. The constants c_i, their standard errors and P-values may be obtained using maximum likelihood. A positive value for c_i indicates that the hazard function increases with x_i; that is, high values of x_i are associated with poorer survival. Keating et al. (1980) give an example of this model in a study of factors affecting duration of remission in acute leukaemia. Also, Hjalmarson et al. (1981) used this method to obtain a significance test for metoprolol versus placebo adjusting for several prognostic factors.

Statistical methods for the analysis of survival data are a fairly recent development. Kalbfleisch and Prentice (1980) give a mathematical account of the various methods, while Peto et al. (1977) discuss many of the practical problems to look out for.

In any survival analysis, one should consider carefully the circumstances regarding patients lost to follow-up. All methods of analysis assume that loss to follow-up is unrelated to the subsequent risk of dying. Hence, if such patients tended to be of better or worse prognosis than the rest, analysis might be misleading. In particular, suspicions should be aroused if the treatments have differing numbers of patients lost to follow-up.

This section has described analysis methods which utilize the actual survival times for each patient. This is usually much better than simply classifying each patient as dead or alive, but there are exceptions to this general rule. If the proportion of patients dying is small and all patients are followed for the same period of time T (with no loss to follow-up), then it may be simpler to concentrate on the numbers dying before time T. For instance, in the metoprolol trial analysis (see sections 13.2–13.3 and 14.1) we have concentrated on whether each patient died within 90 days of randomization. Less than 10% had died so that the fact that a patient had died or survived was more important information than his actual survival time.

14.3 MULTIPLICITY OF DATA

In any clinical trial there is a real danger that so much data are generated that one feels overwhelmed and scarcely knows where to begin analysis. It is then useful to keep an overall perspective as to what is the main purpose of the trial. This may be achieved by defining a *limited number of specific hypotheses* concerning the treatments' relative merits (as should have been done in the study protocol, see section 3.1). One can then sort out those *primary analyses* which are needed to examine such hypotheses. Further exploration of the data may follow in due course, but only as a secondary elaboration once the main results have been studied using relatively straightforward statistical methods.

One fundamental problem is that in any substantial clinical trial it is all too easy to think up a whole multiplicity of hypotheses, each one geared to exploring different aspects of response to treatment. In dealing with this problem of multiplicity I will begin by defining its five main aspects:

(1) *Multiple treatments* Some trials have more than two treatments. The number of possible treatment comparisons increases rapidly with the number of treatments.

(2) *Multiple end-points* There may be many different ways of evaluating how each patient responds to treatment. It is possible to make a separate treatment comparison for each end-point.

(3) *Repeated measurements* In some trials one can monitor each patient's progress by recording his disease state at several fixed time points after start of treatment. One could then produce a separate analysis for each time point.

(4) *Subgroup analyses* One may record prognostic information about each patient prior to treatment. Patients may then be classified into prognostic subgroups and each subgroup analysed separately.

(5) *Interim analyses* In most trials there is a gradual accumulation of data as more and more patients are evaluated. One may undertake repeated interim analyses of the accumulating data while the trial is in progress.

An example may highlight the seriousness of the problem. Suppose a trial for hypertensive patients compared four different hypotensive agents. Each patient had systolic and diastolic BP measured before, during and after a standard exercise test. These measurements were taken weekly over a four-month period. Patients could be classified into subgroups by age, sex and initial blood pressure readings. Interim analyses could be undertaken after every 20 patients were evaluated. This study design could generate literally thousands of hypotheses to be examined. For instance, one could compare

(a) treatments A and B for post-exercise systolic BP after one month for the first 30 male patients or

(b) treatments C and D for pre-exercise diastolic BP after two months for the first 20 such patients under age 60, etc. etc.

Such multiple hypothesis testing, sometimes termed '*data dredging*', is liable to confuse and can impede the correct interpretation of trial findings. In particular, it jeopardizes the validity of significance tests. By definition each test has a 5% chance of producing $P < 0.05$ even if treatments are genuinely equivalent. Hence if one makes excessive use of significance tests a certain number of false-positive findings are bound to arise. Thus, the unscrupulous data analyst will inevitably find some significant treatment differences if the data are manipulated sufficiently. One general way of overcoming this problem is to specify in advance a limited number of major analyses one intends to undertake. Any extra analyses derived after data inspection must then be viewed with considerable caution.

Now, let us return to the five aspects of multiplicity listed above. Problems of subgroup analyses and interim analyses have already been covered in section 14.1 and chapter 10, respectively. Hence, I will consider methods of dealing with the other three aspects:

Multiple Treatments

The majority of trials have just two treatment groups (one of which may be an untreated control group). The feasibility of having more than two treatments was discussed in section 9.5. Here I wish to consider how to analyse the data if one does have more than two treatments.

For example, Lenhard *et al.* (1978) studied tumour response in patients with malignant lymphoma on two-, three- and four-drug chemotherapy, labelled CP, CVP and BCVP, respectively. The results are shown in table 14.8 and indicate that the response rate was lower on CP. Now, how can one use significance tests on these data? The answer depends on what hypotheses the trial was designed to examine.

In this case, CP was the standard therapy so that the intention was to see if CVP or BCVP could produce more responses. Hence, it is sensible to perform two separate χ^2 tests:

$$53\% \text{ on CVP versus } 33\% \text{ on CP, } \chi^2 = 4.71, P < 0.05$$
$$48\% \text{ on BCVP versus } 33\% \text{ on CP, } \chi^2 = 3.00, 0.05 < P < 0.1.$$

This shows that the evidence of a superior response rate is slightly stronger for CVP. Thus, if the trial's purpose is to compare several treatment innovations

Table 14.8. Objective tumour response in a lymphoma trial

| | Treatment | | | |
	CP	CVP	BCVP	Total
Response	22 (33%)	31 (53%)	30 (48%)	83 (44%)
No response	44	28	32	104
Total	66	59	62	187

with a standard control group then there is a logical basis for performing a separate significance test for each innovation versus controls.

However, an alternative argument is that one should first make a single global significance test which examines whether there is evidence to contradict the null hypothesis that *all* the treatments are equivalent. If response is qualitative, as in the lymphoma trial, then one performs a χ^2 test for comparison of several percentages (see Armitage, 1971, section 7.4, for details), while for a quantitative response one would need a one-way analysis of variance (see Armitage, 1971, section 7.1). In this case, $0.05 < P < 0.1$ so that this global test is not quite significant at the 5% level. In practice, I find such a global test of limited use since (a) if statistical significance is achieved this does not give direct evidence about *which* treatments are different, (b) the test lacks power to detect genuine differences and (c) most multiple-treatment trials are designed for direct comparison with controls.

In some multiple-treatment trials one may wish to make a large number of pairwise treatment comparisons. For instance, with four treatments A, B, C, D there are six possible comparisons (A v B, A v C, A v D, B v C, B v D, C v D). Such multiple comparisons increase the chances of getting a false significant difference and so it is advisable to make each significance test more conservative by increasing *P*-values. For a quantitative response the studentized range (Newman-Keuls) method may be used (see Armitage, 1971, section 7.3). One simple method, which overcorrects for multiple comparisons, is to multiply each *P*-value by the number of pairwise comparisons being made. Any treatment differences that remain significant after such correction can be said to be based on reasonably good evidence.

Multiple End-points

There are relatively few trials in which patient response to therapy is assessed by a single outcome measure. One usually has several aspects of response to consider. For instance, the lymphoma trial by Lenhard *et al.* (1978) used tumour response, duration of response, haematologic toxicity and patient survival to evaluate the three drug regimens. Although each end-point was analysed separately, the overall conclusion is a subjective overview of these analyses. In this case, since CVP had longer survival than BCVP and CP, a higher response rate than CP and less toxicity than BCVP it seemed logical to infer that CVP appears to have a better potential for future patients.

Use of significance tests separately for each end-point comparison increases the risk of some false-positives. For instance, consider a crossover trial in which each patient received two antihypertensive drugs for consecutive four-week periods. At the end of each treatment period the patient had pulse rate, systolic and diastolic blood pressure measured (a) before a standard exercise test, (b) during exercise, (c) at the end of exercise and (d) 2 minutes after exercise. This leaves 12 different outcome measures each of which could be analysed as in section 8.3. Now, with this number of treatment comparisons one can almost expect one significant difference even if the drugs were identical. *One simple solution is to multiply every P-value by the number of end-points.* This ensures that if treatments were truly equivalent the trial as a whole would have less than a 5% chance of getting any P-value less than 0.05. That is the overall type I error would be less than 0.05. Hence, in the hypertension trial $P = 0.01$ for any specific comparison (e.g. diastolic BP during exercise) would become $P = 0.12$. Thus, in reducing the overall type I error some results which would be significant when studied alone become non-significant when allowance is made for multiple comparisons. Needleman *et al.* (1979), in an observational study of children with high and low tooth lead, adopted this method when making multiple comparisons for different aspects of measured intelligence. However, this simple increase in P-value is an overcorrection for multiple end-points, particularly if the different measures of patient outcome are strongly associated with one another. There exist more complex methods of multivariate analysis but they are often difficult to apply or interpret.

Having such a large number of end-points all analysed 'on equal terms' may not be a terribly satisfactory way of handling trial data. *It may be preferable to reduce the number of end-points measured or to specify in advance some priority for the various end-points.* For instance, in the hypertension trial one could specify in the study design that the end-of-exercise systolic BP was the measure of greatest interest and would hence be the main end-point in analysis. Other end-points could then be analysed secondarily, with the above multiple comparison adjustment of P-values. Note that the primary end-point must be specified in advance. *Post hoc* selection of the end-point with the most significant treatment difference is a deceitful trick which invariably over-emphasizes a treatment difference.

Another approach is to combine multiple end-points into an overall response score. For instance in trials for depressive illness there are many aspects of depression (e.g. depressed mood, insomnia, anxiety, etc.) which could be evaluated. The Hamilton Psychiatric Scale uses a standardized structured interview to obtain 21 end-points which are combined into an overall numerical score for each patient's depression and has become the most common method of assessing response to antidepressant drugs. The creation of such a global scale for patient assessment is a difficult task which is not usually based on clinical trial results. It may sometimes be developed as a problem of medical diagnosis, e.g. how best to distinguish cases of depressive illness from 'normal' controls.

Repeated Measurements

In many clinical trials each patient's condition is evaluated at regular intervals. For instance, in hypertension or asthma it is a simple matter to record each patient's blood pressure or lung function before treatment starts and at weekly intervals. Such repeated measurement may generate a lot of data so that one needs to think carefully about how it should be analysed.

For example, Feighner (1980) randomized 45 hospitalized patients with primary depression to receive trazodone, imipramine or placebo. Figure 14.2 shows the mean Hamilton scores for each treatment group measured prior to start of treatment and at seven-day intervals thereafter up to 28 days.

Now it appears that patients on trazadone had a greater reduction in Hamilton score than placebo patients, but what significance test(s) is it appropriate to use here? One common approach is to perform separate t tests at each time point, including time 0. However, such multiple comparisons often generate confusion. For instance, trazadone versus placebo showed significant differences at day 7 ($P < 0.05$) and day 28 ($P < 0.01$) but not at days 14 and 21. It is hardly logical to believe that a treatment can be effective at one time point but not at another, so I think it is misguided to perform such multiple tests.

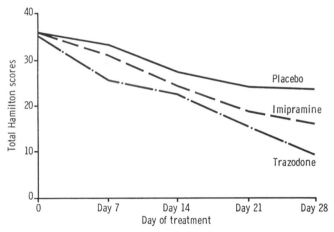

Fig. 14.2. Mean total Hamilton scores at 7-day intervals for three treatment groups of depressed patients

Instead we need to consider what was the underlying purpose of collecting these data. Presumably one wishes to find out whether trazadone does decrease the Hamilton score more than placebo. Furthermore, figure 14.2 and past experience in other trials indicate that whatever treatment is used one generally anticipates that mean Hamilton scores tend to decrease steadily over time. Therefore, it seems most relevant to focus attention on each patient's change in Hamilton score at day 28 compared with day 0. That is, perform just one two-sample t test for the treatment difference in *final − baseline values*, which has $P < 0.01$ in this instance. Further significance tests may be an unnecessary overkill, especially in view of the limited number of patients.

There are one or two alternative possibilities for a significance test. Each patient's Hamilton score will fluctuate from day to day so that the measurement at day 28 may be a rather crude assessment of an individual's response. Hence, *the mean of each patient's last two readings*, i.e. (day 28 score + day 21 score)/2, may provide a more accurate individual score for assessing change from the baseline value.

Another possibility is to take the *mean of all scores on treatment − baseline score* for each patient. It gives equal 'weight' to each time point which may be a good idea if response to treatment is expected to occur early on. If the time-points for assessment are equidistant this is similar to using the 'area under the curve'. Each patient's *minimum* score could be used, but this is likely to exaggerate the effects of all treatments, including placebo.

Fundamentally, *one should aim for a single summary measure of each patient's outcome so that only one significance test is necessary*. It is important to decide on this in advance, indeed specify it in the study protocol, in order to prevent *post hoc* selection of the most highly significant difference.

A more sophisticated analysis of repeated measurements is to use a split-plot analysis of variance (see Armitage, 1971, section 8.5). I find this technique not particularly helpful since it provides only a general test of whether treatments differ over time and it is a baffling procedure not readily understood by non-statisticians. Healy (1981) gives a more theoretical discussion of repeated measurements.

I have emphasized in this section the need to avoid an excessive number of significance tests. Many investigators fail to heed this warning. For instance, Feighner (1980) in his study of 45 depressed patients used over 100 significance tests in describing his results. Such overuse destroys the credibility of each significance test as a method of assessing the strength of evidence for a genuine treatment difference. Tukey (1977) provides further discussion of the multi-plicity problem.

CHAPTER 15

Publication and Interpretation of Findings

The whole purpose of clinical trials is to advance knowledge about the treatment of disease. Accordingly, it is important that a trial's findings be reported in a medical journal so that other interested clinicians can assess the conclusions when determining therapy for future patients. In section 15.1 I discuss the principal issues to consider in publishing a report of high quality. I also emphasize the need for clinicians to make a critical evaluation of published trials in the medical and pharmaceutical literature.

One particularly serious problem in the reporting of clinical trials is the real danger that claims for an advancement in therapy may be erroneous. Section 15.2 assesses the risk of such 'false-positives' and explains why the medical literature tends to be biassed towards an exaggeration of therapeutic effect.

In section 15.3 I discuss the overall strategy that is needed to ensure that the combined effort of all clinical trials for any given disease really does lead to improvements in therapy. One aspect is how to combine evidence from several trials making the same (or similar) therapeutic comparisons. On a more general note, one needs to consider how clinical trials can make a greater impact on improving routine clinical practice.

15.1 TRIAL REPORTS AND THEIR CRITICAL EVALUATION

The usual way of reporting the findings of a clinical trial is in a medical journal. Sometimes additional reports may be produced for:

(1) submission of evidence on drug trials to regulatory bodies such as the British Committee on Safety of Medicines.
(2) more extensive presentation of findings than is possible in a journal article, often just for trial collaborators or a limited circulation to interested groups.
(3) talks at scientific meetings.
(4) advertising by pharmaceutical companies.

However, *articles in medical journals* provide the only reliable means of ensuring that clinical trials become public knowledge.

I now wish to discuss the structure and content of articles on clinical trials firstly in terms of recommendations to authors. This is also relevant to the editors and referees of medical journals who need to decide what constitutes a trial report of acceptable quality. However, journals exist for the benefit of the reader, not the authors, so that my primary concern is how one should interpret wisely the findings of each article. My overall intention is to point out that the reporting of clinical trials does not conform to uniformly high standards and that the reader should be wary of accepting authors' conclusions without questioning their validity. Thus, the following comments are directed both to authors and readers of trial reports.

Writing a Trial Report

In general, articles in medical journals are structured according to the following sequence of sections:

Title	
Summary	
Introduction	Why did you start?
Methods	What did you do?
Results	What did you find?
Discussion	What does it mean?

For clinical trials this sequence is desirable since it provides a convenient means of following the scientific method as previously described in section 1.2 (particularly figure 1.1). That is, the introduction, methods and results sections provide a factual statement of the trial's objectives, design and analysis, respectively, before the authors draw their conclusions in the discussion section.

The *introduction* should present the background to the trial: past evidence which justified the trial being conducted and an explanation of the trial's objectives. The *methods* section is intended to provide an accurate account of the study protocol, as discussed in chapter 3. As in the protocol itself, the main emphasis is on the type of patient eligible for the trial, a description of the treatment regimens to be compared and the methods of evaluating patient response to therapy. However, other aspects of trial design (e.g. randomization, blinding, patient consent procedure, proposed size of trial, plans for statistical analysis, etc.) must also be clearly explained. Essentially, the methods section should include sufficient information to indicate that the trial was properly conducted and is capable of providing a meaningful assessment of treatments. It also forms the basis for detailed comparison with other similar trials.

The *results* section should describe objectively what happened to patients on each treatment. Statistical analysis comparing the treatment regimens is essential here. In addition, some descriptive details (e.g. tables of prognostic factors, the time and place of patient recruitment) should also be given. It is particularly important to report any protocol deviations, especially patient withdrawals (scc chapter 12).

The *discussion* should interpret the results and offer conclusions regarding treatment of future patients. Ideally, the authors should place their findings in the context of previous knowledge so that the article provides a balanced view of the trial's contribution to medical progress. It would also be helpful if authors could display some degree of frankness by pointing out the trial's deficiencies rather than presenting the total success story that is often claimed. The discussion should end with the authors' opinions on therapy and future research.

The *summary* receives greatest attention by the reader. Indeed many busy clinicians will read no further while others need to be tempted to read on by the clarity and interest of the summary. Hence it is of key importance that an accurate précis of the principal findings be achieved. Though a brief interpretation may be warranted and the essence of trial design should be conveyed, the summary should focus primarily on the results. Of course, the *title* needs to be informative, otherwise even the summary may go unread. Thus, the title needs to mention the disease, the treatments and also whether the report concerns a comparative randomized trial.

I do not wish to give extensive details here on what a trial report should contain, since it would largely entail repetition of issues raised throughout this book. The main difficulty is in giving enough details, especially in methods and results, within the tight constraints on the length of published papers. Hence, a clear and condensed style of writing becomes an important aid. Paton (1979), King and Roland (1968) and Thorne (1970) are three general texts on how to write medical articles. For many researchers the act of writing up is a daunting prospect. For instance, Paton says that 'doing the research ... is child's play compared with the moment of truth when you come to write up ... your results'. I think the task is usually made easier by first writing the results section, to be followed by methods, introduction, discussion and summary in that order. Results are the core of any trial report so that it is difficult to make progress with the rest of an article until they are clearly sorted out. In my experience, the ability to write a lucid trial report is a strong indication of whether a research team really has a good grasp of what their clinical trial is about. Unfortunately, there are trial organizers who lack such a clear vision of their research which is why many trial reports are unsatisfactory both in style and content.

Critical Evaluation

One aspect of teaching medical students which I find especially valuable is educating them to become more critical in their assessment of articles in the medical literature. There is a tendency for students, and indeed many clinicians, to treat the medical literature with undue respect. Major journals such as the *Lancet* and the *New England Journal of Medicine* are assumed to present new medical facts which are not to be disputed. Such a naive faith in the 'clinical gospels' is perhaps encouraged by the dogmatic style that many authors adopt, so that the uncertainties inherent in any research project often receive inadequate emphasis in the study report.

So, how can the clinical reader decipher whether a particular clinical trial report is believable or not? Of course, one first has to decide if the trial's findings are of any relevance (i.e. is the article worth reading at all?) and hence a careful reading of the title and summary is a useful preliminary. However, these cannot usually provide enough detail to assess the trial's validity. The real test lies in *careful scrutiny of the methods section*. It is the design of a clinical trial which largely determines whether an unbiased and objective therapeutic comparison can be made. Principal deficiencies to look out for are:

$$\text{inadequate definition of} \begin{cases} \text{eligible patients} \\ \text{treatment schedules} \\ \text{methods of evaluation} \end{cases}$$

lack of an appropriate control group
failure to randomize patients to alternative treatments
lack of objectivity in patient evaluation
failure to use blinding techniques, when appropriate

The methods section often gives insufficient detail to evaluate whether the trial design is satisfactory. In general, I think one should *not* give the authors the benefit of the doubt and one's suspicions should remain until proved otherwise. For instance, if the authors fail to mention randomization one should be inclined to assume that the study is non-randomized and hence may incur serious bias.

If the methods are unsatisfactory then one need not go further: deficiencies in design cannot be corrected by sophisticated analysis and interpretation, so that reliable conclusions are impossible. Indeed, poor design generally leads to exaggerated claims for therapeutic effect.

However, even if the methods section is flawless, there is still *potential for distorting the results*.

Common deficiencies in results are:

too few patients
failure to account for all patients
inappropriate statistical methods
confusing presentation of results
data dredging

It often requires considerable detective skills to pick up problems in the results section. Several enquiries, e.g. Gore *et al.* (1977) and Altman (1982), have demonstrated that statistical errors are a common occurrence in medical journals. However, the two problems I would particularly watch out for are 'failure to account for all patients' (see section 12.3) and 'data dredging' (see section 14.3).

Lastly, one needs to *check that conclusions are justified from the results given*.

Authors have a tendency to give definitive recommendations which sometimes extrapolate beyond what is warranted by their findings on a limited number of patients. In particular, one common over-reaction is to transform an observed therapeutic advantage in a specially selected group of patients into a general recommendation for a much broader class of patients. For example, drug trials for hospital in-patients with chronic depression cannot provide conclusions directly applicable to minor cases of depression seen by general practitioners. Further insight into the critical evaluation of trial reports is given by Sackett (1981), Colton (1974, chapter 13) and Lionel and Herxheimer (1970).

The Need to Improve Editorial Standards

The reasons why readers of medical journals need to exercise caution are:

(1) some authors produce inadequate trial reports
(2) journal editors and referees allow them to be published
(3) journals favour positive findings.

The first reason I have already covered and the third reason is discussed in section 15.2, so that I now wish to discuss the responsibility of editors and referees. I think the editorial standards of some major general medical journals have improved in recent years. For instance, the *British Medical Journal* and the *New England Journal of Medicine* have given greater scrutiny to research methodology, including the use of statistical as well as clinical referees. However, the *Lancet* continues to publish largely without external referees. I fear that the editorial standards in specialist medical journals (where most trials are published) are less critical, so that it remains all too easy for trials of dubious merit to get published. Thus, I feel there is a need for journals to introduce more exacting requirements for evaluating the quality of trial reports, so that misleading articles derived from poor quality research can no longer find an acceptable place in the medical literature. Journals have collaborated in setting stylistic requirements for submitted manuscripts, e.g. International Steering Committee (1978), so that some agreement on research standards should be a feasible proposition.

Mosteller *et al.* (1980) carried out a critical survey of reporting standards for clinical trials. Their conclusion was as follows: 'To encourage authors to include the appropriate descriptions, we recommend that the editor provides a checklist of items expected to be published in a report of a clinical trial. No such list should be cast in bronze, but we believe that editorial expectations will have substantial influence.'

As regards *talks at scientific meetings* and *advertising by pharmaceutical companies*, one needs to be even more sceptical. Neither medium offers the scope for adequate description of research methods, so that the opportunities for bias are enormous.

15.2 AN EXCESS OF 'FALSE-POSITIVES'

Distorted Conclusions

Nowadays it is unlikely that any trial report could conclude that one treatment was better than another without some formal statistical analysis of results. The most widely adopted approach is significance testing: the smaller the P-values the stronger the evidence of a treatment difference. It is a common error for people to interpret statistical significance (e.g. $P < 0.05$) as definitive proof of a treatment difference, whereas a proper interpretation (see section 13.2) should be much more cautious.

Hence, the reader faced with claims of an improvement in therapy should not be overwhelmed by statements of statistical significance. The first task is to look for flaws in the methods and results sections of the paper, as mentioned in section 15.1. In many trials there are sufficiently serious defects in design and/or analysis to suggest that the observed treatment difference may be attributed to bias.

With the improved standards of reporting and editing that exist in some journals today, there is a reasonable chance that one will detect no serious defects. However, *one should still be wary of taking authors' conclusions at face value.* Most clinical trials are undertaken because the trial organizers are enthusiastic about the prospect of making a therapeutic advance. The proper conduct and reporting of a trial is meant to control such enthusiasm, so that the truth (whether positive or negative) is revealed. However, there is always the risk that authors are persuaded towards a greater emphasis on positive findings than is really justified. For instance, there are often many different ways of analysing patient outcomes on two treatments (see section 14.3) and it is tempting for authors to emphasize the significant differences and give scant account, if any, of non-significant analyses. Occasionally, authors may deliberately 'dredge the data to prove a positive' but usually I think such distortion arises quite innocently by authors who are unaware of their subconscious leaning towards the more positive treatment comparisons. Either way, it is up to the reader to compensate for the author's selectivity in reporting of results. Nelson (1979) argues that clinical trials may often resemble pseudoscience 'especially when the report does not contain enough information to enable the reader to determine just what the researcher did do'.

The basic purpose of significance testing is to guard against false claims of a treatment difference. If a properly designed trial has a single treatment comparison which is significant at the 5 % level ($P < 0.05$), then the chances of a truly negative trial producing such a positive finding are 1 in 20. However, many trials have flaws in design or distortion of emphasis in multiple analyses, so that the risk of a false-positive is considerably greater than 1 in 20. This fact alone has serious consequences for the medical literature since it is extremely difficult to sift out those positive claims which are genuine advances in therapy.

Selective Publication

The situation is made worse by the fact that trials with positive findings are more likely to get published. If a trial fails to show any treatment difference, the organizers are inclined to lose interest in writing up their results. Even if they do produce a trial report of their negative findings, medical journals often decline to publish such relatively uninteresting information: after all, it will not lead to any notable medical progress. If a negative trial does get published, it is likely to be in an obscure specialist journal rather than in the major general journals. This *bias against negative articles* by potential authors and editors can seriously mislead the medical profession, particularly when several trials are conducted to evaluate similar therapeutic issues. The more positive trials receive substantial attention in major journals while the negative trials are unpublished or hidden in specialist journals with smaller circulation. Even if all trials were conducted properly, the bias in publication leads to an exaggeration of therapeutic effect.

For instance, Brugarolas and Gosalvez (1980) reported a small, uncontrolled trial of the drug 'norgamem' for treatment of advanced head and neck cancer in which 10 patients all experienced some remission of their disease. These exciting findings also received wide attention in the newspapers: the London *Times* (January 14, 1980) reported a cancer expert as saying that 'if the observations are true, then this is probably the most significant advance since the discovery of methotrexate in 1948'. The European Organization for Research on Treatment of Cancer then undertook a larger phase II trial of norgamem. The results were disappointing: only two out of 31 patients achieved a partial response to therapy. Unfortunately, the report of this trial was not accepted for publication in a major medical journal. Consequently, this negative rebuttal of the earlier positive report could not be made available to such a wide audience.

The Excess of Small Trials

Peto *et al.* (1976) have pointed out that the *bias in publications is made worse by the fact that many clinical trials are of grossly inadequate size*. The logic of their argument, rearranged in terms of one hypothetical example, proceeds as follows. Suppose that standard drug therapy for a certain disease achieves a response in 40% of patients. The pharmaceutical industry would be likely to produce many new drugs with the intention of undertaking randomized controlled trials to find out which drugs can improve on this response rate. Of course, a variety of new drugs can be expected to achieve a whole spectrum of response rates. However, in order to simplify our argument let us suppose that some of the drugs (say 20% of them) were genuine improvements and could increase the response rate to 60% of patients. On the other hand, this leaves 80% of the drugs which were no better than the standard, i.e. they have a response rate of 40%. For only a small proportion of new drugs to improve on standard therapy is quite a common experience in pharmaceutical research. The difficulty is in ensuring that randomized trials are large enough to sift out this minority of effective drugs.

In most diseases the majority of clinical trials involve very few patients and only a small proportion of trials are based on large numbers of patients. For simplicity, suppose there are three sizes of randomized trial comparing new and standard drugs (250 patients, 100 patients and 40 patients) and suppose that the numbers of such trials taking place world-wide are 100, 250 and 1000 respectively. Then, table 15.1 shows the numbers of trials of each size which come up with significant treatment differences, both right and wrong.

Table 15.1. Numbers of trials that will be statistically significant: a hypothetical example

Planned size of trial	Response rates of new and standard drugs	Postulated no. of such trials	Expected no. of trials which are:	
			Non-significant	Significant $(P < 0.05)$
250 patients	40 % v. 40 %	80	76 right	4 wrong
	60 % v. 40 %	20	2 wrong	18 right
100 patients	40 % v. 40 %	200	190 right	10 wrong
	60 % v. 40 %	50	25 wrong	25 right
40 patients	40 % v. 40 %	800	760 right	40 wrong
	60 % v. 40 %	200	150 wrong	50 right

A trial with 250 patients (125 on each treatment) has a 90 % chance of detecting a true response difference of 60 % versus 40 % as being significant at the 5 % level (see section 9.1 for method of calculation). Hence, 18 out of 20 such trials with a genuine treatment difference should achieve a true positive finding. However, four out of 80 trials of equivalent drugs can be expected to come up with a false-positive finding. Still, for trials of this size only a small minority of positives (4/22 = 18 %) will be false-positives.

Each trial with 100 patients has only about a 50 % chance of detecting a 60 % versus 40 % response difference and consequently the proportion of all positive trials which are false-positives becomes 10/35 = 29 %. Worse still, for trials with 40 patients the chances of detecting the response difference are only 1 in 4, so that the false-positive rate becomes 40/90 = 44 %. Since small trials which show no significant difference are unlikely to get published, the medical literature fails to counterbalance these false-positives with the much larger number of negative studies. However, it would be unrealistic and undesirable to have the literature saturated with small negative trials. *The only effective solution is not to publish any small trials*, whether they be negative or positive.

In general, since most studies are on the small side the false-positive rate in the literature is quite high. In this example, the expected totals of true positives and false-positives are 93 and 54, respectively, an overall false-positive rate of 37%. Of course, such a simplified model of trial reporting has its limitations but it should help to emphasize the magnitude of this problem. The above calculation takes no account of the biasses inherent in many trials, so that I think it is reasonable to argue that *perhaps the majority of trial reports claiming a treatment difference are false-positives.*

15.3 COMBINING EVIDENCE AND OVERALL STRATEGY

Replication of Trials

In the previous section I have given a somewhat pessimistic outlook on the medical literature. Essentially, for most diseases it is unrealistic to expect that any single clinical trial can totally resolve a therapeutic issue. The conclusions of any major trial report, no matter how convincingly presented by the authors, are unlikely to be greeted with unanimous agreement by the medical profession. Possible flaws in trial methodology and the statistical uncertainties of any treatment comparison (see section 13.3 on confidence limits) are obvious grounds for concern. In addition, the credibility of any single research project in overcoming previous clinical suspicions and contrary opinions has its limitations. Even the largest and most carefully executed trial may lack persuasiveness if it stands in isolation as the only piece of evidence supporting a certain treatment policy.

Hence, any progress in changing clinical practice is more readily achieved if further clinical trials into the same issue produce similar findings. *Replication of a clinical trial in different circumstances is a valuable step in checking the original's validity.* However, Zelen (1983) points out that 'many journal editors are reluctant to publish articles which are confirmations of earlier published clinical trials. Confirmatory trials are not regarded as being as exciting or innovative as the first report of a therapeutic advance.'

Pooling of Data

Any proper assessment of a therapeutic issue should involve a compilation of all the evidence from published trials. In some circumstances this can be done objectively by *'pooling the data' from several similar trials*, as in the following example:

One major controversy is whether beta-blockers are effective in reducing mortality after myocardial infarction. Baber and Lewis (1982) and Peto (1982) have produced similar reviews of published trials on this topic. Figure 15.1 is derived from Baber and Lewis and summarizes the findings from 17 clinical trials. Each trial was a randomized comparison of mortality for patients on beta-blocker or placebo. For instance, the first trial by Wilcox *et al.* (1980) had

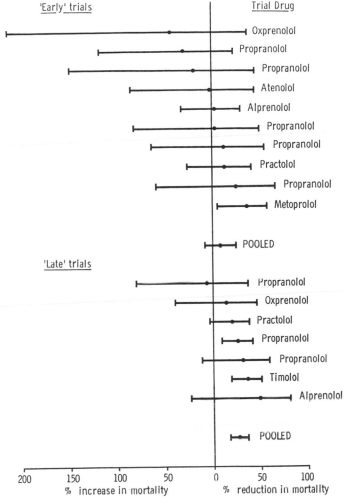

Fig. 15.1. Percentage reduction in mortality (with 95% confidence limits) for 17 beta-blocker postinfarction trials

14/157 (8.9%) patients on oxprenolol dying within six weeks compared with 10/158 (6.3%) on placebo. Thus, the observed proportional increase in mortality on oxprenolol = 41%*. However, this study had too few patients (and hence too few deaths) on each treatment to assess accurately the effect of oxprenolol. In fact, 95% confidence limits for the proportional change in

---

* The apparent mortality increase could have been expressed as a simple difference in percentages = 8.9% − 6.3% = 2.6%. This is not done here since the percentage dying depends heavily on the period of follow-up and the type of patient included in the trial. Instead the proportional change in mortality $= \dfrac{8.9 - 6.3}{6.3} \times 100 = +41\%$ has been used.

mortality on oxprenolol compared with placebo are -37% and $+213\%$, a phenomenally wide range. Note that the confidence intervals overlap 0%, indicating that there was no significant difference between oxprenolol and placebo. In effect, this trial (like many of the others listed) makes little contribution by itself in clarifying the value of beta-blockers.

However, when the results of all seventeen trials are presented simultaneously (as in figure 15.1) certain patterns begin to emerge. Trials were classified as 'early' or 'late' depending on whether treatment was begun within 24 hours of onset of symptoms or not. The ten 'early' trials had a mixture of both increases and reductions in mortality on beta-blocker. Only the metoprolol trial, previously mentioned in chapters 13 and 14, had a significant mortality reduction. The seven 'late' trials appeared more promising: all but one observed a reduction in mortality, which was significant for two trials.

There are statistical methods for pooling the data from several trials to derive an overall estimate of treatment effect; see Peto (1978, Table 1) and Lewis and Ellis (1982) for further details. It is not simply a matter of throwing all the data together, since allowance must be made for the trials' differing patient numbers and differing mortality rates. In this case, the statistical significance of an overall treatment effect can be assessed using the Mantel-Haenszel test described in section 14.1, where each trial contributes its observed and expected deaths towards an overall χ^2.

The end-results of pooling the data are shown in figure 15.1. For 'early' trials and 'late' trials there are estimated overall reductions in mortality of 8% and 26%, respectively. For 'early' trials the pooled confidence limits overlap 0%, so that there is no significant mortality difference between 'early' beta-blockers and placebo. However, 95% confidence limits for the mortality reduction of 'late' beta-blockers are 17% and 35%, which indicates strong evidence in their favour.

Incidentally, this example serves to illustrate the limitation of using significance tests and the advantage of providing confidence limits for treatment effect, as previously mentioned in section 13.3. *I think it would be of benefit if trial reports generally became less obsessed with significance tests, and concentrated more on estimating the possible magnitude of treatment effect.*

I now wish to discuss some of the difficulties inherent in trying to summarize such a collection of clinical trials. The main problem is *the diversity of treatments and trial designs.* In our example, several different drugs were included, on the premise that their common effect, beta-blockade, gave them sufficient similarity for assessment as a single entity. Of course, it may well be that the drugs differ in effectiveness but this would require data on really *huge* numbers of patients which are unlikely to be realized. Also the treatment schedules may differ (e.g. oral versus intravenous therapy, duration and pattern of dosage) and it is a matter of judgement as to how much these variations affect the validity of pooled comparison.

Trials with radically different or inadequate design should not be included, e.g. those trials without placebo controls were excluded here. However, one must be careful not to bias the pooled assessment by rejecting trials on the basis of anomolous results and reasons for exclusion should be provided (e.g. see Lewis and Ellis, 1982).

In reality, the formal pooling of data from related trials can probably only be done for a minority of therapeutic issues, because all too often the measures of patient outcome and the manner of their reporting will not be consistent enough. The potential for pooling data can be applied most readily to mortality studies, as above. Even so, one has to aim for 'all cause' mortality and similar follow-up periods in the different trials. For studies with morbidity outcomes (whether qualitative or quantitative) there is usually less scope for pooling data since criteria of evaluation are likely to be more diverse and less reproducible from one study to another.

Literature Reviews

Hence, reviews of the literature will often need to be less formal than the above example. Nevertheless, expert evaluation of the collected evidence from several trials of a particular therapy is of considerable value, even though they inevitably depend more on personal opinion in interpretation. Henderson and Canellos (1980) is one such review covering many aspects of therapy for breast cancer. They use tabulations of trial results on each issue (e.g. limited versus radical surgery, combination chemotherapy) as a basis for their conclusions. *Such reviews serve an important function: they enable clinicians who have neither the time, knowledge or ability to read all relevant articles to keep informed of current research.*

The validity of any literature review rests on two features: (1) the ability of the reviewer to be reasonably objective in his appraisal of diverse evidence and (2) the extent to which the reviewer is successful in accounting for all relevant trials, whether published or not. This latter aspect can be a particular problem, as pointed out in section 15.2, and is relevant both to pooling of data and more general reviews.

For some issues, such as the above review of beta-blockade post infarction, we may be fortunate in being comprehensive. If a beta-blocker trial is to make a real contribution it has to be a large, collaborative study requiring considerable resources and such studies will get reported. Peto (1982) states that 'a few long term trials have yet to be published, but even if they have been delayed because they happen to indicate a non-significantly opposite effect, no large change in the aggregated results can be expected.'

However, for many diseases evaluation of new treatments is more piecemeal, with a large number of small trials. This is particularly likely for pharmaceutical company sponsored trials of drug therapy for less-serious chronic conditions, as previously mentioned in section 9.3. The arguments in section 15.2 imply that any literature review on such a topic is bound to overstate the effectiveness of new drugs.

The Impact of Clinical Trials on Medical Practice

In considering an overall strategy for clinical trials, one should note that what matters most of all is their ability to improve subsequent treatment practices, not just in those specialist centres conducting trials, but in the medical community as a whole. Spodick (1982) discusses several behavioural pitfalls by trialists and other clinicians which inhibit such progress. Two particular problems he emphasizes are that:

(1) 'General acceptance' of a therapeutic hypothesis is not proof of efficacy, yet physicians traditionally behave as if this were so
(2) Large amounts of poor data tend to preempt any amount of good data

The first quote sums up the fact that objective evidence from clinical trials cannot be expected to make much impact as long as clinicians continue to rely primarily on their collective opinion of which treatments are fashionable. The training of doctors is often conducted as a rather dogmatic transfer of medical facts. This helps to enhance confidence in their abilities which is undoubtedly of value in doctor–patient relationships. Unfortunately, it can also induce undue 'reverence for authority and tradition', a certain 'compulsion to treat' and a 'reluctance to admit doubt' on treatment efficacy. Hence, there is a need for medical education to create a more critical awareness of the uncertainty surrounding many therapies. Only then will physicians have the scientist's attitude of mind which is readily influenced by the findings of properly conducted clinical trials rather than the prejudices of personal opinion.

However, we also need to ensure that the second quote above becomes less applicable to the practice of clinical trials. A critical review of the clinical trials on any specific issue is liable to be a frustrating experience as one discovers the poor quality inherent in much of the work. So, in conclusion I wish to present some of *the main requirements for improvement*:

(1) Better trial design

Many trials lack essential features of design to achieve an unbiassed assessment of therapy. Failure to use randomized controls remains the most crucial deficiency, especially in surgical trials. Other trials may fail due to lack of objectivity in patient evaluation and poor definition of eligible patients or treatments.

(2) More efficient organization

Even a well-designed trial will flounder if there is poor administrative control. Specific problems are protocol violations, poor data handling and lack of patient follow-up. Thus trials require adequate resources as regards finance, staff and experience.

(3) More Patients

One enormous stumbling block is to get enough patients for an accurate treatment comparison. Far too many trials fall woefully short of a realistic sample size. Such trials should not take place and there is a need for greater collaboration so that more multi-centre trials of acceptable size can be achieved.

(4) Improved Presentation of Findings

Trial reports sometimes lack clarity and objectivity. This may be a consequence of inadequate design, but the presentation and interpretation of statistical information is often inadequate or, worse still, biassed. Particular issues are failure to include all patients entered, excessive use of significance testing, undue emphasis on positive findings and actual errors.

(5) Greater Simplicity and Patient Benefit

There is a danger of making trials so complex that they become too unmanageable and expensive. The ultimate emphasis should be towards overall patient benefit and this requires more large-scale trials which focus on general measures of patient outcome (e.g. survival). All too many trials are cluttered with large quantities of patient data which are only of secondary interest.

(6) Reporting of all Clinical Trials

The conclusions so far relate to each individual trial, but we also need to improve overall strategy. The greatest failing is that many trials, especially with negative findings, never become public knowledge. This situation distorts the assessment of therapies but is going to be very difficult to rectify. Perhaps attempts could be made to set up complete registers of active trials in each disease so that there was more scope for obtaining a totality of experience derived from *all* trials of each therapy.

(7) Relevance of Research Effort

Is the direction of clinical trials sufficiently relevant to society's needs? Heart transplants and cures for cancer are likely to capture the public imagination, but a more realistic view of clinical trials suggests that the future lies in making less spectacular gains which are applicable to larger numbers of patients. Furthermore, in areas of major controversy (e.g. oral drugs for diabetes, management of primary breast cancer, multi-vitamin therapy for prevention of neural tube defects) there is resistance by many clinicians to undertake randomized controlled trials. However, unless such trials are allowed to take place adequate evidence to resolve these major issues will never be forthcoming.

References

Abraham, E. P., Chain, E., Fletcher, C. M., *et al.* (1941). Further observations on penicillin. *Lancet*, **ii**, 177–188.

Acute Leukemia Group B (1963). The effect of 6-MP on the duration of steroid-induced remissions in acute leukemia: a model for evaluation of other potentially useful therapy. *Blood*, **62**, 699–716.

Allen, P. A., and Waters, W. E. (1982). Development of an ethical committee and its effect on research design. *Lancet*, **i**, 1233–1236.

Altman, D. G. (1980a). Statistics and ethics in medical research: I. Misuse of statistics is unethical. *Br. Med. J.*, **281**, 1182–1184.

Altman, D. G. (1980b). Statistics and ethics in medical research: III. How large a sample? *Br. Med. J.*, **281**, 1336–1338.

Altman, D. G. (1982). Statistics in medical journals. *Statistics in Medicine*, **1**, 59–71.

Anturane Reinfarction Trial Research Group (1978). Sulfinpyrazone in the prevention of cardiac death after myocardial infarction. *N. Engl. J. Med.*, **298**, 289–295.

Anturane Reinfarction Trial Research Group (1980). Sulfinpyrazone in the prevention of sudden death after myocardial infarction. *N. Engl. J. Med.*, **302**, 250–256.

Armitage, P. (1971). *Statistical Methods in Medical Research*. Oxford: Blackwell.

Armitage, P. (1975). *Sequential Medical Trials*, 2nd edition. Oxford: Blackwell.

Armitage, P. (1980). The analysis of data from clinical trials. *Statistician*, **28**, 171–183.

Armitage, P., and Gehan, E. A. (1974). Statistical methods for the identification and use of prognostic factors. *Int. J. Cancer*, **13**, 16–36.

Armitage, P., and Hills, M. (1982). The two-period crossover trial. *Statistician*, **31**, 119–131.

Armitage, P., McPherson, K., and Rowe, B. C. (1969). Repeated significance tests on accumulating data. *J. R. Statist. Soc. A*, **132**, 235–244.

Armstrong, P. W. (1979). A new design for randomized trials (letter). *N. Engl. J. Med.*, **300**, 786.

Baber, N. S., and Lewis, J. A. (1982). Confidence in results of beta-blocker post-infarction trials. *Br. Med. J.*, **284**, 1749–1750.

Begg, C. B., and Iglewicz, B. (1980). A treatment allocation procedure for clinical trials. *Biometrics*, **36**, 81–90.

Begg, C. B., Carbone, P. P., Elson, P. J., and Zelen, M. (1982). Participation of community hospitals in clinical trials: analysis of five years experience in the Eastern Cooperative Oncology Group. *N. Engl. J. Med.*, **306**, 1076–1080.

Berkson, J. (1978). In dispraise of the exact test. *J. Stat. Planning Inference*, **2**, 27–42.

Bland, J. M., Jones, D. R., Bennett, S., *et al.* (1983). Is the clinical trial evidence for new drugs statistically adequate? Personal communication.

Bodey, G. P., Gehan, E. A., Freireich, E. J., and Frei, E. (1971). Protected

248

environment—prophylactic antibiotic program in the chemotherapy of acute leukemia. *Am. J. Med. Sci.*, **262**, 138–151.

Bonadonna, G., Rossi, A., Valagussa, P., *et al.* (1977). The CMF program for operable breast cancer with positive axillary nodes. *Cancer*, **39**, 2904–2915.

Bonchek, L. I. (1979). Are randomized trials appropriate for evaluating new operations? *N. Engl. J. Med.*, **301**, 44–45.

Brahams, D. (1982). Death of a patient who was unwitting subject of randomized controlled trial of cancer treatment. *Lancet*, **i**, 1028–1029.

Brewin, T. B. (1982). Consent to randomized treatment. *Lancet*, **ii**, 919–921.

British Medical Association (1980). *The Handbook of Medical Ethics.* London: British Medical Association.

British Medical Journal (1970). Double blind or not? (leader) *Br. Med. J.*, **ii**, 597–598.

British Medical Journal (1977). Randomized clinical trials (leader). *Br. Med. J.*, **i**, 1238–1239.

Brown, B. W. (1980). Statistical controversies in the design of clinical trials—some personal views. *Controlled Clin. Trials*, **1**, 13–27.

Brugarolas, A., and Gosalvez, M. (1980). Treatment of cancer by an inducer of reverse transformation. *Lancet*, **i**, 68–70.

Bull, J. P. (1959). The historical development of clinical therapeutic trials. *J. Chron. Dis.*, **10**, 218–248.

Burkhardt, R., and Kienle, G. (1978). Controlled clinical trials and medical ethics. *Lancet*, **ii**, 1356–1359.

Byar, D. (1980). Why data bases should not replace randomized clinical trials. *Biometrics*, **36**, 337–342.

Byar, D. P., Simon, R. M., Friedewald, W. T., *et al.* (1976). Randomized clinical trials: perspectives on some recent ideas. *N. Engl. J. Med.*, **295**, 74–80.

Canadian Cooperative Study Group (1978). A randomized trial of aspirin and sulfinpyrazone in threatened stroke. *N. Engl. J. Med.*, **299**, 53–59.

Cancer Research Campaign Working Party (1980). Trials and tribulations: thoughts on the organisation of multicentre clinical studies. *Br. Med. J.*, **281**, 918–920.

Canner, P. L. (1977). Monitoring treatment differences in long-term clinical trials. *Biometrics*, **33**, 603–615.

Casagrande, J. T., Pike, M. C., and Smith, P. G. (1978). The power function of the exact test for comparing two binomial distributions. *Appl. Statist.*, **27**, 176–180.

Chalmers, T. C. (1972). Randomization and coronary artery surgery. *Ann. Thor. Surg.*, **14**, 323–327.

Chalmers, T. C., and Schroeder, B. (1979). Controls in 'Journal' articles. *N. Engl. J. Med.*, **301**, 1293.

Chalmers, T. C., Block, J. B., and Lee, S. (1972). Controlled studies in clinical cancer research. *N. Engl. J. Med.*, **287**, 75–78.

Chalmers, T. C., Matta, R. J., Smith, H., and Kunzler, A.-M. (1977). Evidence favoring the use of anticoagulants in the hospital phase of acute myocardial infarction. *N. Engl. J. Med.*, **297**, 1091–1096.

Christiansen, C., Rødbro, P., and Sjö, O. (1974). 'Anticonvulsant action' of vitamin D in epileptic patients? A controlled pilot study. *Br. Med. J.*, **ii**, 258–259.

Cochran, W. G., and Cox, G. M. (1957). *Experimental Designs.* New York: Wiley.

Cochrane, A. L. (1972). *Effectiveness and Efficiency: Random Reflections on Health Services.* Oxford: Nuffield Provincial Hospitals Trust.

Cockburn, F., Belton, N. R., Purvis, R. J., *et al.* (1980). Maternal vitamin D intake and mineral metabolism in mothers and their newborn infants. *Br. Med. J.*, **281**, 11–14.

Colebrook, L., and Purdie, A. W. (1937). Treatment of 106 cases of puerperal fever by sulphonilamide. *Lancet*, **ii**, 1237–1242 and 1291–1294.

Colton, T. (1974). *Statistics in Medicine.* Boston: Little Brown.

250

Committee of Principal Investigators (1978). A cooperative trial in the primary prevention of ischaemic heart disease using clofibrate. *Br. Heart J.*, **40**, 1069–1118.

Committee of Principal Investigators (1980). W.H.O. cooperative trial on primary prevention of ischaemic heart disease using clofibrate to lower serum cholesterol: mortality follow-up. *Lancet*, **ii**, 379–385.

Cook, P. J., James, I. M., Hobbs, K. E. F., and Browne, D. R. G. (1982). Controlled comparison of i.m. morphine and buprenorphine for analgesia after abdominal surgery. *Br. J. Anaesth.*, **54**, 285–290.

Costello, W. G. (1974). Phase III study of TIC mustard, DTIC and BCG in malignant melanoma. *Eastern Cooperative Oncology Group Report of Completed Studies*, 195–227.

Cox, D. R. (1958). *Planning of Experiments*. New York: Wiley.

Cox, D. R. (1970). *Analysis of Binary Data*. London: Methuen.

Cox, D. R. (1972). Regression models and life tables. *J. R. Statist. Soc.*, **34**, 187–220.

Cranberg, L. (1979). Do retrospective controls make clinical trials 'inherently fallacious?', *Br. Med. J.*, **ii**, 1265–1266.

D'Angio, G. J., Evans, A. E., Breslow, N., *et al.* (1976). The treatment of Wilms' tumor: results of the National Wilms' Tumor Study. *Cancer*, **38**, 633–646.

Danish Obesity Project (1979). Randomized trial of jejunoileal bypass versus medical treatment in morbid obesity. *Lancet*, **ii**, 1255–1257.

Demets, D. L., and Ware, J. H. (1980). Group sequential methods in clinical trials with a one-sided hypothesis. *Biometrika*, **67**, 651–660.

Diabetic Retinopathy Study Research Group (1976). Preliminary report on effects of photocoagulation therapy. *Am. J. Ophthalmol.*, **81**, 383–396.

Doll, R., and Peto, R. (1980). Randomized controlled trials and retrospective controls. *Br. Med. J.*, **i**, 44.

Douglas, R. B. (1975). Human reflex broncho-constriction as an adjunct to conjunctival sensitivity in defining threshold limit values for irritant gases and vapours. *Ph.D. Thesis*, London University.

Douglass, H. O., Lavin, P. J., Woll, J., *et al.* (1978). Chemotherapy of advanced measurable colon and rectal carcinoma. *Cancer*, **42**, 2538–2545.

Ebbutt, A. F. (1984). Three period crossover designs for two treatments. *Biometrics*, **40**, (in press).

Efron, B. (1971). Forcing a sequential experiment to be balanced. *Biometrika*, **58**, 403–417.

Ehrenkranz, R. A., Bonta, B. W., Ablow, R. C., *et al.* (1978). Amelioration of bronchopulmonary dysplasia after vitamin E administration. *N. Engl. J. Med.*, **299**, 564–569.

Ellison, N. M., Byar, D. P., and Newell, G. R. (1978). Special report on Laetrile: the NCI Laetrile review. *N. Engl. J. Med.*, **229**, 549–552.

Epstein, O., Lee, R. G., Boss, A. M., *et al.* (1981). D-Penicillamine treatment improves survival in primary biliary cirrhosis. *Lancet*, **i**, 1275–1277.

Evans, G. M., and Gaisford, W. F. (1938). Treatment of pneumonia with 2(p-aminobenzene-sulphonamido)pyridine. *Lancet*, **ii**, 14–19.

Ezdinli, E., Pocock, S., Berard, C. W., *et al.* (1976). Comparison of intensive versus moderate chemotherapy of lymphocytic lymphomas: a progress report. *Cancer*, **38**, 1060–1068.

Feighner, J. P. (1980). Trazodone, a triazolopyridine derivative in primary depressive disorder. *J. Clin. Psychiatry*, **41**, 250–255.

Ferguson, F. R., Davey, A. F. C., and Topley, W. W. C. (1927). The value of mixed vaccines in the prevention of the common cold. *J. Hyg.*, **26**, 98–109.

Fibiger, J. (1898). Om Serumbehandling af Difteri. *Hospitalstidende*, **4**, 6, 309 and 337.

Fields, W. S., Maslenikov, V., Meyer, J. S., *et al.* (1970). Joint study of extracranial arterial occlusion. *J. Am. Med. Assoc.*, **211**, 1993–2003.

Fisher, B., Carbone, P., Economou, S. G., *et al.* (1975). L-Phenylalanine mustard (L-Pam) in the management of primary breast cancer: a report of early findings. *N. Engl. J. Med.*, **292**, 117–122.

Fisher, B., Glass, A., and Redmond, C. (1977). L-Phenylalanine mustard (L-Pam) in the management of primary breast cancer. *Cancer*, **39**, 2883–2903.

Fisher, B., Redmond, C., Wolmark, M., *et al.* (1981). Disease-free survival at intervals during the following completion of adjuvant chemotherapy. The NSABP experience from three breast cancer protocols. *Cancer*, **48**, 1273–1280.

Fisher, R. A. (1935). *The Design of Experiments.* Edinburgh: Oliver and Boyd.

Fisher, R. A., and Yates, F. (1974). *Statistical Tables for Biological, Agricultural and Medical Research,* 6th edition. Edinburgh: Oliver and Boyd.

Fleiss, J. L. (1973). *Statistical Methods for Rates and Proportions.* New York: Wiley.

Food and Drug Administration (1977). Bureau of drugs clinical guidelines. U.S. government printing office, Washington.

Foulds, G. A. (1958). Clinical research in psychiatry. *J. Ment. Sci.*, **104**, 259–265.

Francis, T., Korns, R., Voight, R., *et al.* (1955). An evaluation of the 1954 poliomyelitis vaccine trials. *Am. J. Public Health*, **45**, May (part 2), 1–63.

Freedman, L. S. (1980). Problems involved in multi-centre studies of cancer treatment. *Cancer Topics*, **2**, No. 10, 10–11.

Freedman, L. S. (1982). Tables of the number of patients required in clinical trials using the logrank test. *Statistics in Medicine*, **1**, 121–129.

Freedman, L. S., and White, S. J. (1976). On the use of Pocock and Simon's method for balancing treatment numbers over prognostic factors in the controlled clinical trial. *Biometrics*, **32**, 691–694.

Frei, E., Holland, J. F., and Schneiderman, M. A. (1958). A comparative study of two regimens of combination chemotherapy in acute leukemia. *Blood*, **13**, 1126–1148.

Freiman, J. A., Chalmers, T. C., Smith, H., *et al.* (1978). The importance of beta, the type II error and sample size in the design and interpretation of the randomized controlled trial. *N. Engl. J. Med.*, **290**, 690–694.

Friedman, L. M., Furberg, C. D., and Demets, D. L. (1981). *Fundamentals of Clinical Trials.* Boston: Wright.

Gail, M. (1973). The determination of sample size for trials involving several independent 2 × 2 tables. *J. Chron. Dis.*, **26**, 669–673.

Gail, M. H., Demets, D. L., and Slud, E. V. (1982). Simulation studies on increments of the two-sample logrank score test for survival time data, with application to group sequential boundaries. Personal communication.

Garraway, W. M., Akhtar, A. J., Gore, S. M., *et al.* (1976). Observer variation in the clinical assessment of stroke. *Age Ageing*, **5**, 233–240.

Garraway, W. M., Akhtar, A. J., Prescott, R. J., *et al.* (1980). Management of acute stroke in the elderly: preliminary results of a controlled trial. *Br. Med. J.*, **i**, 1040–1043.

Gehan, E. A. (1978). Adjustment for prognostic factors in the analysis of clinical studies. *UICC Tech. Rep. Ser.*, **36**, 35—73.

Gehan, E. A., and Freireich, E. J. (1974). Non-randomized controls in cancer clinical trials. *N. Engl. J. Med.*, **290**, 198–203.

Geigy (1970). *Scientific Tables,* 7th edition. Basle: Geigy.

Gilbert, J. P., Meier, P., Rümke, C. L., *et al.* (1975). Report of the committee for assessment of biometric aspects of controlled trials of hypoglycemic agents. *J. Am. Med. Assoc.*, **231**, 583–608.

Gilbert, J. P., McPeek, B., and Mosteller, F. (1977). Statistics and ethics in surgery and anesthesia. *Science*, **198**, 684–689.

Goldsmith, M. A., and Carter, S. K. (1974). Combination chemotherapy of advanced Hodgkin's disease: a review. *Cancer*, **33**, 1–8.

Gore, S. M. (1981a). Assessing clinical trials—trial size. *Br. Med. J.*, **282**, 1687–1689.

Gore, S. M. (1981b). Assessing clinical trials—record sheets. *Br. Med. J.*, **283**, 296–298.

252

Gore, S. M. (1981c). Assessing methods—transforming the data. *Br. Med. J.*, **283**, 548–550.

Gore, S. M., and Altman, D. G. (1982). *Statistics in Practice*. London: British Medical Association.

Gore, S. M., Jones, I. G., and Rytter, E. C. (1977). Misuse of statistical methods: critical assessment of articles in B.M.J. from January to March 1976. *Br. Med. J.*, **i**, 85–87.

Grace, N. D., Muench, H., and Chalmers, T. C. (1966). The present status of portal hypertension in cirrhosis. *Gastroenterology*, **50**, 684–691.

Grage, T. B. (1981). Prospectively controlled randomized clinical trials—a clinician's views of their advantages and shortcomings and the need for alternative trial designs. Personal communication.

Grage, T. B., and Zelen, M. (1982). The controlled randomized trial in the evaluation of cancer treatment—the dilemma and alternative designs. *UICC Tech. Rep. Ser.*, **70**, 23–47.

Gralla, R. J., Itri, L. M., Pisko, S. E., *et al.* (1981). Antiemetic efficacy of high-dose metoclopramide. *N. Engl. J. Med.*, **305**, 905–909.

Greenwood, M., and Yule, G. U. (1915). The statistics of anti-typhoid and anti-cholera inoculations and the interpretation of such statistics in general. *Proc. R. Soc. Med. 8, Sect. Epidemiol. State Med.*, 113–194.

Gribbin, M. (1981). Placebos: cheapest medicine in the world. *New Sci.*, **89**, 64–65.

Grizzle, J. E. (1967). Continuity correction in the χ^2 test for 2×2 tables. *Am. Statistician*, Oct., 28–32.

Gruer, R. (1976). Evaluation of the Glasgow computerised electrocardiogram interpretation system: addendum to preliminary report. Personal communication.

Halperin, M., Ware, J. H., Byar, D. P., *et al.* (1977). Testing for interaction in an $I \times J \times K$ contingency table. *Biometrika*, **64**, 271–275.

Hampton, J. R. (1981). Presentation and analysis of the results of clinical trials in cardiovascular disease. *Br. Med. J.*, **282**, 1371–1373.

Hansen, R. W. (1979). The pharmaceutical development process: estimates of development costs and times and the effects of proposed regulatory changes. In *Issues in Pharmaceutical Economics* (ed. R. I. Chen), pp. 151–187. D. C. Heath & Co.

Harrison, S. H., Topley, E., and Lennard-Jones, J. (1949). The value of systemic penicillin in finger pulp infections: a controlled trial of 169 cases. *Lancet*, **i**, 425–430.

Hart, F. D., and Huskisson, E. C. (1972). Measurement in rheumatoid arthritis. *Lancet*, **i**, 28–30.

Heady, J. A. (1973). A cooperative trial on the primary prevention of ischaemic heart disease using clofibrate: design, methods, and progress. *Bull. WHO*, **48**, 243–256.

Healy, M. J. R. (1981). Some problems of repeated measurements. In *Perspectives in Medical Statistics* (eds. J. F. Bithell and R. Coppi), pp. 155–171. London: Academic Press.

Henderson, I. C., and Canellos, G. P. (1980). Cancer of the breast: the past decade. *N. Engl. J. Med.*, **302**, 17–30 and 78–90.

Herson, J. (1980). Patient registration in a cooperative oncology group. *Controlled Clin. Trials*, **1**, 99–108.

Hill, Sir A. B. (1962). *Statistical Methods in Clinical and Preventive Medicine*. Edinburgh: Livingstone.

Hill, Sir A. B. (1963). Medical ethics and controlled trials. *Br. Med. J.*, **i**, 1043–1049.

Hills, M., and Armitage, P. (1979). The two-period crossover clinical trial. *Br. J. Clin. Pharmacol.*, **8**, 7–20.

Hjalmarson, A., Herlitz, J., Malek, I., *et al.* (1981). Effect on mortality of metoprolol in acute myocardial infarction. *Lancet*, **ii**, 823–827.

Hjermann, I., Holme, I., Velve Byre, K., *et al.* (1981). Effect of diet and smoking intervention on the incidence of coronary heart disease. *Lancet*, **ii**, 1303–1310.

Holmes, O. W. (1891). Currents and counter currents in medical science. In *Works*, Vol. 9, p. 185.

Ingelfinger, F. J. (1972). The randomized clinical trial. *N. Engl. J. Med.*, **287**, 100–101.

International Steering Committee (1978). Uniform requirements for manuscripts submitted to biomedical journals. *Can. J. Public Health*, **69**, 454–458.

James, I. M., Griffith, D. N. W., Pearson, R. M. *et al.* (1977). Effect of oxprenolol on stage-fright in musicians. *Lancet*, **ii**, 952–954.

Johnstone, E. C., Lawler, P., Stevens, M., *et al.* (1980). The Northwick Park electroconvulsive therapy trial. *Lancet*, **ii**, 1317–1320.

Jones, D., and Whitehead, J. (1979). Sequential forms of the logrank and modified Wilcoxon tests for censored data. *Biometrika*, **66**, 105–113.

Kalbfleisch, J. D., and Prentice, R. L. (1980). *The Statistical Analysis of Failure Time Data*. New York: Wiley.

Karpatkin, M., Porges, R. F., and Karpatkin, S. (1981). Platelet counts in infants of women with autoimmune thrombocytopenia, effect of steroid administration to the mother. *N. Engl. J. Med.*, **305**, 936–937.

Keating, M. J., Smith, T. L., Gehan, E. A., *et al.* (1980). Factors related to length of complete remission in adult acute leukemia. *Cancer*, **45**, 2017–2029.

Kember, N. F. (1982). *An Introduction to Computer Applications in Medicine*. London: Edward Arnold.

Kennedy, I. (1981). *The Unmasking of Medicine*. London: George Allen and Unwin.

King, L. S., and Roland, C. G. (1968). *Scientific Writing*. Chicago: American Medical Association.

Kirk, A. P., Jain, S., Pocock, S., *et al.* (1980). Late results of the Royal Free Hospital prospective controlled trial of prednisolone therapy in hepatitis B surface antigen negative chronic active hepatitis. *Gut*, **21**, 78–83.

Lancet (1979a). Controlled trials: planned deception? (editorial). *Lancet*, **i**, 534–535.

Lancet (1979b). Bypassing obesity (editorial). *Lancet*, **ii**, 1275–1276.

Langlands, A. O., Prescott, R. J., and Hamilton, T. (1980). A clinical trial in the management of operable cancer of the breast. *Br. J Surg.*, **67**, 170–174.

League of Nations Malaria Commission (1937). The treatment of malaria. *Bull. Health Organ. League Nations*, **6**, 895–1033.

Lebacqz, K. (1980). Controlled clinical trials: some ethical issues. *Controlled Clin. Trials*, **1**, 29–36.

Lebrec, D., Corbic, M., Nouel, O., *et al.* (1980). Propranolol —a medical treatment for portal hypertension? *Lancet*, **ii**, 180–182.

Lebrec, D., Poynard, T., Hillon, P., *et al.* (1981). Propranolol for prevention of recurrent gastro-intestinal bleeding in patients with cirrhosis: a controlled study. *N. Engl. J. Med.*, **305**, 1371–1374.

Lellouch, J., and Schwartz, D. (1971). L'essai thérapeutique: éthique individuelle ou éthique collective? *Rev. Inst. Int. Statist.*, **39**, 127–136.

Lenhard, R. E., Ezdinli, E. Z., Costello, W., *et al.* (1978). Treatment of histiocytic and mixed lymphomas: a comparison of two, three and four drug chemotherapy. *Cancer*, **42**, 41–52.

Lewis, J. A., and Ellis, S. H. (1982). A statistical appraisal of post-infarction beta-blocker trials. *Primary Cardiol. Suppl.*, No. 1, 31–37.

Lind, J. (1753). *A Treatise of the Scurvy*. Edinburgh: Sands Murray & Cochran.

Lionel, N. D. W., and Herxheimer, A. (1970). Assessing reports of therapeutic trials. *Br. Med. J.*, **ii**, 637–640.

Lister, J. (1870). On the effects of the antiseptic system upon the salubrity of a surgical hospital. *Lancet*, **i**, 4 and 40.

Louis, P. C. A. (1834). *Essay on Clinical Instruction* (translated by P. Martin). London: S. Highley.

Louis, P. C. A. (1835). *Recherches sur les Effets de la Saignée*. Paris: De Mignaret.

Makuch, R., and Simon, R. (1978). Sample size requirements for evaluating a conservative therapy. *Cancer Treat. Rep.*, **62**, 1037–1040.

Mantel, N., and Haenszel, W. (1959). Statistical aspects of the analysis of data from retrospective studies of disease. *J. Nat. Cancer Inst.*, **22**, 719–748.

Mather, H. G., Morgan, D. C., Pearson, N. G., *et al.* (1976). Myocardial infarction: a comparison between home and hospital care for patients. *Br. Med. J.*, **i**, 925–929.

McPherson, K. (1974). Statistics: the problem of examining accumulating data more than once. *N. Engl. J. Med.*, **290**, 501–502.

McPherson, K. (1982). On choosing the number of interim analysis in clinical trials. *Statistics in Medicine*, **1**, 25–36.

Medical Research Council (1948). Streptomycin treatment of pulmonary tuberculosis. *Br. Med. J.*, **ii**, 769–782.

Medical Research Council (1950). Clinical trials of antihistaminic drugs in the prevention and treatment of the common cold. *Br. Med. J.*, **ii**, 425–429.

Medical Research Council Working Party (1977). Randomized controlled trial of treatment for mild hypertension: design and pilot trial. *Br. Med. J.*, **i**, 1437–1440.

Meier, P. (1972). The biggest public health experiment ever: the 1954 field trial of the Salk poliomyelitis vaccine. In *Statistics: A Guide to The Unknown* (ed. J. M. Tanur), pp. 2–13. San Francisco: Holden-Day.

Meier, P. (1975). Statistics and medical experimentation. *Biometrics*, **31**, 511–529.

Miller, R. G., Efron, B., Brown, B. W., *et al.* (1980). *Biostatistics Casebook*. New York: Wiley.

Moertel, C. G., and Reitemeier, R. J. (1969). *Advanced Gastrointestinal Cancer: Clinical Management and Chemotherapy*. New York: Hoerber.

Moertel, C. G., Fleming, T. R., Rubin, J., *et al.* (1982). A clinical trial of amygdalin (Laetrile) in the treatment of human cancer. *N. Engl. J. Med.*, **306**, 201–206.

Mosteller, F., Gilbert, J. P., and McPeek, B. (1980). Reporting standards and research strategies for controlled trials. *Controlled Clin. Trials*, **1**, 37–58.

Needleman, H. L., Gunnoe, C., Leviton, A., *et al.* (1979). Deficits in psychologic and classroom performance of children with elevated dentine lead levels. *N. Engl. J. Med.*, **300**, 689–695.

Nelson, R. B. (1979). Are clinical trials pseudoscience? *Forum Med.*, **2**, 594–600.

O'Brien, P. C., and Fleming, T. R. (1979). A multiple testing procedure for clinical trials. *Biometrics*, **35**, 549–556.

Paton, A. (1979). Write a paper. In *How to Do It*. London: British Medical Association.

Peto, R. (1978). Clinical trial methodology. *Biomedicine Special Issue*, **28**, 24–36.

Peto, R. (1980). Aspirin after myocardial infarction (editorial). *Lancet*, **i**, 1172–1173.

Peto, R. (1982). Long-term and short-term beta-blockade after myocardial infarction. *Lancet*, **i**, 1159–1161.

Peto, R., Pike, M. C., Armitage, P., *et al.* (1976). Design and analysis of randomized clinical trials requiring prolonged observation of each patient: I. Introduction and design. *Br. J. Cancer*, **34**, 585–612.

Peto, R., Pike, M. C., Armitage, P., *et al.* (1977). Design and analysis of randomized clinical trials requiring prolonged observation of each patient: II. Analysis and examples. *Br. J. Cancer*, **35**, 1–39.

Pocock, S. J. (1976). The combination of randomized and historical controls in clinical trials. *J. Chron. Dis.*, **29**, 175–188.

Pocock, S. J. (1977a). Group sequential methods in the design and analysis of clinical trials. *Biometrika*, **64**, 191–199.

Pocock, S. J. (1977b). Randomized clinical trials (letter). *Br. Med. J.*, **i**, 1661.

Pocock, S. J. (1978). The size of cancer clinical trials and stopping rules. *Br. J. Cancer*, **38**, 757–766.

Pocock, S. J. (1979). Allocation of patients to treatment in clinical trials. *Biometrics*, **35**, 183–197.

Pocock, S. J. (1982). Interim analysis for randomized clinical trials: the group sequential approach. *Biometrics*, **38**, 153–162.

Pocock, S. J., and Lagakos, S. W. (1982). Practical experience of randomization in cancer trials: an international survey. *Br. J. Cancer*, **46**, 368–375.

Pocock, S. J., and Simon, R. (1975). Sequential treatment assignment with balancing for prognostic factors in the controlled clinical trial. *Biometrics*, **31**, 103–115.

Pocock, S. J., Armitage, P., and Galton, D. A. G. (1978). The size of cancer clinical trials: an international survey. *UICC Tech. Rep. Ser.*, **36**, 5–34.

Rawles, J. M., and Kenmure, A. C. F. (1980). The coronary care controversy. *Br. Med. J.*, **281**, 783–786.

Ritter, J. M. (1980). Placebo-controlled double-blind clinical trials can impede medical progress. *Lancet*, **i**, 1126–1127.

Robinson, B. N., Anderson, G. D., Cohen, E., *et al.* (1980). *S.I.R. (Scientific Information Retrieval) User's Manual Version 2.* Evanston Illinois: S.I.R. Inc.

Rose, G. A., Holland, W. W., and Crawley, E. A. (1964). A sphygmomanometer for epidemiologists. *Lancet*, **i**, 296–300.

Rose, G. A., Blackburn, H., Gillum, R. F., and Prineas, R. J. (1982). *Cardiovascular Survey Methods.* Geneva: World Health Organization.

Rush, B. (1794). *An Account of the Bilious Remitting Yellow Fever as it Appeared in the City of Philadelphia in 1793.* Philadelphia: Dobson.

Sackett, D. L. (1981). How to read clinical journals: I. Why to read them and how to start reading them critically. V. To distinguish useful from useless or even harmful therapy. *Can. Med. Assoc. J.*, **124**, 555–558 and 1156–1162.

Sackett, D. L., and Gent, M. (1979). Controversy in counting and attributing events in clinical trials. *N. Engl. J. Med.*, **301**, 1410–1412.

Schoenfeld, D. A., and Gelber, R. D. (1979). Designing and analysing clinical trials which allow institutions to randomize patients to a subset of the treatments under study. *Biometrics*, **35**, 825–829.

Schwartz, D., and Lellouch, J. (1967). Explanatory and pragmatic attitudes in therapeutic trials. *J. Chron Dis.*, **20**, 637–648.

Schwartz, D., Flamant, R., and Lellouch, J. (1980). *Clinical Trials.* London: Academic Press.

Shaper, A. G., Ashby, D., and Pocock, S. J. (1983). The relationship between alcohol consumption and serum biochemistry and haematology. Personal communication.

Siegel, S. (1956) *Nonparametric Statistics for the Behavioral Sciences.* New York: McGraw-Hill.

Simon, R. (1979). Restricted randomization designs in clinical trials. *Biometrics*, **35**, 503–512.

Simpson, R. J., Tiplady, B., and Skegg, D. C. G. (1980). Event recording in a clinical trial of a new medicine. *Br. Med. J.*, **i**, 1133–1134.

Smith, R. N. (1977). Ethical aspects of drug evaluation. In *Clinical Trials* (eds. F. N. and S. Johnson). Oxford: Blackwell.

Smithells, R. W., Sheppard, S., Schorah, C. J., *et al.* (1980). Possible prevention of neural-tube defects by periconceptional vitamin supplementation. *Lancet*, **i**, 339–340.

Spodick, D. H. (1982). Randomized controlled clinical trials: the behavioral case. *J. Am. Med. Assoc.*, **247**, 2258–2260.

Stanley, K. E. (1980). Prognostic factors for survival in patients with inoperable lung cancer. *J. Natl. Cancer Inst.*, **65**, 25–32.

Starmer, C. F., Rosati, R. A., and McNeer, J. F. (1974). Data bank use in management of chronic disease. *Comput. Biomed. Res.*, **7**, 111–116.

Stott, N. C. H. (1982). Clinical trial in general practice? *Br. Med. J.*, **285**, 941–944.

Student (1931). The Lanarkshire milk experiment. *Biometrika*, **23**, 398–406.

Sutton, H. G. (1865). Cases of rheumatic fever treated for the most part by mint water. *Guy's Hosp. Rep.*, **2**, 392.

256

Swedish Study Group (1982). Cefuroxime versus ampicillin and chloramphenicol for the treatment of bacterial meningitis. *Lancet*, i, 295–298.

Swinscow, T. D. V. (1977). *Statistics at Square One*. London: British Medical Association.

Sylvester, R. J., Pinedo, H. M., De Pauw, M., *et al.* (1981). Quality of institutional participation in multicenter clinical trials. *N. Engl. J. Med.*, **305**, 852–855.

Tate, H. C., Rawlinson, J. B., and Freedman, L. S. (1979). Randomized comparative studies in the treatment of cancer in the United Kingdom: room for improvement? *Lancet*, ii, 623–625.

Thorne, C. (1970). *Better Medical Writing*. London: Pitman.

Truelove, S. C. (1960). Stilboestrol. phenobarbitone and diet in chronic duodenal ulcer: a factorial therapeutic trial. *Br. Med. J.*, ii, 559–566.

Tukey, J. W. (1977). Some thoughts on clinical trials, especially problems of multiplicity. *Science*, **198**, 679–684.

Turpeinen, O., Karvonen, M. J., Pekkarinen, M., *et al.* (1979). Dietary prevention of coronary heart disease: the Finnish mental hospital study. *Int. J. Epidemiol.*, **8**, 99–118.

van der Linden, W. (1980). Pitfalls in randomized surgical trials. *Surgery*, **87**, 258–262.

Walker, S. H., and Duncan, D. B. (1967). Estimation of the probability of an event as a function of several independent variables. *Biometrika*, **54**, 167–179.

Warlow, C. (1979). Design and protocol of the UK-TIA Aspirin Study. In *Drug Treatment and Prevention in Cerebrovascular Disorders* (eds. G. Tognoni and S. Garattini). Amsterdam: Elsevier/North-Holland.

White, S. J., and Freedman, L. S. (1978). Allocation of patients to treatment groups in a controlled clinical study. *Br. J. Cancer*, **37**, 849–857.

Whitehead, J. (1982). *The Design and Analysis of Sequential Clinical Trials*. Chichester: Ellis Horwood.

Wilcox, R. G., Hampton, J. R., Rowley, J. M., *et al.* (1980). Randomized placebo-controlled trial comparing oxprenolol with disopyramide phosphate in immediate treatment of suspected myocardial infarction. *Lancet*, ii, 765–769.

Willey, R. F., Grant, I. W. B., and Pocock, S. J. (1976). Comparison of cardiorespiratory effects of oral salbutamol and pirbuterol in patients with bronchial asthma. *Br. J. Clin. Pharmacol.*, **3**, 595–600.

Williams, C. J., and Carter, S. K. (1978). Management of trials in the development of cancer chemotherapy. *Br. J. Cancer*, **37**, 434–447.

Wolf, G. T., and Makuch, R. W. (1980). A classification system for protocol deviations in clinical trials. *Cancer Clin. Trials*, **3**, 101–103.

Wright, I. S., Marple, C. D., and Beck, D. F. (1948). Report of committee for evaluation of anticoagulants in treatment of coronary thrombosis with myocardial infarction. *Am. Heart J.*, **36**, 801–815.

Wright, P., and Haybittle, J. (1979). Design of forms for clinical trials (3 articles). *Br. Med. J.*, **2**, 529–530, 590–592 and 650–651.

Yanchinski, S. (1980). What next for interferon? *New Sci.*, **87**, 917–921.

Zelen, M. (1974). The randomization and stratification of patients to clinical trials. *J. Chron. Dis.*, **27**, 365–375.

Zelen, M. (1979). A new design for randomized clinical trials. *N. Engl. J. Med.*, **300**, 1242–1245.

Zelen, M. (1983). Guidelines for publishing papers on cancer clinical trials: responsibilities of editors and authors. *J. Clin. Oncology* **1**, 164–169.

Index

Accrual of patients, *see* Selection of patients, Size of trial
Administration, 31–35, 246
multi-centre trial, 135–137
Adverse events, *see* Side effects
Age, eligibility, 37
recording date of birth, 165
stratification, 82–84
subgroup analysis, 215
Anaesthetics, 16, 64
Analgesics trial, patient withdrawals, 185–186
Analysis, *see* Statistical analysis
Analysis of covariance, *see* Multiple regression
Analysis of variance, 230, 233
Animal studies, pharmaceutical industry, 4, 26
Anticoagulants, 24, 60
Antidepressant trial, repeated measurements, 231–233
withdrawal of patients, 182
Antidepressants, side effects, 44
Antiemetics, 196
Antihistamines, randomized controlled trial for common cold, 17–18
Antihypertensive drugs, *see* Hypertension, Beta-blocking drugs, Diuretics
Antimalarial drugs, 16–17
Antiseptics, 16
Anturane Reinfarction Trial, control group, 5–6
selection of patients, 178–179
size of trial, 123–125, 132
withdrawal of patients, 184
Aspirin trials, 24–25, 31, 140–141
Assessments, clinical, 46–47
Asthma trial, carry-over effect, 113
crossover design, 112–113

informed patient consent, 107
repeated measurement of peak flow rate, 191
statistical analysis, 117–118
Attitude of patients, effect of placebo, 90–93
Auto-immune thrombocytopenia, Wilcoxon test, 202–204

Bacterial meningitis, 5–6
Balanced incomplete block design, crossover trials, 121
Balancing for institution in randomization, 86–87
Baseline data, 42, 45, 72
crossover trials, 119
form design, 161–166
statistical analysis, 188, 190, 211–221, 232–233
stratified randomization, 81
Benefit of patients, 247
Beta-blocking drugs, long term effect in hypertension, 43, 136–137
pooling of trial data, 242–244
side effects, 44
see also Metoprolol trial
Bias, 7, 103–104
avoidance, 7, 9, 50, 64–65, 90–92, 97–99, 176
historical control groups, 54–60
in publications, 236–237, 239–242
non-blinded trials, 90–92
non-randomized trials, 50–63
protocol deviations, 176
significance tests, 205
withdrawal of patients, 182–186
Biassed coin method, 79–80
Bleeding, treatment of yellow fever, 15
Blinded evaluation, 48, 99

257

Blinding, 16, 90–99
see also Double blind trials
BMDP, 172
Breast cancer, 5–6, 7–13, 22–23, 58, 82–85, 89
L-Pam trial, 7–13, 22
British Medical Association, *Handbook of Medical Ethics*, 102
Bronchodilators, dose escalation studies, 121
Bronchopulmonary dysplasia, neonatal, 60

Cancer chemotherapy, adjuvant trials, 22
consent of patients, 107–109
co-operative groups, 21–24, 137
data handling, 161, 171–172
eligibility of patients, 177
historical control group, 57–58
interim analyses, 149–150
optional crossover trial, 114
response criteria, 43, 189
size of trial, 126
treatment schedules, 8, 39–40
trials in USA, 21–24
uncontrolled trials, 51–53
Cancer patients, informed consent, 106–108
Cancer trials, inadequate size, 133–134
Card punch operator, 169–170
Care of patients, ethics, 100–108
double-blind trials, 40, 90–93
historical controls, 55
treatment definition, 40
Carotid stenosis, bilateral, 183
Carry-over effect, crossover trials, 113
statistical analysis, 116–117
Case studies, 2
Chi-squared test, 197–200
adjusting for prognostic factors, 220–221
for trend in proportions, 200
interpretation, 204–205
multiple treatment trials, 229–230
size of trial estimation, 123–127
subgroup analyses, 215
Yates correction, 127, 200
Cholesterol, clofibrate trial, 43–44
dietary intervention, 114
Cirrhosis, primary biliary, 89, 154–155
Classification of clinical trials, 2
Clinical assessments, 46–47
Clinical trial, *see under specific items*

Clofibrate trial, 43–44
size of trial, 126
withdrawal of patients, 186
Closed sequential plans, stopping rule, 156
Collective ethics, 104–105
Colorectal cancer trial, historical controls, 55
patient selection criteria, 37
randomized control group, 5–6
treatment schedules, 39–40
see also Rectal cancer
Combined modality trials, cancer treatments, 22
Committee on Safety of Medicines, 26, 102, 138
Common cold, trial of antihistamines, 17–18
Common cold vaccines, single blind trial, 16
Comparability of treatment groups, 212–213
Compliance of patients, 40
checking, 180–181
double blind trials, 96
Phase I/II trials, 186
Computers, data management, 168–175
statistical packages, 172–174
Conclusions, validity, 237–239
Confidence limits, 187, 206–210
crossover trial, 114–115
interpretation, 207–208
means, 208–210
multiple logistic model, 219
multiple regression, 218
percentages, 206–209, 242–244
Confidentiality, interim results, 145–146
Confirmatory trials, 242
Consent of patients, 10, 66, 68, 100–102, 105–109
Continuous sequential designs, 155–159
Control groups, 4–6, 8–9
historical, 54–60
non-randomized, 54–63
randomized, 63–65
Co-operative groups, cancer chemotherapy, 21–24
multi-centre trials, 137
Coordinating centre, 34, 136
data management, 167
randomization, 70
Coordination, 33–34
Coronary care units, clinical trials, 25–26, 41, 178

Coronary heart disease, *see* Myocardial infarction

Costs, multi-centre trials, 135
National Institutes of Health (US), 23, 25
pharmaceutical industry, 26–27
see also Funding

Critical evaluation, trial reports, 236–238

Crossover trials, 110–122
design, 112–114, 119–122
double blind, 96–97
multi-period, 119–122
rationale, 110–112
statistical analysis, 114–119
two-period, 112–119
withdrawal of patients, 119

Cumulative frequency distributions, data display, 194–195

Cytotoxic drugs, *see* Cancer chemotherapy

Danish Obesity Project, 64, 108

Data analysis, *see* Statistical analysis

Data banks, information for treatment comparison, 62–63

Data checking, 166–168, 170

Data collection, 31, 166–168, 188
historical control groups, 55
multi-centre trials, 135

Data display, graphical, 193–197, 210

Data description, 188–197

Data dredging, 229

Data handling, 31, 45, 143, 166–168
computers, 169–175
form design, 45, 160–166
interim analysis, 144
multi-centre trials, 135

Data managers, 167–168

Data multiplicity, 228–233

Data pooling, 24–25, 242–245

Data transfer, computing for clinical trials, 169–170

Data transformation, interpretation of results, 196

Data types, 41–49, 188–191

Database management computer packages, 172

Death, *see* Survival data

Decision-making process, interim analysis, 145

Declaration of Helsinki, 100–102
informed patient consent, 105

Definition, clinical trial, 2
eligible patients, 35–38

objectives, 29–30
response criteria, 41–49
treatment schedules, 38–41

Degrees of freedom, paired differences t test, 115
two-sample t test, 202

Delayed response, interim analyses, 150–151, 159

Depression, Hamilton rating scale, 47, 231–233
repeated measurements, 231–233
side effects of treatment, 44
withdrawal of patients, 182

Descriptive statistics, 187–197

Design of trial, 28–30, 246
crossover trials, 112–114, 119–122
plans for statistical analysis, 31, 188

Diabetes, UGDP trial, 19–21

Diabetic Retinopathy Study, 99, 111

Dietary intervention, coronary heart disease, 41, 114

Diphtheria trial, 16

Disease free interval, 8–13, 83–84
see also Survival data

Diuretics, long term effect in hypertension, 43, 136–137

Documentation, patient entry, 71–72
study protocol, 28–31
see also Form design, Publication

Dose-escalation studies, 3, 121

Double blind trials, 9, 17, 40, 90–99
breaking the code, 94–96
comparison of active drugs, 96–97
conduct, 93–97
feasibility, 97–99
justification, 90–93
randomization, 70–71, 94

D-penicillamine, cirrhosis trial, 89, 154–155

Drop-outs, *see* Withdrawal of patients

Drug trials, classification, 2–4
definition of treatment schedules, 38–40

Drugs, development costs, 26–27
dose modification, 39
dose schedule, 39
formulation, 39
non-compliance, 180
packaging and distribution, 40

Duodenal ulcer, factorial trial, 139–140

Dummy variables, multiple logistic model, 218
multiple regression, 216

Duration of treatment, 39
crossover design, 112–113

Eastern Cooperative Oncology Group, 22–23, 89, 126
Editorial standards, 238
Electroconvulsive therapy, double blind trial, 97
Eligibility of patients, 35–38, 176–179, 188
  checking, 67, 117
  multi-centre trials, 135, 177, 179
End-points, see Evaluation of patient response
Epilepsy, crossover trial of vitamin D, 111
Errors, see Type I error, Type II error
Ethical committees, 29, 102
Ethics, 100–109
  collective, 104–105
  crossover trial, 114
  double blind trials, 97–98
  guidelines, 100–103
  individual, 104–105
  interim analyses, 143–144
  locally based trials, 33
  patient consent, 10, 68, 105–109
  poor scientific and organizational standards, 103–105
  randomization, 63–64, 105
  randomized consent design, 108–109
  surgical trials, 41, 64
  stopping rules, 20, 143–144, 149
Evaluation of patient response, 30, 41–49
  blinding, 48, 99
  criteria of response, 42–45, 188–191
  forms, 161
  frequency, 49
  historical control groups, 55
  incomplete data, 181–182
  interim analyses, 144
  sequential designs, 158
  types of data, 188–191
Explanatory approach, data analysis, 182, 186

Factorial design, two or more therapeutic comparisons, 139–141
Factors for stratification, 81
False-negative findings, 125, 241
False-positive findings, significance testing, 125, 148, 204, 230–231, 239–242
Field trials, vaccines, 2, 18–19
Fisher's exact test, 127, 200
Flow sheets for patient evaluation, 161
Follow-up studies, 49
  data handling, 171–172
  patients lost to follow-up, 227

trial size, 129
  see also Survival data
Food and Drug Administration (USA), 26–27, 114
  guidelines for drug development programmes, 3–4, 26, 32
Form design, 31, 160–166
Forms, registration of patients, 68–69, 71
Frequency distribution, quantitative response data, 192–197
Funding, 31–33
  see also Costs

General practitioners, 33
Geometric mean, 196
GGTP, log transform, 196–197
Graphical data display, 193–197, 210
Group sequential design, 147–155

Hamilton Psychiatric Scale, 47, 231–233
Health education, 41
Hepatitis trial, analysis of survival data, 221–226
Histograms, data display, 194–195
Historical control groups, 24, 54–60
Historical development of clinical trials, 14–27
Hodgkins lymphoma, qualitative response data, 189
Hypertension, crossover trial, 113–119
  form design, 162–166
  long term effect of drugs, 43
  multi-centre controlled trial, 5–6, 29, 38, 43, 136–137
  multiplicity of trial data, 228–229
  patient entry requirements, 38
  response data, 189–190
Hypoglycaemic agents, UGDP trial, 19–21
Hypothesis testing, see Significance tests

Identification of patients, forms, 163
Impact of trials on medical practice, 246
Individual ethics, 104–105
Ineligible patients, 176–179
Informed patient consent, see Consent of patients
Instructions, form completion, 162, 166
  patient compliance, 180
  study protocol, 28–31
  writing publications, 236
Interactions, significance tests, 213–215
Interim analyses, 10, 142–159
  confidentiality, 10, 145–146

continuous sequential designs, 155–159
data preparation, 143–144, 151, 168
frequency, 152–153
group sequential designs, 147–155
stopping rules, 146–159
Interferon, uncontrolled trials, 52
Invalidation of patients, 176–186
historical controls, 55

Judgement assignment, problems, 61–63

Kaplan–Meier life table estimation, 223
Key-to-disk, 170

Labelling, effect on compliance, 180
Laetrile, uncontrolled trials, 51–52
Latin square design, crossover trials, 120–122
Leukemia trials, first use of randomization, 21
matched controls, 58–59
stopping rules, 156–158
Life tables, analysis of survival data, 11–12, 221–224
Literature, see Publication
Literature controls, validity, 56–57
Literature reviews, 245
Log odds, multiple logistic model, 219
Log sheet for randomization, 68–69
Log transformation, skew data, 196–197
Logistic coefficients, multiple logistic model, 219
Logrank test, 224–226
size of trial, 129
stopping rule, 151, 158
Long term effects, drug trials, 43–44
Loss to follow-up, see Survival data, Withdrawal of patients
L-Pam trial in primary breast cancer, 7–13, 22
Lung cancer trials, prognostic factors, 81
unequal randomization, 89
Lymphoma chemotherapy trial, confidence limits, 208
haematological toxicity, 189
histological classification, 47
interim analyses, 149–151
multiple end points, 230
multiple treatments, 229–230
patient response, 189, 191–192
significance tests, 200

Management of patients, randomized trials for, 2, 5–6, 25–26, 41

Mann-Whitney U Test, 204
Matching, historical controls, 58–59
sequential designs, 158
Mantel-Haenszel Test, 220–221
Means, confidence limits, 208–210
crossover trial, 115–119
geometric, 196
graphical display, 209–210
significance tests, 200–202
skew data problem, 196
subgroup analyses, 212–214
summary of quantitative response, 192–193
Measurements, error reduction, 46
frequency, 49
see also Evaluation of patient response
Median, summary of quantitative data, 196
Medical care, clinical trials, 2, 25–26, 41
Medical ethics, see Ethics
Medical literature, see Publication
Medical practice, impact of clinical trials, 246
Medical progress, ethical issues, 100–102
Medical Research Council, first randomized trial, 17–18, 63, 98–99
funding, 32–33
hypertension trial, 5–6, 29, 38, 43, 136–137
Melanoma trial, 184–185
Metoprolol trial, statistical analysis, 198–200, 204, 206–208, 212–213, 215, 227, 244
Microcomputers, 174
Minimization method, stratification, 84–87
Monitoring patients, 45
forms, 161–163
Monitoring trial progress, see Interim analyses
Mortality, see Survival data
Multi-centre trials, 134–138
data management, 167–168
examples, 7–13, 21–24, 136–137
funding, 32–33
interim results, 145–146, 151
motivation of participants, 35, 135
protocol deviations, 179
randomization, 67–72, 86–87
trial size, 131
Multiperiod crossover trials, 119–122
Multiple endpoints, 228, 230–231
Multiple hypothesis testing, 228–233

Multiple logistic model, qualitative response, 218–220
Multiple regression analysis, quantitative response, 216–218
Multiple treatments, 138–141, 228–230
Multiplicity of data, 228–233
Myocardial infarction trials, anticoagulant therapy, 24, 60
  aspirin, 24–25
  beta-blocking drugs, 242–245
  clinical diagnosis, 45, 47
  control groups, 5–6, 24, 55, 60
  coronary care units, 25–26, 41, 178
  informed patient consent, 107
  patient eligibility, 178–179
  patient withdrawals, 184, 186
  prevention, 41, 43–44, 126
  randomized v. historical controls, 24, 55
  response criteria, 45, 47, 189, 191
  trial size, 123–126, 132

National Cancer Institute (US), 9, 21, 23, 51
National Institutes of Health (US), funding for clinical trials, 23, 25, 32–33
Negative trials, bias against publication, 240
  determination of trial size, 129–130
Neonatal hypocalcaemia, see Vitamin D trial of neonatal hypocalcaemia
Neural tube defects trial, ethics, 102
  judgement in treatment assignment, 62
Newman–Keuls method, paired treatment comparisons, 230
Nominal significance levels, 148–154
Non-compliance with protocol, 40, 179–181, 186
Non-drug therapy, 2, 5–6, 41
Non-parametric tests, 204
Non-randomized controlled trials, problems, 19, 24, 54–63, 205
Non-randomized patients, exclusion from randomized trials, 178
Null hypothesis, 11, 198–199, 201, 203, 214, 220, 224
Number of patients, see Size of trial
Number of treatments, 138–141
Numerical method, assessment of therapies, 15

Obesity, 64, 108
Objectives, 29–30
Observations, see Evaluation of patient response

Observer variation, 46
On-study data, see Baseline data
On-study form, 66, 72, 161–166
One-sided significance testing, 127, 155, 205–206
Open sequential plans, stopping rule, 156
Opinion of patients, response evaluation, 47–48
Ophthalmology, simultaneous comparison of different treatments to each eye, 111
Oral drug therapy, double blind trials, 93–97
  non-compliance, 180
Organization, 28–49, 246
  data management, 166–168
  ethics, 103–104
  multi-centre trials, 135–137
Outcome, see Evaluation of patient response
Overall response score, combined multiple endpoints, 231
Overall significance level, multiple endpoints, 231
  stopping rules, 148–154
Oxprenolol: crossover trial in nervous musicians, 112

$P < 0.05$, interpretation, 199, 204–206
  excessive use of significance tests, 229
  interim analyses, 147
P-values, 198–206
Pain measurement, 47–48, 190
Pairing, continuous sequential designs, 156–158
Patient, see under specific items
Penicillin, early trials, 17
Percentages, chi-squared test, 198–200, 204–205
  confidence limits, 206–208
  data description, 191–192
  multiple treatments, 229–230
  standard error, 206–207
  subgroup analyses, 215
Performance status, stratification, 81, 83–85
Pharmaceutical industry, 2–3, 26–27, 32, 137–138
  classification of drug trials, 2–3
  computing needs, 175
  funding for clinical trials, 32
  multiple trials of same drug, 137–138
  organization, 26–28

Pharmaceutical Manufacturers Association, 26
Pharmacist, role in double blind trials, 70, 94
Phase I trials, 2–3, 120–122, 186
Phase II trials, 3, 120–122, 186
  historical controls, 59
  uncontrolled, 52–53, 57
Phase III trials, 3–4, 52, 137
Phase IV trials, pharmaceutical industry, 3
  uncontrolled, 54
Photocoagulation therapy, 99, 111
Placebos, 9, 16, 90–99
Planning, clinical trial, 28–49
  statistical analysis, 31, 188
Platelet-active drugs, coronary artery disease, 24–25
Polio field trials of Salk Vaccine, 18–19
Pooling of trial data, 24–25, 242–245
Portacaval shunt operation, value of controlled trials, 53–54
Postoperative care, randomized trials, 2, 41
Power, 125–129, 132–133
  group sequential designs, 152–154, 156
Power calculations, 125–129, 131–133
  group sequential designs, 152–153
Pragmatic approach, data analysis, 182, 186
Preventive medicine, myocardial infarction, 41, 43–44, 126
  vaccines, 2, 18–19
Prognostic factors, 188, 211–221
  comparable treatment groups, 212–213
  historical controls, 58–59
  multiple logistic model, 218–220
  multiple regression, 216–218
  statistical analysis, 211–221
  stratified randomization, 80–87
  subgroup analyses, 213–216, 228–229
  survival data, 226–227
  see also Baseline data
Progress of trial, monitoring, 142–147
Proportional hazard model, survival data analysis, 227
Protocol, 9, 28–31
  deviations, 31, 176–186
  non-compliance, 142, 179–181
Psychiatric illness, clinical assessment, 46–47
  uncontrolled trials, 54
  see also Depression
Psychological effects, double blind trials, 90–91

Publication of trial reports, 234–247
  critical evaluation, 236–239
  failure to publish, 103, 138, 240–241
  pharmaceutical industry, 138
Punch cards, 169
Purpose of trial, definition, 29–30

Qualitative response data, 188–192
  multiple logistic model, 218–220
  statistical method for determining trial size, 124–127
  see also Percentages
Quality control, multi-centre trials, 135
Quantitative response data, 188, 190–197
  multiple regression, 216–218
  statistical method for determining trial size, 127–129
  see also Means
Question design, trial forms, 163–166

Radiotherapy trials, problems, 60, 61
Random permuted blocks, 76–79
  block size, 77, 82
  within strata, 82–84, 87
Randomization, 5, 30, 50–65, 66–89
  biassed coin method, 79–80
  crossover trial, 113–114
  double blind trial, 70–71, 94
  efficiency and reliability, 72–73
  ethics, 63–64, 105
  feasibility, 63–65
  first randomized trial, 17
  justification, 50–65
  minimization, 84–87
  organization, 66–73
  permuted blocks, 76–79, 82–84, 87
  statistical methods, 73–89
  stratified, 80–87
  unequal, 59–60, 87–89
  unstratified, 73–81
Randomized consent design, 108–109
Randomized v. historical controls, 24, 54–60
Rare diseases, historical control groups, 59
Rationale of clinical trials, 1–13
Rectal cancer, death of patient, 104
  radiotherapy, 60
  see also Colorectal cancer trial
Records, form design, 31, 160–166
  registration of patients, 68–69, 71, 179
Recruitment, see Selection of patients, Size of trial
Registration of patients, 30, 66–73, 177

Regression coefficients, multiple regression analysis, 216–218
Relapse data, *see* Survival data
Relevance of trials to society's needs, 247
Repeated measurements, statistical analysis, 191, 228, 231–233
Repeated significance tests, interim analyses, 146–157
Replacement randomization, 76
Replication of trials, 242
Reports of trial findings, *see* Publication of trial reports
Representative sample of patients, 1, 35–36, 52, 178–179, 208
Response criteria, *see* Evaluation of patient response
Response data, *see* Evaluation of patient response
Restricted randomization, 76–80
Results, *see* Publication, Statistical analysis
Retrospective controls, 2, 24, 54–60
Reviews of literature, 245
Rheumatic fever, trial of mint water, 15–16
Rheumatoid arthritis trials, assessment of pain relief, 47–48, 190
informed patient consent, 107
Run-in period, crossover trials, 113

Salk polio vaccine, field trials, 18–19
Sample of patients, representativeness, 1, 35–36, 52, 178–179, 208
SAS, 172, 174
Scatter diagrams, 190
Scientific design, trial protocol, 29
Scientific method, application to clinical trials, 4–7
Scientific requirements, trial size, 123, 131–133
Scientific standards, ethics, 103–105
Scurvy, comparative trial, 14–15
Sealed envelopes, randomization, 70
Selection of patients, 35–38, 66–67
historical controls, 54–55
ineligibility, 37, 67, 176–179
representative sample, 1, 35–36, 52, 178–179, 208
Selective publication, trial results, 240
Sequential analysis, *see* Interim analyses
Short-term effects of treatment, 43
crossover trials, 110
Side effects, 39–40, 44–45, 95–96
dose modification, 39–40, 180
double blind trials, 95–96

L-Pam trial, 13, 95–96
monitoring, 143
Phase I trials, 3, 122
recording methods, 44–45
withdrawal of patients, 39, 180–185
Significance tests, 7, 11, 187, 197–206
adjustment for prognostic factors, 216–221
crossover trials, 114–119
false-positive findings, 125, 148, 204, 230–231, 239–242
interactions, 213–215
interpretation, 204–206, 239
limitations, 244
link with confidence limits, 208
means, 200–202
multiple hypothesis testing, 228–233
non-parametric, 204
non-randomized trials, 205
one sided *v.* two sided, 127, 155, 205–206
percentages, 198–200
stopping rules, 146–159
subgroup analysis, 213–216
survival data, 221, 224–227
see also under names of individual tests
Single centre trials, organization, 33
patient registration, 71
small number of patients, 33, 131
SIR, 172
Size of trial, 7, 30, 123–141, 147, 247
effect of interim analyses, 147, 152–153
ethics, 103
factorial designs, 139–141
follow-up studies, 129
multi-centre trials, 134–138
negative trials, 129–130
number of treatments, 138–139
percentages, 124–127
power calculations, 123–129, 131–133
problem of small trials, 133–134, 240–242, 247
realistic assessment, 130–133
statistical methods for estimation, 123–133
Skewness, problem for *t* tests, 119, 202
transformations, 196–216
use of log transform, 196–197
Wilcoxon tests, 119, 202–204
Small trials, ethics, 103
hand analysis, 174
inadequacy, 133–134, 144–145, 240–242, 247
value of historical controls, 59

Smoking education, coronary heart disease, 41
Source of patient recruitment, 36
Split-plot analysis of variance, 233
SPSS, 172–173
Staffing, 33–35
  data manager, 167–168
Standard deviation, 193, 209–210
  paired t test, 115, 118–119
  two-sample t test, 201–202
Standard error, difference in means, 201–202
  difference in percentages, 198–199, 207
  logistic coefficients, 219
  mean, 208–209
  mean of paired differences, 115
  percentage, 206–207
  regression coefficients, 216–218
  subgroup analyses, 214
Standard error of prediction, multiple regression analysis, 218
Statistical analysis, 7, 187–210, 211–233
  computers, 172–175
  confidence limits, 187, 206–210
  crossover trials, 114–119
  data description, 187–197
  ineligible patients, 178
  interim results, 142–159
  multiplicity of data, 228–233
  patient withdrawals, 182–186
  planning, 31, 188
  prognostic factors, 211–221
  significance tests, 187, 197–206
  survival data, 221–227
Statistical findings, communication, 210
Statistical methods, determination of trial size, 123–130
  retrospective adjustment for historical control groups, 58
Statistical packages, 172–174
Statistical properties, sequential designs, 159
Statistician, role in trial design and co-ordination, 35
Stopping rules, 146–159
  see also Interim analyses
Stratified analysis, see Prognostic factors
Stratified randomization, 80–87
  balancing for institution, 86–87
  justification, 80–82, 213
  minimization method, 84–87
  random permuted blocks within strata, 82–84, 87

Streptomycin, randomized controlled trial, 17, 63, 98–99
Stroke, clinical assessment, 47, 120
  factorial trial, 140–141
  preventive trials, 31, 43, 140–141, 183–184
  randomized trial of patient management, 5–6
Studentized range, paired treatment comparisons, 230
Subgroup analyses, 213–226, 228–229
Sulphonamides, clinical trials, 16
Surgical procedures, clinical trials, 2, 41, 64–65, 108, 183
Survival data, 10–12, 191
  adjusting for prognostic factors, 226–227
  interim analyses, 145, 151, 158
  life tables, 222–224
  logrank test, 224–226
  proportional hazard model, 227
  size of trial, 129
  statistical analysis, 191, 221–227
  see also Follow-up studies
Systematic assignment of treatment, 60–61

t tests, crossover trials, 115–119
  degrees of freedom, 115, 202
  interaction test, 214
  paired differences, 115
  repeated measurements, 232
  skew data, 119, 196, 202
  subgroup analyses, 213–214
  two-sample, 196, 200–202
Time to relapse, see Survival data
Transient ischaemic attack, aspirin trial, 31
Treatment, cessation or modification, 39–40, 180–181
  duration, 39, 112–113
Treatment groups, 2, 4
  comparability, 212–213
Treatment-period interaction, crossover trials, 116–117
Treatment schedules, 38–41
Treatment team, attitudes in double blind trial, 91
Treatments, number for inclusion in trial, 138–141
Trial, see under specific items
Tuberculosis, streptomycin trial, 17, 63, 98–99
Two-period crossover design, 112–119

Type I error, 125–129, 132–133
  repeated significance tests, 148–149,
    152–154, 156
  see also False-positive findings
Type II error, 125–129, 132–133, 152–154,
    156

Uncontrolled trials, problems, 51–54
Unequal randomization, 59–60, 87–88
University Group Diabetes Program, 19–
    21

Vaccines, 2, 18–19
Vitamin D treatment of epilepsy, cross-
    over trial, 111
Vitamin D trial for neonatal hypocal-
    caemia, determination of trial size,
    127–129
  statistical analysis, 192–196, 200–202,
    205, 208–210, 213–214, 216–218
  systematic assignment of patients, 61,
    205
Vitamin E for bronchopulmonary dys-
    plasia patients, 60–61

Vitamin supplements, neural tube defects
    trial, 62, 102
Volunteer studies, 1–3, 120–122
Volunteer effect, field trial of polio vac-
    cine, 19

Wash-out period, crossover trials, 113
Wilcoxon test, modified for survival data,
    12
  paired differences for crossover trial,
    119
  two-sample, 202–204
Wilm's tumour, randomized trial, 59
Withdrawal of patients, 39, 179–186
  crossover trials, 119
  statistical analysis, 10, 119, 182–186,
    188
Within-patient studies, 110–122
World Medical Association, Declaration
    of Helsinki, 100–102

Yellow fever, treatment by bleeding, 15